Addressing Challenges in Child Mental Health: Research and Strategies for Comprehensive Development

Addressing Challenges in Child Mental Health: Research and Strategies for Comprehensive Development

Guest Editors

Ignasi Navarro-Soria
Tíscar Rodríguez-Jiménez

MDPI

Basel • Beijing • Wuhan • Barcelona • Belgrade • Novi Sad • Cluj • Manchester

Guest Editors
Ignasi Navarro-Soria
Department of Developmental Psychology and Didactics
University of Alacant
Alicante
Spain

Tíscar Rodríguez-Jiménez
Department of Psychology and Sociology
University of Zaragoza
Teruel
Spain

Editorial Office
MDPI AG
Grosspeteranlage 5
4052 Basel, Switzerland

This is a reprint of the Special Issue, published open access by the journal *Children* (ISSN 2227-9067), freely accessible at: https://www.mdpi.com/journal/children/special_issues/51H9G9SF00.

For citation purposes, cite each article independently as indicated on the article page online and as indicated below:

Lastname, A.A.; Lastname, B.B. Article Title. *Journal Name* **Year**, *Volume Number*, Page Range.

ISBN 978-3-7258-6240-5 (Hbk)
ISBN 978-3-7258-6241-2 (PDF)
https://doi.org/10.3390/books978-3-7258-6241-2

Contents

About the Editors

Ignasi Navarro-Soria

Ignasi Navarro-Soria is an Associate Professor in the Department of Developmental Psychology and Didactics at the University of Alicante, Spain. His research focuses on attention deficit hyperactivity disorder (ADHD), executive function, emotional regulation, attachment, and social inclusion. He has directed and participated in national and international research projects and published extensive research on child and adolescent development.

Tíscar Rodríguez-Jiménez

Tíscar Rodríguez-Jiménez is a Professor in the Department of Psychology and Sociology at the University of Zaragoza, Spain. Her research addresses child and adolescent mental health, with a focus on emotional disorders, autism spectrum disorder, suicide prevention, and clinical interventions. She has led various funded projects and contributed to scientific networks on developmental psychopathology and mental health promotion.

Preface

This Reprint, Addressing Challenges in Child Mental Health: Research and Strategies for Comprehensive Development, brings together international contributions focused on the prevention, assessment, and intervention regarding mental health problems in children and adolescents. The aim is to provide both a scientific and applied overview that highlights the complexity of child development and the urgent need for comprehensive approaches to care. We hope this work will support researchers, clinicians, educators, and policymakers in their efforts to improve child and adolescent mental health worldwide.

Ignasi Navarro-Soria and Tíscar Rodríguez-Jiménez
Guest Editors

children

Editorial

Addressing the Child and Adolescent Mental Health Gap After the Pandemic: Why Translational, Practice-Oriented Research Matters

Ignasi Navarro-Soria * and Boglarka Adorjan

Departamento de Psicología Evolutiva y Didáctica, Facultad de Educación, Universidad de Alicante, Carretera San Vicente del Raspeig s/n, San Vicente del Raspeig, 03690 Alicante, Spain; bogi.adorjan@gmail.com
* Correspondence: ignasi.navarro@ua.es

The global disruption caused by COVID-19 has drawn renewed attention to an already pressing reality: child and adolescent mental health requires sustained, system-level investment and high-quality evidence to guide practice. Even before the pandemic, mental health conditions were among the leading causes of disability in young people worldwide. The Lancet Commission on Global Mental Health and Sustainable Development urged a decisive shift toward closing the science-to-service gap and scaling evidence-based interventions across systems of care [1]. The pandemic then acted as a stress test for families, schools, and services: meta-analyses and national surveillance studies showed meaningful increases in internalizing symptoms and service needs among children and adolescents, with disparities concentrated in vulnerable groups [2–4].

Against this backdrop, the current Special Issue brings together empirical studies and practice-oriented innovations spanning early childhood through adolescence. Collectively, these contributions foreground three cross-cutting priorities: (a) early detection and monitoring of developmental-mental health needs in real-world settings; (b) feasible, scalable supports embedded in natural ecologies (families, classrooms, community); and (c) technology-enabled solutions that complement (not replace) human relationships at the heart of mental health care.

1. Early Childhood: From Developmental Risk to Protective Classrooms

A consistent lesson from developmental science is that risk and protection co-accumulate over time. In early childhood, language, pragmatic communication, self-regulation, and classroom climate interact bidirectionally with socio-emotional development. Pragmatic language challenges can undermine peer relations and teacher–child interactions, while supportive, predictable classroom environments buffer risk and foster competence. Evidence accumulated over the last decade indicates that strengthening protective factors at the classroom level (e.g., warm teacher–child relationships, clear routines, emotionally attuned feedback) can yield measurable improvements in child adjustment, especially when adversity is present [5–7].

The studies in this collection that examine preschool communication and early years' classroom supports align with this translational aspiration: they employ real-world samples and focus on feasible practices (e.g., coaching, structured routines, targeted small-group supports). Such work advances the field by moving beyond efficacy trials to effectiveness and implementation questions—what works, for whom, and under which classroom conditions—while keeping sight of equity considerations.

2. Middle Childhood and Adolescence: Executive Functions, Digital Behaviors, and Life Satisfaction

During middle childhood and adolescence, executive functions (working memory, inhibition, and cognitive flexibility) are tightly coupled with academic outcomes, emotion regulation, and risk behaviors. In that developmental window, problematic technology use can co-occur with anxiety and cyberbullying and may both reflect and exacerbate self-regulatory difficulties. Recent studies, including those represented in the Special Issue, underscore that profiles of executive functioning are not simply correlates of mental health; they are tractable intervention targets with classroom-level impact [8–10].

Physical education and active pedagogies appear to be promising contexts for promoting subjective well-being and life satisfaction, especially when teachers explicitly link bodily engagement with self-awareness and regulation strategies [11]. This aligns with broader evidence that school-based programs with active ingredients, emotion coaching, behavioral rehearsal, goal setting, and peer collaboration produce small-to-moderate gains in mental health and learning when delivered with fidelity in supportive climates [6].

3. Neurodevelopmental Conditions and Somatic Comorbidity: A Systems Lens

Neurodevelopmental disorders often present with complex constellations of somatic or connective-tissue-related symptoms, sleep disturbances, and sensory processing differences [12]. Far from being accidental, these features may shape stress physiology, pain sensitivity, and participation in learning, thereby influencing mental health trajectories. The Special Issue includes exploratory designs that invite a more integrative systems lens, one that weaves together neurodevelopmental profiles, embodied experience, and family/school accommodations. Such a lens helps translate clinical insight into practical screening, referral, and support pathways across health and education.

4. Digital Mental Health: Opportunity with Guardrails

Digital approaches, mobile apps, teleconsultation, and AI-enabled tools can expand reach, offer just-in-time self-help, and amplify scarce specialist capacity. Systematic meta-reviews show that digital mental health supports can be acceptable and beneficial for youth, particularly when they are human-supported, embedded in services, and underpinned by solid clinical content [13]. The Special Issue features work on mobile consultation and toolkits that exemplify this "digital-plus-human" model. Yet, the pandemic also reminded us that technology can amplify inequities and does not uniformly benefit all learners. A prudent way forward is to treat digital tools as adjuncts that enhance, not replace, relationship-based care, with attention to accessibility, privacy, and cultural fit [13,14].

5. Suicide Risk, Self-Harm, and the Urgency of Pathways to Care

Emergency presentations for suicidal behavior and non-suicidal self-injury rose in several settings during and after the pandemic [2,15]. Retrospective cohort approaches, like those included in this Special Issue, provide needed signals about age, sex, and contextual correlates of acute risk. However, signals must translate into pathways: (a) routine, developmentally appropriate screening in schools and primary care; (b) rapid access to stepped care; and (c) continuity across crisis, outpatient follow-up, and school reentry. Strengthening these pathways requires intersectoral collaboration and data systems that track outcomes beyond discharge.

6. A Unifying Thread: Translation to Practice and Policy

What binds the contributions of this collection is not a single methodology, but a shared commitment to usable knowledge: measures that teachers can administer; classroom strategies that fit the school day; family-centered practices that respect caregiver load; and digital resources that are simple, secure, and clinically grounded. This is precisely the translational ethos advocated by the global mental health movement, connecting rigorous evidence with scalable delivery in the settings where children grow and learn [1].

At the same time, the field must address persistent evidence gaps. First, effectiveness in diverse, under-resourced contexts remains underexplored; much of the literature is still anchored in high-income settings [1,16]. Second, heterogeneity is the rule: subgroup analyses by sex/gender, neurodevelopmental profile, socioeconomic status, and cultural community are essential to avoid one-size-fits-all recommendations. Third, implementation matters: fidelity, training load, and teacher well-being are not side issues but mediators of impact.

7. Where Do We Go from Here?

A pragmatic agenda emerges from the studies gathered in this Special Issue and the wider literature:

1. Detect earlier, support sooner. Embed brief, valid screeners for social-emotional development, language/pragmatics, and executive functions into routine educational workflows, with clear referral pathways and feedback loops to families and teachers [5,6,9].
2. Invest in protective classrooms. Scale professional learning that helps teachers create emotionally supportive, structured, and culturally responsive environments; prioritize low-burden practices that are demonstrably linked to student mental health and engagement [6,7].
3. Couple digital with human supports. Leverage apps and teleconsultation to expand access, but ensure clinician oversight, data protection, and attention to digital equity; evaluate not only efficacy but also uptake and sustained use in everyday life [13,14].
4. Bridge health and education. Co-design stepped-care pathways that span school, primary care, and specialized services, with protocols for crisis risk, re-entry after hospitalization, and ongoing accommodations for neurodevelopmental diversity [2,15].
5. Measure what matters. Beyond symptom change, track functional outcomes: attendance, peer relationships, life satisfaction, and participation, outcomes that families, students, and teachers recognize as meaningful [11,16].

None of this is easy. But a decade of calls, from global commissions to national strategies, converges on the same point: children's mental health is foundational to learning, development, and social cohesion [1]. The studies in this Special Issue, though diverse in scope and method, move the needle by keeping the focus where it belongs: early, feasible, relational, and equitable supports [16].

Acknowledgments: I would like to thank the authors and reviewers whose thoughtful work and constructive dialog made this Special Issue possible, and the editorial office of *Children* for their consistent support throughout the process. My special appreciation goes to the educators, families, and young people who contributed their time and perspectives to the research featured here.

Conflicts of Interest: The authors declare no conflict of interest.

References

1. Patel, V.; Saxena, S.; Lund, C.; Thornicroft, G.; Baingana, F.; Bolton, P.; Chisholm, D.; Collins, P.Y.; Cooper, J.L.; Eaton, J.; et al. The Lancet Commission on global mental health and sustainable development. *Lancet* **2018**, *392*, 1553–1598. [CrossRef] [PubMed]
2. Racine, N.; McArthur, B.A.; Cooke, J.E.; Eirich, R.; Zhu, J.; Madigan, S. Global prevalence of depressive and anxiety symptoms in children and adolescents during COVID-19: A meta-analysis. *JAMA Pediatr.* **2021**, *175*, 1142–1150. [CrossRef] [PubMed]
3. Newlove-Delgado, T.; McManus, S.; Sadler, K.; Thandi, S.; Vizard, T.; Cartwright Ford, T. Child mental health in England before and during the COVID-19 lockdown. *Lancet Psychiatry* **2021**, *8*, 353–354. [CrossRef] [PubMed]
4. Loades, M.E.; Chatburn, E.; Higson-Sweeney, N.; Reynolds, S.; Shafran, R.; Brigden, A.; Linney, C.; McManus, M.N.; Borwick, C.; Crawley, E. Rapid systematic review: The impact of social isolation and loneliness on the mental health of children and adolescents in the context of COVID-19. *J. Am. Acad. Child Adolesc. Psychiatry* **2020**, *59*, 1218–1239.e3. [CrossRef] [PubMed]
5. Justice, L.M.; Petscher, Y.; Schatschneider, C.; Mashburn, A. Peer effects in preschool classrooms: Is children's language growth associated with their classmates' skills? *Child Dev.* **2011**, *82*, 1768–1777. [CrossRef] [PubMed]
6. Durlak, J.A.; Weissberg, R.P.; Dymnicki, A.B.; Taylor, R.D.; Schellinger, K.B. The impact of enhancing students' social and emotional learning: A meta-analysis of school-based universal interventions. *Child Dev.* **2011**, *82*, 405–432. [CrossRef] [PubMed]
7. Pianta, R.C.; Hamre, B.K.; Allen, J. Teacher–student relationships and engagement: Conceptualizing, measuring, and improving the capacity of classroom interactions. In *Handbook of Research on Student Engagement*; Christenson, S.L., Reschly, A.L., Wylie, C., Eds.; Springer: Boston, MA, USA, 2012; pp. 365–386. [CrossRef]
8. Zelazo, P.D.; Blair, C.; Willoughby, M.T. *Executive Function: Implications for Education (NCER 2016-3)*; U.S. Department of Education: Washington, DC, USA, 2016.
9. Kofler, M.J.; Irwin, L.N.; Soto, E.F.; Groves, N.B.; Harmon, S.L.; Sarver, D.E. Executive functioning heterogeneity in pediatric ADHD. *J. Abnorm. Child Psychol.* **2019**, *47*, 273–286. [CrossRef] [PubMed]
10. Treier, A.K.; Döpfner, M.; Ravens-Sieberer, U.; Görtz-Dorten, A.; Boecker, M.; Goldbeck, C.; Banaschewski, T.; Aggensteiner, P.M.; Hanisch, C.; Ritschel, A.; et al. Screening for affective dysregulation in school-aged children: Relationship with comprehensive measures of affective dysregulation and related mental disorders. *Eur. Child Adolesc. Psychiatry* **2024**, *33*, 381–390. [CrossRef] [PubMed]
11. Marques, A.; Peralta, M.; Santos, T.; Martins, J.; Gaspar de Matos, M. Self-rated health and health-related quality of life are related with adolescents' healthy lifestyle. *Public Health* **2019**, *170*, 89–94. [CrossRef] [PubMed]
12. Murphy, J.; Brewer, R.; Catmur, C.; Bird, G. Interoception and psychopathology: A developmental neuroscience perspective. *Dev. Cogn. Neurosci.* **2017**, *23*, 4–56. [CrossRef] [PubMed]
13. Hollis, C.; Falconer, C.J.; Martin, J.L.; Whittington, C.; Stockton, S.; Glazebrook, C.; Davies, E.B. Annual Research Review: Digital health interventions for children and young people with mental health problems—A systematic and meta-review. *J. Child Psychol. Psychiatry* **2017**, *58*, 474–503. [CrossRef] [PubMed]
14. Ebert, D.D.; Van Daele, T.; Nordgreen, T.; Karekla, M.; Compare, A.; Zarbo, C.; Brugnera, A.; Øverland, S.; Trebbi, G.; Jensen, K.L.; et al. Internet- and mobile-based psychological interventions: Applications, efficacy, and potential for improving mental health. *Eur. Psychol.* **2018**, *23*, 167–187. [CrossRef]
15. Yard, E.; Radhakrishnan, L.; Ballesteros, M.F.; Sheppard, M.; Gates, A.; Stein, Z.; Hartnett, K.; Kite-Powell, A.; Rodgers, L.; Adjemian, J.; et al. Emergency department visits for suspected suicide attempts among persons aged 12–25 years before and during the COVID-19 pandemic—United States, January 2019–May 2021. *MMWR Morb. Mortal. Wkly. Rep.* **2021**, *70*, 888–894. [CrossRef] [PubMed]
16. World Health Organization. *World Mental Health Report: Transforming Mental Health for All*; WHO: Geneva, Switzerland, 2022. Available online: https://www.who.int/publications/i/item/9789240049338 (accessed on 26 November 2025).

children

Article

Development of Language and Pragmatic Communication Skills in Preschool Children with Developmental Language Disorder in a Speech Therapy Kindergarten—A Real-World Study

Dieter Ullrich [1,*] and Magret Marten [2]

1 Medical Practice Pediatric/ENT, Wedemarkstr. 83, 30900 Wedemark, Germany
2 Logopaedic Kindergarten, An der Autobahn 2, 30851 Langenhagen, Germany; magretmarten@gmx.de
* Correspondence: ullrich-dieter@t-online.de

Abstract: Background: Several studies document the importance of communicative abilities for children's development. Especially in recent years verbal communication in preschool children with developmental language disorder (DLD) has been studied, relying heavily on statistical analysis, outcome measures, or/and parents' reports. Purpose: This explorative study investigates the effects of speech therapy on the development of language and verbal communication skills in preschool children with DLD within their peer group in a day-to-day setting using objective video-documentation. Hypothesis: Speech therapy leads to improvement of language, communication, and possibly to concurrent development of both language and verbal communication skills in preschool children. Methods: Preliminary prospective study to assess language and verbal communications skills of nine preschool children (seven boys, two girls, 4–6 y) with DLD in a speech therapy kindergarten using video recordings over a one-year therapy period. The communicative participation of the members of the peer group was assessed and included the verbal address (Av) and the ratio of "verbal address/verbal reaction" (Av/Rv). Results: The investigation results in evidence for two outcome groups: One group with suspected preferential verbal communication disorders ($n = 4$) was characterised by a high Av/Rv value, meaning they were scored to have a normal or high verbal address (Av) and a low verbal response (Rv) (predominantly interpersonal communication related disorder). This group showed minimal changes in the short term but demonstrated improvement after 5 years of schooling; thus, pedagogical activities seemed to be particularly effective for these children. The second group showed a balanced Av/Rv ratio (predominantly language related disorder) (n = 5); but after five years they demonstrated a partial need for special school support measures. This group may therefore particularly benefit from speech therapy. Conclusions: The present study clearly shows that even with speech-language therapy, the linguistic ability of DLD-disturbed children does not necessarily develop simultaneously with their communication ability. Rather, the investigations provide evidence for two groups of preschool children with DLD and communication disorder: One group demonstrated a predominantly verbal communication related disorder, where pedagogical intervention might be the more important treatment. The second group showed predominantly DLD, therefore making speech therapy the more effective intervention. In this study, all children expressed their desire to communicate with their peers. To the authors' best knowledge, this is the first study determining the ability to communicate in a preschool cohort with DLD using characterisation with video documentation in a follow-up for 1 year.

Keywords: verbal communication development; preschool children with speech-language disorder; communicative participation; logopaedic kindergarten; importance of SL-therapy and educational measures

 https://doi.org/10.3390/children12070921

1. Introduction

Human communication involves the interpersonal exchange of ideas, wishes, and feelings among people [1–3]. The development of social and verbal communication skills is a significant developmental step for infants and children and is critical for their intelligence, the development of cognition, their future communicative participation, and thus for their future lives [2,4]. Earlier research has primarily investigated children's speech and language skills, but in recent years the importance of pragmatic communicative skills has been recognised [1–8]. The scientific and educational importance of communication skills is reflected in the introduction of social (pragmatic) communication disorder as a new category in the fifth edition of the *Diagnostic and Statistical Manual of Mental Disorders* [9]. The importance of communication is also emphasised in the International Classification of Functioning, Disability and Health (ICF) [10]. Nevertheless, uncertainties and unanswered questions remain [11].

The concept of communication is complex. An infant's smiling and crying represent the first type of communication [12]. Andalo et al. [13] documented that the development of language and communication is partially based on physical motoric development. According to Piaget et al. [14] and Zollinger [15], the development of communication is linked to the child's ability to play, recognise symbols, and triangulate. In recent years, numerous publications and reviews on child communication have appeared and contributed to a better understanding [6,16–19]. However, it should not be overlooked that individual elements of communication do not necessarily reflect communicative participation. Ultimately, however, it is communicative participation that is of crucial importance [7,11].

To assess communication skills in preschool children, some studies attempted caregiver questionnaires. The FOCUS (*Focus on the Outcomes of Communication Under Six*) questionnaire examines the communicative skills of subjects under the age of six years and is also used to correlate communication and DLD development in children [20]. In the vast majority of all studies, the development of communication is assessed on the analysis of various test procedures or questionnaires and, furthermore, on patient-reported outcome measures or parents' reports concerning communicative skills [16]. These approaches often only provide indirect (evaluative) and/or retrospective information regarding communication skills. However, communicative skills do not necessarily equate to possessing the ability for "communicative participation" [7,11,18]. To our best knowledge currently there exist no objective testing methods to characterise communicative abilities in preschool children.

In Germany, specialised logopaedic/speech therapy kindergartens exist. The concept of logopaedic kindergartens is founded on scientific evidence showing that children with speech and language impairments benefit from appropriate therapy. The multimodal approach of these kindergartens involving the participation of specialised educators, speech therapists, occupational therapists, and psychologists aims to help the children to integrate into mainstream schools and pursue vocational training later in life [21,22].

Prior to admission to a speech therapy kindergarten, other significant impairments apart from speech development disorders must be excluded. Furthermore, children must have received 30 h or more of unsuccessful outpatient speech therapy. Upon admission, children are aged between 4 and 6 years, and the average duration of therapy is 18 months. The ratio of children to educators in the logopaedic kindergarten is 8:1.5, thus significantly better than that in regular kindergarten with a ratio of 25:3.

Pedagogical research [23,24] has shown that objective skills such as a high IQ (hard skill) do not necessarily guarantee success or stimulate optimal development. Instead, soft skills, such as the environment or intensive practice (life skills), seem to be crucial for a positive long-term development. The authors suggest that this situation might be comparable for speech-language development. This implies that, in agreement with Cunningham et al. [7,18], individual language skills, such as articulation, vocabulary, or phonological awareness (hard skills) or single communicative skills alone are not sufficient for children's language or communicative development and participation outcome. It is important that soft skills, such as interindividual communication and language practice, must be further developed. Enhancing these soft skills could potentially improve the long-term prognosis of children with DLD and communication disorders.

Consequently, this explorative study investigated verbal interpersonal communication of preschool children with their peers as an important aspect of communicative participation behaviour in young children with DLD. Additionally, we introduced video analysis as a novel method to analyse communicative development and participation in preschool children. One important research hypothesis investigates whether speech-language therapy will improve DLD and communication concurrently.

2. Methods

2.1. Study Design

The authors present a prospective observational study with preschool children in a speech therapy kindergarten in Hanover, Germany, over one therapy year (2016 to 2017). As part of the admission process, parents were required to consent to various examinations, possible scientific analyses, and publications. This informed consent was obtained from parents and caregivers prior to enrolment. No additional examinations were conducted specifically for this study.

2.2. Participants

Nine preschool children (7 boys, 2 girls) (Table 1) with DLD were included in the study. At study enrolment, the children were aged 4–6 years. All children had a pronounced developmental language disorder (ICD-10: F 80.9) and minor additional disorders, such as problems associated with the oral musculature (ICD-10: F 82) [25] (see Appendix A). Table 1 summarises the characteristics of the study participants, including age, native family language, IQ, number of siblings, and characterisation of SL-disorder according to ICD [25]. Five children came from non-native German-speaking families (Child: D1, P, D2, J1, E). However, German was also the everyday language in these households. Logopaedic speech therapy assessment established that the extent of German language problems was comparable in all study participants, regardless of their language background (Appendix A). For children of a non-German-speaking background, caregiver feedback confirmed the similarities of speech problems in both languages. The details on the different logopaedic criteria and the language status before and after therapy are presented in Appendix A.

Table 1. Characterisation of the children.

Child	Age (y) *1	Native Family Language	IQ (SON-R) *2 [26]	Number of Siblings	ICD-10 *3 [25]
D1	6	Polish	h	1	F80-9
N	5	German	a	1	F80.9

Table 1. *Cont.*

Child	Age (y) *1	Native Family Language	IQ (SON-R) *2 [26]	Number of Siblings	ICD-10 *3 [25]
L	5	German	a	1	F80.9, F82.9
P	5	Russian	a(b), borderline	0	F80.9
K	5	German	a	1	F80.9
D2	5	Polish	a	1	F80.9, F82.9
J1	5	Russian	h	9	F80.9
J2	5	German	a	1	F80.9, F82.9
E	4	Russian	a	1	F80.9

*1: Beginning of the study; *2: a (average; 90–110), b (below average, <90), h (higher than average, >110); *3: International Classification of Diseases.

All children underwent a psychological and a speech-therapy assessment upon admission. Within the therapy year all children were routinely tested 4 times per therapy year with regard to their language skills and 2 to 3 times per year regarding their overall development. Similar to the initial assessments, these examinations are based on various validated test procedures (Table 2), which were individually conducted by experienced examiners under optimal conditions. After evaluation and additional consideration of the individual assessments by educators and therapists (Tables 2 and 3; Appendices A–D), the further logopaedic and pedagogical treatment concept was developed and adapted.

Table 2. Test procedures in the logopaedic kindergarten.

Skills	Test Procedure	Validated
Language + Speech	SETK—3–5 Test for language/speech development of children 3–5 years [27]	yes
	AWST-R—Vocabulary test for children 3–5 years [28]	yes
	PDSS—Patholinguistic diagnostics for speech-language-impaired children [29]	yes
Cognition	Kaufmann Assessment Battery for Children II (KABC-II 2015) [30]	yes
	SON-R2.5–7—Non-verbal IQ test for children 2.5–7 years [26]	yes
Motor skills + Movement	MOT 4–6—Test for children 4–6 years [31]	yes

Table 3. Linguistic abilities at the beginning and the end of the therapy year based on logopaedic and educational assessment.

Child	Linguistic Skills Before Therapy	Linguistic Skills After Therapy
D1	hardly any dialogue ability	partially good dialogue ability
N	hardly any dialogue ability	good dialogue ability
L	limited dialogue ability	good dialogue ability
P	good dialogue ability	good dialogue ability
K	good dialogue ability	good dialogue ability
D2	limited dialogue ability	good dialogue ability

Table 3. *Cont.*

Child	Linguistic Skills Before Therapy	Linguistic Skills After Therapy
J1	limited dialogue ability	good dialogue ability
J2	limited dialogue ability	good dialogue ability
E	hardly any dialogue ability	good dialogue ability

The assessment data on the children's various abilities and characteristics and the changes in some of these during the therapy year are shown in condensed form in Table 3 and in Appendices A–D.

2.3. Methods and Analysis of Communication Skills

The authors developed an internal assessment protocol for communication evaluation previously unreported.

Based on this protocol, the children's communication behaviour was assessed qualitatively or semi-quantitatively by educators and speech therapists using standardised methodology on admission and at regular intervals of 3 to 4 months (Tables 2 and 3; Appendices A and B).

Given the children's frequent difficulties in passing objective tests, all children in the study groups were also routinely assessed using Zollinger's developmental profiles (Appendix B). Zollinger's [15] non-standardised developmental profiles are qualitative assessments of four skills (i.e., practical-gnostic, symbolic, linguistic, social-communicative criteria) which have shown to be present in approximately 80% of children aged 9 to 42 months. However, Zollinger's test results in the present study are limited by the fact that the children analysed are significantly older than 42 months. But the developmental profiles were a valuable aid for a pedagogical-therapeutic routine.

In general, it is evident that all standardised and non-standardised test procedures can only characterise single aspects of the children's abilities and/or disorders. Thus, multiple, simultaneous testing procedures—as conducted in this study—most accurately reflect the abilities and limitations of the different children.

2.4. Pedagogical Principles

As described above, all children were extensively tested when they started kindergarten and individual support plans were created based on the results. The criteria for these examinations included self-confidence, social skills, knowledge of materials, and motor skills (Appendices C and D). The development of these abilities, which were either missing or not fully developed according to age, was then specifically supported by pedagogical means. Typically, a pedagogic review was conducted four times during the therapy year and the support measures were adjusted accordingly. As stated, pedagogical principles for the children focused on the criteria "temperament and personality functions", "energy and drive functions", "basic learning", and "general tasks and demands"(ICF-CY 2007) [32].

The specialised educators (1.5 educators for 8 children) tried to improve the children's abilities with targeted measures, entertained them, and sang with them. Reading aloud was not possible due to the children's impaired abilities. In contrast to the speech therapists, the educators did not correct the children in their speech—linguistic corrections were made only by the speech therapists. The specialised educators and one speech therapist were available to provide long-term care for these nine children. In addition, one psychologist and one motopedist were sometimes available.

2.5. Video Documentation and Analysis

The individual quantitative examinations of communication behaviour were performed using video analyses of the children at the beginning of the therapy year (0 months) and after 3, 7, and 10 months. Speech, behaviour, and verbal communication skills of all children in the study group were documented for one hour, starting from 8:15 to 9:15 a.m. During this observation period, the children acted autonomously without intervention from teachers and/or therapists.

Evaluation of the recordings was conducted by a speech-language therapist, an educator specialised in speech-language therapy, and a paediatric medical expert specialising in treatment of children with language impairment. In borderline situations, the assessment of the majority of assessors was accepted.

The verbal communication behaviour of the children involved was analysed for a duration of 10 s every 2 min. The three assessors categorised the quantitative communication behaviour of the children as "verbal expressive action" (Av) and the language reaction or answer as "verbal responsive action" (Rv). In addition, "non-verbal expressive action" (An), such as hand gestures or facial expressions, "non-verbal responsive action" (Rn), and "no interaction" (D0) were evaluated. The criteria for the assessment of non-verbal responsive actions were observable gestures, movement, and significant facial expressions. Highly subtle reactions, such as a wink, were neglected due to the scope of this investigation. However, it has previously been shown that these reactions are significant in the assessment of communication skills [33].

The communication activities Av, Rv, An, Rn, and D0 were extrapolated for the observation hours and presented as percentage proportions per hour (%/h). Consequently, 28 to 30 evaluations per hour were conducted for each child, and a total of 4 observation hours were recorded at 0, 3, 7, and 10 months throughout the therapy year.

In 2022, five years after discharge, a telephone follow-up survey was conducted to evaluate the study participants, including their current level of school education (Figure 1).

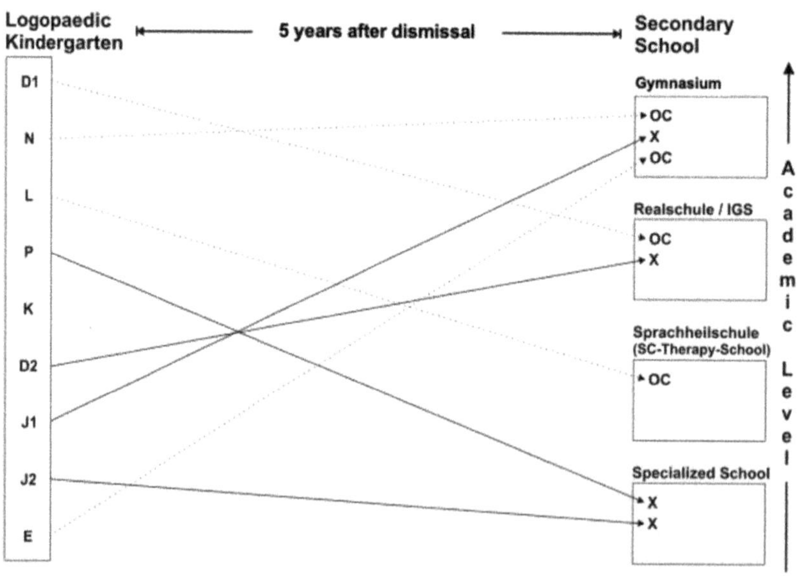

Figure 1. Long-term school development of the children (OC: children with predominantly communication problems: D1, N, L, E); X: children with predominantly speech-language problems: P, D2, J1, J2) (Appendix E).

The primary outcome measure was the quantitative and qualitative change in interpersonal speech-language (SL) and communication behaviour in the kindergarten group (peer group) over the course of one therapy year, as measured by standardised test procedures, but also judged by subjective assessments of the therapy team. An objective method to assess communication was video documentation.

Secondary outcome measures included the level of secondary schooling achieved and language skills at the time of, and following, discharge from the kindergarten.

2.6. Problems Concerning Statistical Analysis

Three assessors (a speech-language therapist, an educator specialised in speech-language therapy, and a paediatric medical expert) conducted the video analysis. All three evaluators were involved in the study and were informed about the study parameter "communication". There was consensus in almost all cases in the video assessment of the children's communication behaviour. However, despite best efforts, experimenter bias cannot be completely ruled out.

Further statistical peculiarities: The present study is a "psychological study" with the known peculiarities and limitations of a small number of subjects. Statistical and assessment problems in psychological studies can arise, among other things, from differences between laboratory and field studies, experimenter bias, problems of generalisability, individual differences and subjective problems of the subjects, and effects of confounding factors. In addition, the effect size of the phenomenon under investigation (e.g., Cohen's effect size) also plays a role in psychological studies, as this can, among other things, provide a measure of the significance of an observed effect. However, the statistical analysis of the various influences requires a control group or larger study groups, which is not the case in the present study. Even though no statistical data is available, the observed effect size of the parameter "communication" appears to be high in the present investigation.

2.7. Significance of Other Influencing Factors

The authors are aware that certain factors influencing language and communication development were not considered in this study that may alter results. Examples include the children's IQ, the number of siblings, or similar variables. Among others, Alons et al. [16] and Cunningham et al. [8] have documented a wide range of such influencing factors.

The authors believe that, despite (or perhaps because of) the data reduction performed, the study results provide important insights into children's development of language and communication skills.

In terms of study design, this exploratory study involves a small number of subjects, making statistical analysis mathematically inappropriate.

3. Results

All study participants demonstrated verbal communication disorders to varying degrees and with different problems (Appendix A). Figure 2 summarises verbal address (Av) and shows that all the children communicated or tried to communicate to varying degrees regardless of their individual disorders. Within the therapy year no systematic development is detectable.

The ratio between Av (active verbal expressive action) and Rv (verbal responsive action) was defined as an indicator for individual social communication (communicative participation) of the children. The authors classified the Av/Rv ratio with a range between ≤ 0.9 and 1.1 as "normal", indicating an appropriate balance between verbal expression and reaction. An Av/Rv ratio of more than 1.1 due to a low Rv was classified as "irregular, less communicative".

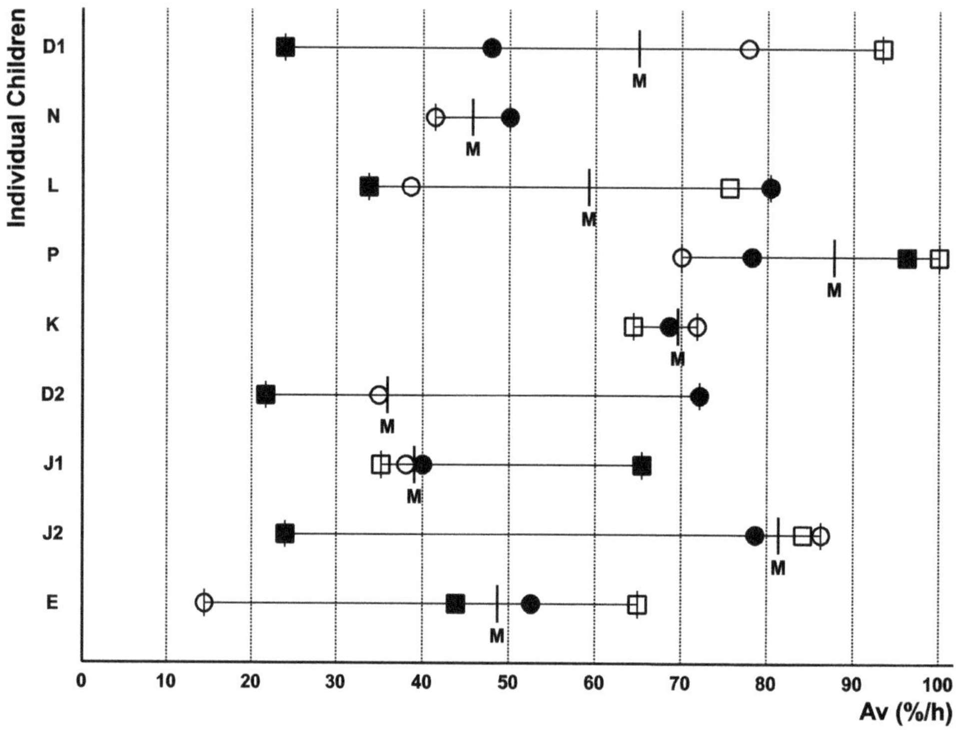

Figure 2. Verbal address Av in percentage per hour (%/h) of the various children at the observation times, 0 (○), 3 (•), 7 (□), and 10 (■) months; median: (M).

A general correlation was observed between expressive Av (%/h) and responsive Rv (%/h) action with a Pearson correlation coefficient of r = 0.881. The correlation between An (%/h) and Rn (%/h) for the corresponding non-verbal communication behaviour was considerably lower, with a Pearson correlation coefficient of r = 0.475.

The balance between "verbal expressive action" and "responsive reaction" is thought to be important for verbal interpersonal communication. The authors expressed this via repeated evaluation of the Av/Rv ratio (i.e., the ratio of verbal expressive action to verbal response), as shown in Figure 3. This Av/Rv ratio proved to be a useful method for quantifying communication behaviour, although it varies significantly throughout the year. The median Av/Rv ratio correlated with the additional assessments of communication behaviour (Figure 4, Table 3, and Appendices A and B). During these video investigations, children acted independently of adult presence and influence, thus being able to solely communicate with their peers. It has previously been shown that the presence of adults alters communication behaviour in preschool children [3,34,35].

Figure 3 demonstrates a median Av/Rv ratio greater than 1.1 for children D1, N, L, and E. The authors interpreted this ratio as non-reciprocal communication behaviour, displaying a large amount of verbal share Av (in part without the apparent intention to communicate) and a low reactive share Rv. Children P, K, D2, J1, and J2 with an Av/Rv ratio between ≤0.9 and 1.1 appeared to have predominantly "normal" communication behaviour, with equally weighted proportions of responsive and reactive verbal behaviour, therefore displaying a "give and take" behaviour. In the present study the Av/Rv ratio fluctuated substantially over the course of the study year.

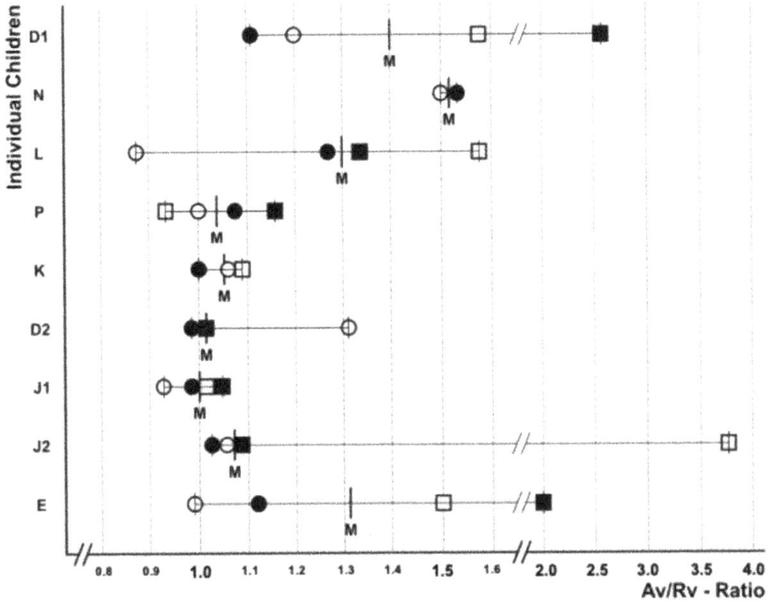

Figure 3. Av/Rv-ratio (verbal address/verbal response) of the various children at the observation times, 0 (○), 3 (•), 7 (□), and 10 (■) months; median: (M).

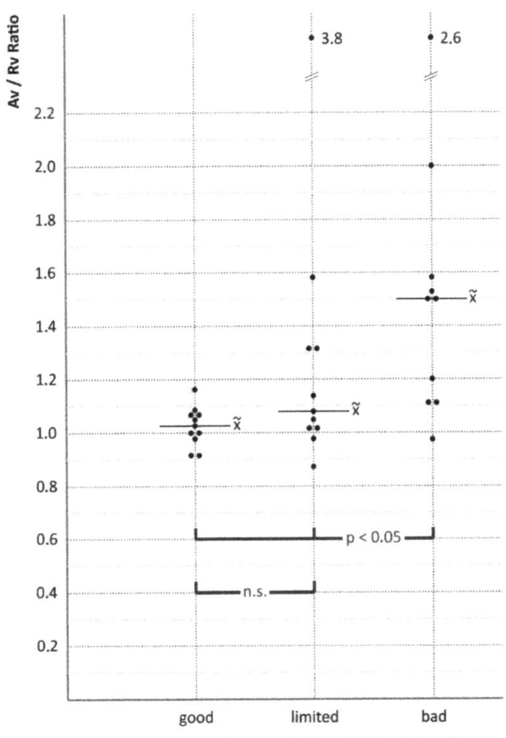

Figure 4. Relations between Av/Rv-ratios during therapy period and "communication abilities before therapy" (based on assessment of speech therapists and educators), with median $\tilde{x}$.

Clearly observable non-verbal communication (consisting of actions (An) and non-verbal reactions (Rn)) was rarely detected, with a median of 5% per hour (range: 2–12.5% per hour).

According to the assessment of speech therapists, educators, and test procedures in general, the children's linguistic phonological, phonetic, and grammatical progress was better than their verbal communicative progress over the course of the therapy year (Figure 4, Table 3, Appendix A).

In a telephone follow-up five years after discharge, three (D1, N, E) of the four children (D1, N, E, L) with a high Av/Rv ratio (Av/Rv $\geq$ 1.1) and the assessment "pronounced communication disorder" were attending a "high-level secondary school" (German "Gymnasium"/"Realschule"/IGS; characterised by the academic level, these refer to types of secondary schools) (Figure 1; characterisation of school types in Germany: see Appendix E). In comparison, two (P, J2) of four children (P, D2, J1, J2) with significant speech-language impairment and presumed "normal" communication behaviour (based on Av/Rv < 1.1) were attending a "specialised school" with distinct support measures.

In the present study two (L, J2) of three children with DLD and oral dysfunction (L, D2, J2) had to attend a "specialised school" or "speech therapy school" in the long term.

4. Discussion

In this study all examined preschool children suffered from DLD and all of them expressed their desire to communicate with their peers. The verbal communication behaviour of the children as core competence for their individual development and communicative participation was determined by their peer group without adult influence. Children's communication amongst their peers varies from that displayed in the presence of adults [3,35], in particular in young children developing language skills and children with language disorders. Research findings give some evidence that not necessarily logopaedic therapy methods, but practice and environment might be decisive for a successful development [8,11,18] similar to pedagogical development [23,24].

All children in this study showed varying degrees of improvement in linguistic aspects such as phonology, phonetics, and/or grammar during the therapy year, as determined by test procedures and the assessment of therapists. This result is in agreement with the studies of Cunningham et al. [3,35], Levickis [11], and Law et al. [36]. In contrast, unexpectedly, the examined children showed no significant changes or development in communicative verbal address (Av) or in the ratio Av/Rv as measured by objective video documentation throughout the year. Presumably, the ratio Av/Rv is an important hint for individual and interpersonal communication abilities/communicative participation. These observations were interpreted as a long-term verbal communication disorder and are consistent with the published literature [37]. According to Buzhardt et al. [38] the simultaneous impairments in speech-language and communication may be an indicator for increased risk for autism spectrum disorder. However, in the present study all children with communicative problems analysed gave no evidence for autism spectrum disorder and even showed positive speech/language and communicative development in the long term.

For the participation and development of children, linguistic abilities as well as communication skills and social abilities are highly important [1,5,39]. Whilst very often therapy differentiates between linguistic and communicative abilities, linguistic abilities are an important prerequisite for communication. Linguistic abilities can be supported and improved by intensive speech therapy [40]. For the development of communication skills and communicative participation, the authors believe that in addition to the linguistic skills, a combination of exercise and environment are crucial and that logopaedic and pedagogical support are important additional measures. This interpretation of the study findings is in concurrence with other studies [7,8,23].

In the present study, all preschool children with DLD showed a strong desire to communicate with one another, despite their speech and communication challenges. This finding shows how children use their communication abilities to engage with others and seems to indicate a strong individual intrinsic motivation [7,10,11,41,42].

Although no significant improvement in children with mainly communication skills was observed during the therapy period, the children's long-term development seemed surprisingly successful, illustrated by their attendance at regular secondary schools. In comparison to the above group, the long-term academic development of the children with predominant DLD and "normal" communicative behaviour was less accomplished.

The observation of a positive development of communication after intensive pedagogical care during preschool age also corresponds to the observations of Mortensen et al. [43], Whitehouse et al. [44], Dickinson et al. [45], and others. It is debatable whether social, educational, or physical problems or a lack of educational support are critical determinants of the long-term problems of children with language development and communication disorders, as described by Botting et al. [46], Maggio et al. [47], and Johnson et al. [48]. From the pedagogical aspect Stamm [23,24] emphasises the importance of practice and a positive environment, which is in accordance with the findings of Cunningham et al. [8] and Alons [16].

The present study offers valuable insights to the children's perspective to use communication for engagement in life, but also has certain limitations. It is a prospective, long-term observational study focused on the communication behaviour of preschool children with DLD in a speech therapy kindergarten. Unlike many studies that rely on questionnaires, this research aims to provide a more direct objective and comprehensive understanding through video documentation, various tests, and evaluations by specialised professionals. However, the sample size is small, with just nine children who vary significantly in their individual conditions, such as number of siblings, mother tongue, and others. The data was assessed and summarised by three examiners as described above (a speech-language therapist, an educator specialised in speech-language therapy, and a paediatric medical expert). Additional limitations include the intra-observer reliability of grading, the socio-economic context of the kindergarten studied, and potential linguistic characteristics unique to the German language.

In conclusion, although the study was limited by a small sample size and a simplified model, the findings suggest that the speech-language and communication environment plays a crucial role for the development of children. Results indicate that all children have a strong desire to engage in communicative participation with their peers. There is also some evidence that the first signs of communication problems can be recognised early in young children. In addition, we believe that video documentation and subsequent computerised analysis (for example, utilising machine learning or artificial intelligence) can also be a significant aid in the future assessment of possible communicative disorders in preschool children with DLD.

Ethics Considerations of This Study

This study involved a secondary analysis of pseudonymised data originally collected during routine diagnostic and therapeutic speech therapy procedures in a kindergarten. No additional diagnostic interventions were conducted for research purposes, and all video recordings were deleted prior to analysis. Parental consent was obtained at admission for data use in diagnostic documentation and for specific therapeutic video recordings. No identifiable information was retained, and the research posed no additional risk to participants. The Ethics Committee of the Lower Saxony Medical Association was consulted after the study concluded and declined to issue a retrospective opinion, citing ambiguity regarding the need for prior consultation in such cases. Although no ethical violations occurred and the Ethics Committee raised no significant concerns, in future work we will seek formal ethics approval prior to the start of data collection, regardless of the perceived level of risk, to ensure alignment with best research practices.

5. Conclusions

This study is a prospective study in which we expected a continuous, largely parallel improvement of speech and verbal communication due to continuous therapy. However, findings show that linguistic ability of speech-language-disturbed children does not necessarily develop simultaneously with their communication ability. Evidence suggests that two groups with different disorder foci emerged, and they differed over the course of the therapy year. The present study suggests that children with mostly DLD problems predominantly require speech therapy. Children with a predominant verbal communication problem could have an incipient or existing "social (pragmatic) communication disorder". According to the current literature, a combination of educational and speech therapy seems to be helpful for this type of disorder. Overall, our findings show that an improvement in language skills does not necessarily lead immediately to improved communication behaviour.

Despite the aforementioned limitations and the small, heterogeneous group of children with DLD studied—along with the resulting statistical challenges—the authors believe that further large-scale studies would be beneficial.

What This Paper Adds

Little is known about the relations between language and verbal communication development in preschool children with DLD. In general, it is assumed that language and verbal communication development occur largely in parallel.

In the present study, evidence suggests that young children can be divided into two distinct groups: one group primarily exhibits language disorders, while the other shows predominantly verbal communication difficulties. However, independent of their impairment, all children want to engage in communication/communicative participation with their peers. It is important to note that speech-language therapy may not lead to simultaneous improvements in speech-language and communication skills.

The authors suggest that speech therapy should be sought for preschool children with a speech disorder, and a combination of educational and speech therapy interventions should be used for children with a verbal communication disorder.

Author Contributions: Conceptualisation, D.U. and M.M.; Methodology, D.U. and M.M.; Validation, D.U.; Formal analysis, D.U.; Investigation, D.U. and M.M.; Resources, M.M.; Data curation, D.U.; Writing—original draft, D.U.; Writing—review and editing, M.M. All authors have read and agreed to the published version of the manuscript.

Funding: This research received no external funding.

Institutional Review Board Statement: This study involved a secondary analysis of pseudonymised data originally collected during routine diagnostic and therapeutic speech therapy procedures in a kindergarten.

Informed Consent Statement: Written informed consent has been obtained from the patient(s) to publish this paper.

Data Availability Statement: The original contributions presented in this study are included in the article. Further inquiries can be directed to the corresponding author(s).

Conflicts of Interest: The authors declare no conflict of interest.

Appendix A

Table A1. Speech-language development status at the beginning (B) and end (E) of speech therapy in the logopaedic kindergarten (based on assessment by SL teachers).

	D1 B E	N B E	L B E	P B E	K B E	D2 B E	J1 B E	J2 B E	E B E
Articulation	6 4	5 3	4 3	4 3	4 3	4 3	5 2	5 4	4 4
Orofacial complex	4 4	4 2	3 2	4 2	3 3	3 2	3 2	4 3	1 1
Semantic lexical	5 5	4 3	3 1	4 3	4 3	5 3	4 1	5 1	4 4
Grammar Syntax	6 4	6 2	4 2	4 3	5 3	5 3	4 2	4 3	5 4
Grammar Morphology	6 4	6 4	4 3	4 3	3 3	4 3	4 3	4 3	6 4
Language understanding	5 4	4 2	2 1	4 3	4 3	3 2	3 1	3 1	5 3
Auditory Processing	6 3	5 3	5 3	4 3	3 3	4 3	3 3	4 2	4 3
Communicative pragmatic	6 4	5 2	4 2	3 3	4 3	5 3	4 3	4 3	5 2

1: age-appropriate, trouble-free; 2: slightly conspicuous; 3: partially, still defective; 4: defective, multiple; limited; 5: considerably disturbed, severe; 6: not assessable, not present.

Appendix B

Table A2. Skills necessary for speech-language development before and after therapy (according to Zollinger [15]. The data refer to individual abilities compared to normally developed 3.5-year-old children. Legend: (↓)↓: (strongly) impaired; Ø: average; ↑: enhanced.

Name	IQ	Before Therapy				Age (Years)	After Therapy			
		Practical-Gnostic	Symbolic	Linguistic	Social Communicative		Social Communicative	Linguistic	Symbolic	Practical-Gnostic
D1	↑	↓↓	Ø	↓↓	↓↓	6	↓↓	Ø	Ø	Ø
N	Ø	Ø	Ø	↓↓	↓↓	5	↓↓	↓↓	Ø	Ø
L	Ø	Ø	Ø	↓↓	↓	5	Ø	↓↓	Ø	Ø
P	↓	Ø	Ø	↓↓	↓↓	5	↓↓	Ø	Ø	Ø
K	Ø	Ø	Ø	↓	Ø	5	Ø	↓	Ø	Ø
D2		Ø	Ø	↓↓	↓↓	5	↓↓	↓↓	Ø	Ø
J1	↑	Ø	Ø	Ø	Ø	5	Ø	Ø	Ø	Ø
J2		Ø	Ø	↓↓	↓	5	Ø	Ø	Ø	Ø
E	Ø	Ø	↓	↓	Ø	4	Ø	Ø	↓Ø	Ø

Appendix C

Table A3. Non-verbal parameter for the assessment of emotional and social qualities (assessed by educators).

Parameters	Assessment Score		
	Below Average	Average	Above Average
Frustration tolerance	1	2	3
Ability to accept criticism	1	2	3
Social competence	1	2	3
Compliance with rules	1	2	3
Ability to form relationships	1	2	3
Maximum points			15
Average points		10	
Minimum points	5		

Appendix D

Table A4. Assessment of social and emotional qualities of the various children by educators and therapists. Criteria as shown in Table A3.

	Child								
	D1	N	L	P	K	D2	J1	J2	E
Frustration tolerance	1	2	2	1	2	1	2	3	1
Ability to accept criticism	2	2	2	2	2	2	3	2	1
Social competence	2	3	2	1	2	3	3	3	2
Compliance with rules	3	3	2	1	2	3	3	1	2
Ability to form relationships	1	1	3	3	2	2	1	2	1
Total Points	9	11	11	8	10	11	12	11	7

Appendix E. Characterisation of School Types in Germany

The German "Gymnasium" specifically refers to a type of secondary high school that prepares students for university education.

"Realschule" refers to a type of secondary school that provides a more practical and vocational education compared to the academically focused Gymnasium, typically for students aged around 10 to 16.

The "IGS" integrates various educational tracks, offering a range of academic and vocational courses within the same institution, allowing students to choose different pathways based on their abilities and interests.

References

1. Hood, N. Communication in the Early Years: An Introduction. ECE Resources. White, A, Ed. 2019. Available online: https://theeducationhub.org.nz/communication-in-the-early-years-an-introduction (accessed on 23 April 2022).
2. Hickman, M. The pragmatics of reference in child language: Some issues in developmental theory. In *Social and Functional Approaches to Language and Thought*; Hickman, M., Ed.; Academic Press: New York, NY, USA, 1987; pp. 165–184.
3. Falkum, I.L. Pragmatic development: Learning to use language to communicate. In *International Handbook of Language Acquisition*; Horst, J.S., von Koss Torkildsen, J., Eds.; Project: Acquiring Figurative Meanings: A Study in Developmental Pragmatics 2018; accessed 10 February 2021; Routledge/Taylor & Francis Group: New York, NY, USA, 2019.
4. Cutting, A.L.; Dunn, J. Theory of mind, emotion understanding, language and family background: Individual differences and interrelations. *Child Dev.* **1999**, *70*, 853–865. [CrossRef] [PubMed]
5. Barron, B. When smart groups fail. *J. Learn. Sci.* **2003**, *12*, 307–359. [CrossRef]

6. Schoon, I.; Parsons, S.; Rush, R.; Law, J. Childhood language skills and adult literacy: A 29-years follow-up study. *Pediatrics* **2010**, *125*, e459–e466. [CrossRef]
7. Cunningham, B.J.; Thomas-Stonell, N.; Rosenbaum, P. Assessing Communicative Participation in Preschool Children with the Focus on the Outcomes of Communication Under Six: A Scoping Review. *Dev. Med. Child Neurol.* **2020**, *63*, 47–53. [CrossRef]
8. Cunningham, B.J.; Hanna, S.E.; Rosenbaum, P.; Thomas-Stonell, N.; Oddson, B. Factors Contributing to Preschooler's Communicative Participation Outcomes: Findings from a Population-Based Longitudinal Cohort Study in Ontario, Canada. *Am. J. Speech Lang. Pathol.* **2018**, *27*, 737–750. Available online: https://ir.lib.uwo.ca/precisepreschoolpubs/7 (accessed on 20 April 2022). [CrossRef] [PubMed]
9. American Psychiatric Association. *Diagnostic and Statistical Manual of Mental Disorders*, 5th ed.; Text Revision, DSM-5-TR; American Psychiatric Association: Washington, DC, USA, 2013.
10. World Health Organization. *International Classification of Functioning, Disability and Health (ICF)*; World Health Organisation: Geneva, Switzerland, 2001.
11. Levickis, P. Measuring communicative participation in population-based sample of children with speech and language difficulties. *Dev. Med. Child Neurol.* **2017**, *59*, 993–994. [CrossRef]
12. Schneider-Antrich, P. Entwicklung und Themen früher Peerbeziehungen. Erschienen 2011. Available online: http://www.kita-fachtexte.de (accessed on 20 July 2021).
13. Andalò, B.; Rigo, F.; Rossi, G.; Majorano, M.; Lavelli, M. Do motor skills impact on language development between 18 and 30 months of age? *Infant Behav. Dev.* **2022**, *66*, 101667. [CrossRef] [PubMed]
14. Piaget, J.; Stöber, N.; Loch, W. *Sprechen und Denken des Kindes*; Pädagogischer Verlag Schwann: Düsseldorf, Germany, 1975.
15. Zollinger, B. *Die Entdeckung der Sprache 1975*, 9th ed.; Haupt: Bern, Switzerland, 2015.
16. Alons, E.; Brauner, L.; Luinge, M.; Terwee, C.B.; van Ewijk, L.; Gerrits, E. Review Article Identifying Relevant Concepts for the Development of a Communicative Participation Item Bank for Children and Adolescents: A Systematic Review of Existing Instruments. *J. Speech Lang. Hear. Res.* **2024**, *67*, 1186–1205. [CrossRef]
17. Doove, B.M.; Feron, F.J.M.; van Os, J.; Drukker, M. Preschool Communication: Early Identification of Concerns About Preschool Language Development and Social Participation. *Front. Public Health* **2021**, *8*, 546536. [CrossRef]
18. Cunningham, B.J.; Hanna, S.E.; Oddson, B.; Thomas-Stonell, N.; Rosenbaum, P. A population-based study of communicative participation in preschool children with speech-language impairments. *Dev. Med. Child Neurol.* **2017**, *59*, 1049–1055. [CrossRef]
19. Martynenko, I. State of Communication Activity of Elder Reschool Children with Developmental Language Disorders. *Int. J. Pedagog. Innov. New Technol.* **2016**, *3*, 1207089. [CrossRef]
20. Thomas-Stonell, N.; Oddson, B.E.; Robertson, B.; Rosenbaum, P.L. Development of the FOCUS (Focus on the Outcomes of Communication Under Six), a Communication Outcome Measure for Preschool Children. *Dev. Med. Child Neurol.* **2010**, *52*, 47–53. [CrossRef] [PubMed]
21. Flöther, M.; Schlüter, E.; Bruns, T. Multidisciplinary Assessment and management of children with hearing and language disorders—An assessment of the effectiveness of a concept from Lower Saxony, Germany. *LOGOS Interdiszip.* **2011**, *19*, 282–292.
22. Ullrich, D.; Ullrich, K.; Marten, M. A longitudinal assessment of early childhood education with integrated speech therapy for children with significant language impairment in Germany. *Int J. Lang. Commun. Disord.* **2014**, *49*, 558–566. [CrossRef]
23. Stamm, M. Begabung, Kultur und Schule. Mythen, Gegenmythen und Wissenschaftliche Erkenntnisse zu den Grundlagen der Begabtenförderung. *Z. Int. Bild. Entwicklungspädagogik* **2010**, *33*, 25–33.
24. Stamm, M. Lebenskompetenz Schlägt Intelligenz. Dossier 24/1, Swiss Education 2024. Available online: https://margritstamm.ch/dokumente/dossiers/292-lebenskompetenz-def/file/.html (accessed on 16 July 2024).
25. WHO. *ICD-10, International Statistical Classification of Diseases and Related Health Problems, 10th Revision*, 5th ed.; WHO: Geneva, Switzerland, 2016.
26. Snijders-Oomen. *Non-Verbal Intelligence Test SON-R 2,5-7*; Hild, P., Winkel, M., Wijnberg-Williams, B., Laros, J., Eds.; Swets & Zeitlinger B.V.: Lisse, The Netherland, 1997.
27. Grimme, H. *SETK 3-5: Sprachentwicklungstest für 3-5jährige Kinder*; Hogrefe: Göttingen, Germany, 2001.
28. Kiese-Himmel, C. *AWST-R: Aktiver Wortschatztest für 3-5jährige Kinder*; Hogrefe: Göttingen, Germany, 2005.
29. Kauschke, C.; Siegmülle, J. *Patholinguistische Diagnostik bei Sprachentwicklungsstörungen*, 2nd ed.; Hogrefe: Göttingen, Germany, 2009.
30. *KABC-II—Kaufman Assessment Battery for Children*, 2nd ed.; Kaufman, A.S., Kaufman, N.L., Eds.; Deutsche Bearbeitung Hrsg; Melchers, P., Melchers, M.; Hogrefe: Göttingen, Germany, 2015.
31. Zimmer, R.; Volkamer, M. *MOT4-6: Motoriktest für vier-bis Sechsjährige Kinder*, 2nd ed.; Verlag Weinheim: Landsberg, Germany, 1987.
32. WHO. *ICF-CY International Classification of Functioning, Disability and Health—Children + Youth Version*; WHO: Geneva, Switzerland, 2007.
33. Boyatzis, C.; Satyaprasad, C. Children's facial and gestural decoding and encoding: Relations between skills and with popularity. *J. Nonverbal Behav.* **1994**, *18*, 37–55. [CrossRef]

34. Randhawa, E. Das Frühkindliche Selbstkonzept. Struktur, Entwicklung, Korrelate und Einflußfaktoren. Dissertation 2012. Available online: https://opus.ph-heidelberg.de/frontdoor/index/docld/42/file/Randdhawa_Dissertation_Selbstkonzept (accessed on 1 November 2019).
35. Lloyd-Esenkaya, A.; Russell, J.; St Clair, M.C. What Are the Peer Interaction Strengths Difficulties in Children with Developmental Language Disorder? A Systematic Review. *Int. J. Environ. Resfr. Public Health* **2020**, *17*, 3140. [CrossRef]
36. Law, J.; Garrett, Z.; Nye, C. Speech and language therapy interventions for children with primary speech and language delay or disorder. *Cochrane Database Syst. Rev.* **2003**, *3*, CD004110. [CrossRef]
37. Timm, A. *Sprache und Interaktion im Kindergarten. Eine Quantitativ-Qualitative Analyse der Sprachlichen und Kommunikativen Kompetenzen von drei- bis Sechsjährigen Kindern*; Julius Klinkhard: Bad Heilbrunn, Germany, 2009.
38. Buzhardt, J.; Wallisch, A.; Irvin, D.; Boyd, B.; Salley, B.; Jia, F. Exploring Growth in Expressive Communication of Infants and Toddlers with Autism Spectrum Disorder. *J. Early Interv.* **2022**, *44*, 3–22. [CrossRef]
39. Heckman, J.J. Investing in disadvantaged young children is an economically efficient policy. In *Building the Economic Case for Investments in Preschool*; accessed 2015; Committee for Economic Development: New York, NY, USA, 2006.
40. Gallagher, A.L.; Chiat, S. Evaluation of speech and language therapy interventions for pre-school children with specific language impairment: A comparison of outcomes following specialist intensive, nursery-based and no intervention. *Int. J. Lang. Commun. Disord.* **2009**, *44*, 616–638. [CrossRef]
41. Coombes, L.; Bristowe, K.; Ellis-Smith, C.; Aworinde, J.; Fraser, L.K.; Downing, J.; Bluebond-Langener, M.; Chambers, L.; Murtagh, F.E.M.; Harding, R. Enhancing validity, reliability and participation in self-reported health outcome for children and young people: A systematic review of recall period, response scale format, and administration modality. *Qual. Life Res.* **2021**, *30*, 1803–1832. [CrossRef]
42. Khadka, J.; Kwon, J.; Petrou, S.; Lancsar, E.; Ratcliffe, J. Mind the (inter-rater) gap. An investigation of self-reported versus proxy-reported assessments in the derivation of childhood utility values for economic evaluation: A systematic review. *Soc. Sci. Med.* **2019**, *240*, 112543. [CrossRef] [PubMed]
43. Mortensen, J.A.; Barnet, M.A. Teacher-child interactions in Infant/toddler child care and socioemotional development. *Early Educ. Dev.* **2015**, *26*, 209–229. [CrossRef]
44. Whitehouse, A.J.O.; Varcin, K.J.; Pilar, S.; Billingham, W.; Alvares, G.A.; Barbaro, J.; Bent, C.A.; Blenkley, D.; Boutrus, M.; Chee, A.; et al. Effect of Preemptive Intervention on Developmental Outcomes Among Infants Showing Early Signs of Autism. A Randomized Clinical Trial of Outcomes to Diagnosis. *JAMA Pediatr.* **2021**, *175*, e213298. [CrossRef] [PubMed]
45. Dickinson, D.K.; Porche, M.V. Relation between language experiences in preschool classrooms and children's kindergarten and fourth-grade language and reading abilities. *Child Dev.* **2011**, *82*, 870–886. [CrossRef]
46. Botting, N.; Conti-Ramsden, G. Social and Behavioural Difficulties in Children with Language Impairment. *Child Lang. Teach. Ther.* **2000**, *16*, 105–120. [CrossRef]
47. Maggio, V.; Grana, N.E.; Richaudeau, A.; Torres, S.; Giannotti, A.; Suburo, A.M. Behavior Problems in Children with Specific Language Impairment. *J. Child Neurol.* **2014**, *29*, 194–202. [CrossRef]
48. Johnson, C.J.; Beitchman, J.H.; Brownlie, E.B. Twenty-Year Follow-up of Children with and Without Speech-Language-Impairments: Family, Educational, Occupational, and Quality of Life Outcomes. *Am. J. Speech Lang. Pathol.* **2010**, *19*, 51–65. [CrossRef]

children

MDPI

Article

Strengthening Early Childhood Protective Factors Through Safe and Supportive Classrooms: Findings from Jump Start + COVID Support

Ruby Natale [1], Tara Kenworthy LaMarca [1], Yue Pan [2], Elizabeth Howe [1], Yaray Agosto [1], Rebecca J. Bulotsky-Shearer [3], Sara M. St. George [2], Tanha Rahman [1], Carolina Velasquez [1] and Jason F. Jent [1,*]

1 Mailman Center for Child Development, School of Medicine, University of Miami Miller, Miami, FL 33136, USA; rnatale@med.miami.edu (R.N.); tlk38@med.miami.edu (T.K.L.); ewfxhowe@gmail.com (E.H.); yagosto@med.miami.edu (Y.A.); txr321@med.miami.edu (T.R.); cxv308@med.miami.edu (C.V.)

2 Department of Public Health Sciences, School of Medicine, University of Miami Miller, Miami, FL 33136, USA; panyue@med.miami.edu (Y.P.); s.stgeorge@med.miami.edu (S.M.S.G.)

3 Department of Psychology, University of Miami, Coral Gables, FL 33146, USA; rshearer@miami.edu

* Correspondence: jjent@med.miami.edu

Abstract: Background/Objectives: Early care and education programs promote children's social–emotional development, predicting later school success. The COVID-19 pandemic worsened an existing youth mental health crisis and increased teacher stress. Therefore, we applied an infant and early childhood mental health consultation model, Jump Start Plus COVID Support (JS+CS), aiming to decrease behavioral problems in children post-pandemic. Methods: A cluster randomized controlled trial compared JS+CS to an active control, Healthy Caregivers–Healthy Children (HC2), at 30 ECE centers in low-income areas in South Florida. Participants were not blinded to group assignment. Teachers reported on children's social–emotional development at baseline and post-intervention using the Devereux Early Childhood Assessment and Strengths and Difficulties Questionnaire. We assessed whether teacher stress, classroom practices, and self-efficacy mediated the relationship between JS+CS and child outcomes. We also explored whether baseline behavior problems moderated JS+CS effects on child protective factors, relative to HC2. Results: Direct group-by-time differences between JS+CS and HC2 were limited. However, JS+CS demonstrated significant within-group improvements in teacher-reported child protective factors, behavior support practices, and classroom safety practices. Classroom safety practices consistently mediated positive changes in child behaviors, including the DECA total protective factor score and subdomains of initiative and self-regulation. Additionally, teacher perceptions of behavior support mediated gains in child attachment. Conclusions: JS+CS shows promise in building protective systems around children through intentional support for teachers, underscoring the value of whole-child, whole-environment approaches in early intervention.

Keywords: infant and early childhood mental health consultation; protective factors; behavior problems; social–emotional development; COVID-19

1. Introduction

Early childhood is a critical period of development, as children's environments and experiences shape later outcomes [1,2]. Social–emotional development is especially important, as it is a powerful indicator of young children's future success in school and

https://doi.org/10.3390/children12070812

into adulthood [3–5]. Most children spend some time daily in some form of early care and education (ECE) program [6,7], many for at least 35 h per week [8]. These programs foster the learning and development of critical academic and social–emotional skills. However, children with poor or delayed social–emotional skills are more likely to engage in challenging behaviors, which puts them at risk for suspension and expulsion from ECE programs [9,10]. In fact, it is far more likely that children will be suspended from ECE centers than K-12 programs [11].

Attendance in an ECE program is particularly important for young children who are from minoritized racial and ethnic backgrounds, as they may experience higher levels of risk factors related to their development. For example, social environments in which children or families experience racial discrimination can negatively influence both health and behavioral outcomes [12]. Yet, suspensions and expulsions are higher in boys and Black and Hispanic children relative to their White peers [13,14]. The suspension and expulsion of these young children both limit their educational opportunities in the short term and are linked to long-term negative impacts on their social–emotional development and the risk of permanent school dropout years later [15]. It is therefore critical to identify alternative interventions to manage child behaviors in the classroom. Interventions implemented within ECE programs and the systems that surround them, such as high-quality learning programs and infant and early childhood mental health consultation, have demonstrated success in improving outcomes for marginalized youth in multiple domains (e.g., social–emotional, cognitive, and physical) [16–19].

Efforts to promote young children's positive social–emotional development have become even more critical post-COVID-19 [20,21]. The initial impact and sequelae of the pandemic, including lockdowns, social isolation, and increased family stressors, have contributed to a crisis in children's mental health [22] that has persisted in the years post-pandemic [23]. It is therefore imperative to provide ECE programs and teachers with the knowledge and skills for teaching emotional regulation and other resiliency skills during this post-pandemic period [17,24,25].

The COVID-19 pandemic also negatively impacted childcare centers, particularly in poor counties that were epidemic hotspots, like Miami-Dade in Florida [26]. In 2020, a third of Miami's childcare centers permanently closed [27], which led to an urgent need to help the remaining centers maintain high-quality care while adapting to critical safety requirements [28–30]. The Centers for Disease Control and Prevention (CDC) published public health guidelines to improve physical safety, but these guidelines were costly, complex, and frequently changing, leading to implementation barriers for many community-based childcare centers. These additional job demands were among many stressors for early childhood teachers during COVID-19 [31,32], in a profession where burnout and turnover were already common [33]. Furthermore, there are negative outcomes for children when teachers are stressed in ECE settings. For example, workplace stress is related to increased conflict in teacher–child relationships [34], and teacher emotional health and well-being are negatively associated with exclusionary practices [35]. It is therefore essential to support teachers and foster an environment at the center level that promotes growth during stressful times.

Jump Start Plus COVID Support (JS+CS) [36] is an infant and early childhood mental health consultation (IECMHC) program that adapted the Georgetown Model of IECMHC for the COVID-19 pandemic [37,38]. Bronfenbrenner's Bioecological Systems Theory serves as the foundation for the Georgetown Model of IECMHC. According to this paradigm, children develop within nested environmental systems, such as their families, schools, and larger cultural contexts. The Georgetown Model employs multilevel interventions (center, teacher, and child) that target systemic concerns rather than concentrating only on individual children [39,40]. This strategy, which has been modified for Jump Start, acknowledges that difficult behaviors frequently result from external circumstances, including poor teacher communication, difficulties at the center director level, and/or high teacher turnover brought on by work-related stress. Multilevel interventions that focus on the larger ecological system surrounding the child are therefore required [41]. Within the Jump Start IECMHC model, the teacher's skills and practices are the focus of the intervention as a means to improve child outcomes. The goal of IECMHC is to increase teacher capacity to manage challenging behaviors and promote social–emotional skills in children [42]. Master-level mental health consultants trained in IECMHC practices meet with teachers on a weekly basis to help them address their professional development goals related to promoting young children's social competence [38]. There is a strong evidence-base for the effectiveness of IECMHC for improving children's social–emotional well-being [43] and growing evidence that IECMHC promotes social–emotional learning in both children and their teachers [44]. We expect that children with more behavioral problems will benefit more from the intervention, as high-quality classroom practices offer greater benefits for children with behavioral risk factors [45–47]. Yet, the mediating factors associated with child outcomes have not been studied. A 2010 research synthesis called for a better understanding of the extent to which teachers' skills or classroom practices mediate the relationship between mental health consultation interventions and child outcomes [48]. This information is crucial to understand, especially in the context of public health crises such as COVID-19, so that interventions can be designed to support teachers in keeping children safe.

The purpose of this study was to explore how JS+CS, an IECMHC program adapted for public health crises like COVID-19, improved child social–emotional outcomes. JS+CS was adapted by promoting self-care and improving coping strategies by teachers within childcare centers to support children's needs during a public health crisis (see Figure 1 for program model overview) [36]. The theoretical underpinnings are based on the Georgetown Model of IECMHC (REF). Based on this framework, we posit that improved child psychosocial functioning (reduced internalizing/externalizing behaviors and increased prosocial behaviors) will improve via improvements in teachers' practices (e.g., use of trauma-focused behavior management), self-efficacy in handling challenging behaviors (attitudes), and beliefs (support from center directors) [38,49]. Thus we hypothesized that JS+CS would lead to (1) improved child protective factors as measured by the overall social–emotional protective factors on the Devereux Early Childhood Assessment (DECA; comprising three subscales: initiative, attachment, and self-regulation), (2) reduced child problem behaviors, (3) effects of JS+CS on child social–emotional and problem behaviors being mediated by teacher classroom practices and teacher stress, and (4) problem behaviors moderating the relationship between JS+CS practices and child protective factors, relative to an active control group and controlling for sociodemographic characteristics. Our study aimed to answer the following research questions:

1. Was the teacher's implementation of JS+CS practices effective in increasing children's protective factors over time, as mediated by teacher stress, teacher self-efficacy, and classroom practices, relative to the active control?
2. Was the teacher's implementation of JS+CS practices effective in decreasing children's problematic behaviors over time, as mediated by teacher stress, teacher self-efficacy, and classroom practices, relative to the active control?
3. To what extent do child externalizing and internalizing behaviors at baseline moderate the relationship between JS+CS practices and improvements in children's protective factors over time, relative to the active control?

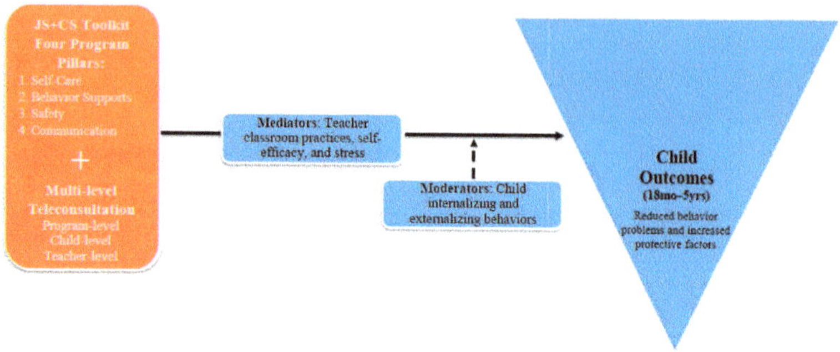

Figure 1. Program model overview.

2. Materials and Methods

2.1. Setting

This study took place in 30 ECE centers in South Florida, United States. The center inclusion criteria were as follows: (1) have ≥50 children (≥30 of whom are 18 months–3 years old); (2) be located in the low-income census tract, with at least 50% of families receiving childcare subsidies; (3) serve at least 60% Hispanic or 60% Non-Hispanic Black families; (4) have directors, teachers, and parents who agree to participate; and (5) have no prior enrollment in an early childhood mental health consultation program.

2.2. Participants

A total of 608 children and 190 teachers participated in this study (see Table 1 for child demographics and Table 2 for teacher demographics). This study was approved by the university's Institutional Review Board (IRB) and is currently registered with ClinicalTrials.gov (NCT05445518). The teacher participants and parents/guardians of the child participants signed informed consent forms prior to participating.

Table 1. Child demographic characteristics by intervention group.

Characteristic	JS+CS (n = 287)	HC2 (n = 317)	Total (N = 608)	Test Statistic	p-Value
Age (years)					
Mean (SD)	3.59 (1.18)	3.34 (1.15)	3.46 (1.17)	$F(1, 606) = 7.37$	0.007
Gender				$\chi^2(1) = 7.23$	0.007
Female	160 (55.7%)	142 (44.8%)	302 (50.0%)		
Male	127 (44.3%)	175 (55.2%)	302 (50.0%)		
Race				$\chi^2(5) = 13.25$	0.021
White	206 (74.1%)	198 (64.5%)	404 (69.1%)		
Black	48 (17.3%)	87 (28.3%)	135 (23.1%)		
Native American	4 (1.4%)	4 (1.3%)	8 (1.4%)		
Asian Pacific Islander	1 (0.4%)	0 (0.0%)	1 (0.2%)		
Multiracial	14 (5.0%)	9 (2.9%)	23 (3.9%)		
Other	5 (1.8%)	9 (2.9%)	14 (2.4%)		
Ethnicity				$\chi^2(4) = 20.62$	<0.001
Hispanic	238 (83.8%)	217 (68.9%)	455 (76.0%)		
Non-Hispanic White	11 (3.9%)	16 (5.1%)	27 (4.5%)		
Non-Hispanic Black	24 (8.5%)	60 (19.0%)	84 (14.0%)		
Haitian	7 (2.5%)	18 (5.7%)	25 (4.2%)		
Other	4 (1.4%)	4 (1.3%)	8 (1.3%)		

Table 1. *Cont.*

Characteristic	JS+CS (n = 287)	HC2 (n = 317)	Total (N = 608)	Test Statistic	p-Value
English Proficiency				$\chi^2(1) = 4.90$	0.027
Yes	174 (61.5%)	218 (70.1%)	392 (66.0%)		
No	109 (38.5%)	93 (29.9%)	202 (34.0%)		
Primary Language				$\chi^2(2) = 16.63$	<0.001
English	90 (31.6%)	151 (47.6%)	241 (40.0%)		
Spanish	194 (68.1%)	164 (51.7%)	358 (59.5%)		
Creole	1 (0.4%)	2 (0.6%)	3 (0.5%)		
Secondary Language				$\chi^2(3) = 8.45$	0.038
English	173 (65.5%)	149 (55.6%)	322 (60.5%)		
Spanish	80 (30.3%)	95 (35.4%)	175 (32.9%)		
Creole	8 (3.0%)	14 (5.2%)	22 (4.1%)		
Other	3 (1.1%)	10 (3.7%)	13 (2.4%)		

Note: Percentages for each characteristic are calculated within treatment groups. JS+CS = intervention group; HC2 = Healthy Caregivers–Healthy Children comparison group. Some categories may not sum to the total N due to missing data.

Table 2. Teacher demographic characteristics by treatment group.

Characteristic	JS+CS (n = 86)	HC2 (n = 104)	Total (n = 190)	Test Statistic	p-Value
Age (years)					
Mean (SD)	46.09 (12.58)	42.94 (13.67)	44.39 (13.24)	$F(1, 184) = 2.65$	0.105
Gender				$\chi^2(1) = 0.06$	0.811
Female	84 (97.7%)	101 (97.1%)	185 (97.4%)		
Male	2 (2.3%)	3 (2.9%)	5 (2.6%)		
Race				$\chi^2(4) = 1.71$	0.79
White	66 (76.7%)	74 (72.5%)	140 (74.5%)		
Black	12 (14.0%)	21 (20.6%)	33 (17.6%)		
Native American	1 (1.2%)	1 (1.0%)	2 (1.1%)		
Multiracial	4 (4.7%)	3 (2.9%)	7 (3.7%)		
Other	3 (3.5%)	3 (2.9%)	6 (3.2%)		
Ethnicity				$\chi^2(2) = 10.03$	0.007
Hispanic	76 (90.5%)	81 (77.9%)	157 (83.5%)		
Non-Hispanic White	1 (1.2%)	7 (6.7%)	8 (4.3%)		
Non-Hispanic Black	3 (3.6%)	9 (8.7%)	12 (6.4%)		
Haitian	0 (0.0%)	5 (4.8%)	5 (2.7%)		
Other	4 (4.8%)	2 (1.9%)	6 (3.2%)		
English Proficiency				$\chi^2(1) = 6.53$	0.011
Yes	32 (37.2%)	57 (55.9%)	89 (47.3%)		
No	54 (62.8%)	45 (44.1%)	99 (52.7%)		
Secondary Language				$\chi^2(3) = 6.74$	0.081
English	48 (64.0%)	44 (51.2%)	92 (57.1%)		
Spanish	21 (28.0%)	28 (32.6%)	49 (30.4%)		
Creole	0 (0.0%)	6 (7.0%)	6 (3.7%)		
Other	6 (8.0%)	8 (9.3%)	14 (8.7%)		
Education Level				$\chi^2(7) = 6.86$	0.443
Elementary or Less	0 (0.0%)	1 (1.0%)	1 (0.5%)		
Some High School	2 (2.4%)	3 (2.9%)	5 (2.7%)		
High School/GED	16 (19.5%)	19 (18.4%)	35 (18.9%)		
Technical Training	9 (11.0%)	4 (3.9%)	13 (7.0%)		
Some College	15 (18.3%)	21 (20.4%)	36 (19.5%)		
Associate Degree	8 (9.8%)	14 (13.6%)	22 (11.9%)		
Bachelor's Degree	25 (30.5%)	37 (35.9%)	62 (33.5%)		
Graduate Degree	7 (8.5%)	4 (3.9%)	11 (5.9%)		

Table 2. Cont.

Characteristic	JS+CS (n = 86)	HC2 (n = 104)	Total (n = 190)	Test Statistic	p-Value
Professional Experience	M (SD)	M (SD)	M (SD)		
Years as Childcare Professional	11.30 (10.18)	11.24 (8.40)	11.27 (9.17)	$F(1, 162) = 0.00$	0.967
Years at Current Program	8.59 (8.75)	6.28 (7.01)	7.28 (7.87)	$F(1, 139) = 3.03$	0.084
Children Enrolled in Classroom	13.39 (6.15)	12.13 (5.61)	12.70 (5.88)	$F(1, 187) = 2.14$	0.145

Note: Percentages are calculated within intervention groups. JS+CS = intervention group; HC2 = comparison group. Sample sizes vary by characteristic due to missing data.

2.3. Measures

2.3.1. Demographics

Parents completed a 33-item intake form that collected sociodemographic information about themselves and their child. Child-specific items included age, gender, race, ethnicity, English proficiency, preferred language, and health insurance coverage. Teachers completed both an intake form and a classroom demographics form, which collected information about themselves as early childcare professionals, the makeup of their classroom, and suspension and expulsion practices.

2.3.2. Child Protective Factors

The Devereux Early Childhood Assessment (DECA) for Infants and Toddlers (DECA-I/T) [50] and the DECA for Preschoolers, Second Edition (DECA-P2) [51], are validated, reliable parent and teacher report measures of protective factors that promote resilience in children ages 1 month through 5 years [52,53]. In this study, we focus on the teacher report scale. These measures are standardized and norm-referenced. There are 36 items on the DECA-I/T and 38 items on the DECA-P2 that are rated on a 5-point scale from "never" (0) to "very frequently" (4). The measures yield three subscales: initiative (i.e., the ability to use independent thoughts and actions to meet needs), self-regulation (i.e., the ability to express emotions and behaviors in healthy ways), and attachment/relationships (i.e., a mutual, strong, long-lasting relationship between children and significant adults). Example items include "try to clean up after herself/himself", "adjust to changes in routine", and "act happy when praised" (DECA-I/T), as well as "show an interest in learning new things", "show affection for familiar adults", and "play well with others" (DECA-P2). These measures yield subscale scores as well as a total protective factor (TPF) score. The DECA measures have adequate internal consistency in English- and Spanish-speaking, low-income, and diverse samples [54]. In this study, the internal consistency for the DECA total protective factors scale was a = 0.975.

2.3.3. Child Externalizing and Internalizing Behaviors

The Strengths and Difficulties Questionnaire (SDQ) is a 25-item behavioral screening measure for youth ages 2–17, with versions for 2–4-year-olds and 4–17-year-olds. The SDQ has also shown promising reliability for 12–24-month-old children, though reliability was better for externalizing than internalizing subscales [55]. There are both parent and teacher report versions, and the teacher report is used for this study. Items are rated on a 3-point Likert scale ranging from "not true" (0) to "somewhat true" (1) and "certainly true" (2). The items are divided into five scales in the following domains: emotional symptoms, conduct problems, hyperactivity/inattention, peer relationship problems, and prosocial behavior. Example items include "Often loses temper" (conduct), "Helpful if someone is hurt, upset or feeling ill" (prosocial), and "Many fears, easily scared" (emotional). The conduct problems and hyperactivity/inattention scales are summed for an externalizing score; the emotional and peer problems scales are summed to create an internalizing score. Based on published SDQ scoring categories, children's scores for total problems, externalizing problems, and internalizing problems were categorized as being within the normal, borderline, high, or very high range. The SDQ has established validity and reliability [56]. In this study, the internal consistency for the SDQ total problem scale was $\alpha = 0.860$.

2.3.4. Teacher Implementation of JS+CS Model

The Health Environment Rating Scale-Classroom (HERS-C) is a 30 min classroom observation developed by the study investigators that measures the extent to which teachers implement practices and policies within the classroom related to the JS+CS intervention model. The observation comprises four domains: safety, behavioral supports, communication, and resiliency coping. These domains align with core national standards for health and safety in ECE programs [57], map onto the JS+CS pillars, and allow for the measurement of expected areas of change in the control centers' obesity prevention intervention (nutrition and physical activity). Items reflect key classroom practices such as the "number of times children are taken outside for active play per 8 h day" and how often "high sugar/high fat snacks such as chips, cake, pastry, doughnuts and ice cream are served". This measure is scored on a 7-point Likert scale rated from "little or no implementation" (1) to "excellent implementation" (7). In this study, internal consistency of the HERS-C subscales ranged from adequate to good, with Cronbach's a coefficients of 0.62 for safety, 0.85 for behavior management, 0.71 for communication, and 0.70 for resiliency. All four pillars were examined.

2.3.5. Teacher Self-Efficacy

The Teacher Opinion Survey is a 12-item self-report measure of teachers' confidence in their ability to manage challenging child behaviors [58]. Example items include "If a student in my class became disruptive and noisy, I feel pretty sure that I'd know how to respond effectively" and "I have enough training to deal with almost any classroom situation". It is rated on a Likert scale from "strongly disagree" (1) to "strongly agree" (5), with higher scores representing higher perceptions of teachers' confidence in managing children's behaviors. The total score for this measure in this study had adequate internal consistency ($\alpha = 0.785$).

The Brief Resilient Coping Scale is a 4-item measure of the tendency to cope with stress in an adaptive manner, with demonstrated reliability and validity [59]. Representative items include "I look for creative ways to alter difficult situations" and "Regardless of what happens to me, I believe I can control my reaction to it". Items are rated on a 5-point scale from "does not describe me at all" (1) to "describes me very well" (5) and are summed to identify low (4–13 points), medium (14–16 points), and high (17–20 points) resilient copers. In this study, the internal consistency for the Brief Resilient Coping Scale was $\alpha = 0.835$.

2.3.6. Teacher Stress

The Everyday Stressors Index (ESI) is a 20-item measure of common life stressors such as family, housing, transportation, and employment [60]. Items reflect experiences, for example, "having too many responsibilities" and "not enough money for basic necessities, such as clothing, housing, food, and health care". The ESI has shown good reliability and validity with low-income and Hispanic populations [61]. It is rated on a Likert scale from "not bothered at all" (1) to "bothered a great deal" (4), with higher ratings indicating more worry, upset, or bother from problems. There was also an option to select "don't know" (0). In this study, the internal consistency for the Everyday Stressors Index was $\alpha = 0.868$.

The Child Care Worker Job Stress Inventory is a 51-item measure of workplace stress for childcare center workers, with established reliability and validity [62]. This measure consists of three 17-item scales: job demands, job control, and job resources. The job demand and job resource scales include questions that begin with the stem "How often do the following things happen at work?" which includes "I have to work long hours" and "I feel respected for the work that I do" and are rated on a Likert scale from "rarely/never" (1) to "most of the time" (5). The job control scale items begin with the stem "How much control do you have over the following things at work?" which includes "the types of daily activities that you do" and are rated from "very little" (1) to "very much" (5). In this study, internal consistency of the Childcare Worker Stress Inventory subscales was excellent, with Cronbach's a coefficients of 0.83 for job demands, 0.87 for job control, and 0.94 for job resources.

2.4. Procedures

Details of the study design and procedures have been described elsewhere [17], but briefly, similar to [63], as the intervention is multilevel and center-wide, we randomly assigned centers (N = 24) to one of two groups (intervention or attention control). In cluster randomized controlled trials such as this, clusters (i.e., childcare centers) rather than individuals are randomized to intervention or control groups, and outcomes are measured on individuals within those clusters. The intervention group received the JS+CS program (n = 12). The attention control group (n = 12) was an active, time-matched group that was placed in the HC2 [63] obesity prevention program, a program unrelated to JS+CS. The implementation phase lasted approximately 14 weeks for both groups. Demographic data and outcome measures were collected at baseline and immediately post-intervention via paper surveys or an online database, REDCap [64], based on participant preference. Virtual telepresence robots were utilized to complete classroom observational measures (i.e., HERS-C).

2.4.1. Jump Start Plus COVID Support (JS+CS)

JS+CS is an IECMHC program modeled after Georgetown University's IECMHC model to improve children's social, emotional, and behavioral development, prevent behavioral challenges, and reduce suspension and expulsion. JS+CS incorporates *Caring for Our Children National Health and Safety Standards* [57], CDC COVID-19 guidelines for childcare centers [65], and evidence-based practices for building social competence in children [66]. It is organized into four pillars: self-care, trauma-informed behavior support, safety, and communication. It is delivered by mental health consultants at the program (to directors), classroom (to teachers), and child (to parents) levels [36]. Given that the pandemic led childcare centers to restrict visitors at times, consultations were applied in a hybrid model, both in person and via virtual telepresence robotic consultation [63]. In addition, teachers received multiple resources, including 24 infographics covering each of the program's four pillars.

2.4.2. Healthy Caregivers–Healthy Children (HC2)

HC2 is an existing, evidence-based obesity prevention program that targets childcare centers' nutrition and physical activity environments and has been delivered by mental health consultants in settings similar to this study [67–69]. The HC2 toolkit is organized around four program policies: (1) snack, which emphasizes serving fresh fruits, vegetables, and whole grains over sweets and high-fat foods; (2) beverage, which involves offering low-fat or non-fat milk, limiting juice, and promoting water; (3) physical activity, which encourages providing at least 90 min of physical activity daily; and (4) screen time, which limits screen use to under 30 min per week. Like JS+CS, HC2 was implemented over 14 weeks with a minimum of one hour per week using the same multilevel approach (program, classroom, and child), but was delivered by trained research assistants through in-person visits or virtual telepresence robots. Teachers received weekly lesson plans tailored to each policy, along with Supplementary Materials (e.g., puppets, soccer balls, and parachutes). Control centers received the same pre- and post-intervention measures and incentives as the JS+CS sites to ensure retention.

2.5. Analysis

To evaluate the effectiveness of the JS+CS program compared to the HC2 control group, we first conducted generalized estimating equation (GEE) analyses for each child outcome. Seven outcome variables were examined, including four DECA subscales—total protective factors, attachment/relationships, self-regulation, and initiative—and three SDQ subscales: total difficulties and externalizing and internalizing problems. Each outcome was modeled as a function of treatment group (JS+CS vs. HC2), time (baseline vs. follow-up), and their interaction, adjusting for child age. Repeated measures were accounted for using an exchangeable correlation structure, with child ID specified as the repeated subject. These models allowed us to estimate the time-specific effects of JS+CS and determine whether outcomes improved more in the intervention group relative to the control group. We used an intent-to-treat (ITT) approach that retained all participants with baseline data and applied robust standard errors to mitigate potential biases. We also conducted sensitivity analyses by comparing models restricted to complete cases to examine the robustness of our findings.

To investigate potential mechanisms through which JS+CS exerts its effects, we implemented a longitudinal mediation analysis using the GEE framework. For each of the seven outcomes and ten proposed mediators (e.g., teacher stress, teacher efficacy, and classroom practices), we conducted a three-step mediation procedure. Step 1 estimated the total effect (Path C) of JS+CS on the outcome. Step 2 estimated the effect of JS+CS on the mediator (Path A). Step 3 included both the treatment and the mediator to estimate the direct effect of treatment (Path C') and the mediator's effect on the outcome (Path B). Indirect effects were computed as the product of coefficients $A \times B$, and standard errors were calculated using the delta method. Mediation was classified as full, partial, or none based on the significance of the indirect effect and comparison between total and direct effects. Full mediation was defined as a statistically significant indirect effect accompanied by a non-significant direct effect (Path C'), indicating that the mediator fully explains the treatment–outcome relationship. Partial mediation was defined as both the indirect and direct effects being significant, suggesting that the mediator accounts for part, but not all, of the intervention's effect. This longitudinal GEE approach leveraged the repeated measures design to account for within-subject correlations and produce population-averaged estimates.

In parallel, we conducted a change score-based mediation analysis using linear regression models to examine how changes in mediators contributed to changes in child outcomes (See Figure 2). For each outcome–mediator pair, we computed difference scores from baseline until follow-up. We then estimated Path A (effect of JS+CS on change in the mediator), Path B (effect of mediator change on outcome change, controlling for treatment), and Path C (total effect of JS+CS on outcome change). Indirect effects were calculated as the product of treatment $\rightarrow$ mediator and mediator $\rightarrow$ outcome paths.

Significance was determined via Z-tests, and mediation was classified as full, partial, or none depending on whether indirect and/or direct effects were statistically significant. The same definitions of full and partial mediation were applied: full mediation required a significant indirect effect and a non-significant direct effect, while partial mediation required both paths to be significant. This approach provides a straightforward interpretation of change over time, directly focusing on pre–post differences attributable to the intervention. The GEE method leveraged repeated measures for robust population-averaged estimates, while the change score method isolated treatment-driven within-subject differences. Results from both approaches were compared to ensure consistency and to enhance the validity of conclusions regarding mediation.

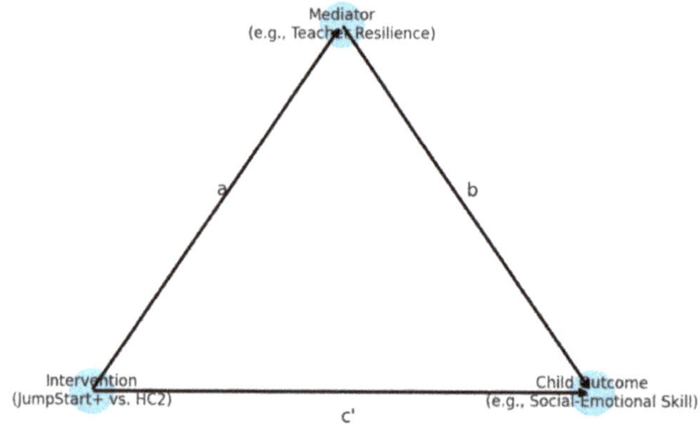

Figure 2. Conceptual mediation model for JS+CS analysis.

We also examined potential moderation by baseline SDQ risk categories by including three-way interactions (e.g., treatment × time × SDQ category), with SDQ total, externalizing, and internalizing classifications included as moderators in separate models.

All models reported parameter estimates, robust standard errors, *p*-values, and 95% confidence intervals. All statistical analyses were conducted using SAS (version 9.4), with supplemental data cleaning, visualization, and descriptive statistics conducted in R (version 4.4.2) using the base, Hmisc, dplyr, tidyr, lme4, and emmeans packages [70–74].

3. Results

3.1. Effectiveness of JS+CS

Analysis of the data revealed several significant findings regarding the treatment groups and changes over time (See Table 3). Although children were randomized to intervention conditions at the childcare center level, teacher reports indicated significant differences in protective factors and problem behaviors between intervention groups. Children in the JS+CS group were rated by teachers as demonstrating significantly lower protective factors on the DECA compared to the HC2 group, indicating worse overall protective factors ($\beta = -5.3576$, $p < 0.0001$), attachment/relationships ($\beta = -2.4879$, $p < 0.0001$), self-regulation ($\beta = -4.1818$, $p < 0.0001$), and initiative ($\beta = -6.5743$, $p < 0.0001$). Additionally, the JS+CS group exhibited significantly higher SDQ total problems (estimate = 2.0777, $p < 0.0001$) and externalizing scores (estimate = 1.6939, $p < 0.0001$) relative to the HC2 group, reflecting more problematic behavioral concerns as perceived by their teachers. However, no significant difference was observed between groups on SDQ internalizing scores ($\beta = 0.3805$, $p = 0.0901$).

As it relates to within-subject changes over time, both children in the JS+CS and HC2 groups demonstrate significant improvements in DECA attachment/relationships scores ($\beta = 3.8329$, $p < 0.0001$), and total protective factors ($\beta = 1.9311$, $p = 0.0309$) were observed from baseline to follow-up. Other DECA subscales did not show significant changes over the study period. Further, there were no significant changes over time in teacher perceptions of children's problem behaviors as measured by the SDQ.

Table 3. Child outcome measures by intervention condition at baseline and follow-up.

	JS+CS (Intervention)		HC2 (Comparison)		Effect	Estimate	Std. Error	p-Value
	Baseline (N = 304)	Follow-Up (N = 304)	Baseline (N = 367)	Follow-Up (N = 367)				
DECA Total Protective Factors Mean (SD)	51.5 (10.7)	53.1 (10.1)	55.6 (12.5)	57.1 (10.5)	Treatment (JS+CS)	−5.3576	1.065	<0.0001
Missing	82 (27.0%)	104 (34.2%)	137 (37.3%)	213 (58.0%)	Time (Follow-Up vs. Baseline)	1.9311	0.8948	0.0309
					Interaction (JS+CS × Follow-Up)	0.199	1.2054	0.8689
DECA Attachment/Relationships Mean (SD)	49.3 (11.2)	51.8 (9.58)	50.5 (11.9)	53.7 (10.5)	Treatment (JS+CS)	−2.4879	0.9724	0.0105
Missing	67 (22.0%)	90 (29.6%)	116 (31.6%)	187 (51.0%)	Time (Follow-Up vs. Baseline)	3.8329	0.818	<0.0001
					Interaction (JS+CS × Follow-Up)	−0.864	1.1522	0.4533
DECA Self-Regulation Mean (SD)	52.8 (10.6)	52.9 (10.1)	56.2 (11.9)	56.0 (10.6)	Treatment (JS+CS)	−4.1818	1.0208	<0.0001
Missing	64 (21.1%)	88 (28.9%)	126 (34.3%)	192 (52.3%)	Time (Follow-Up vs. Baseline)	0.3181	0.8269	0.7004
					Interaction (JS+CS × Follow-Up)	0.1974	1.1162	0.8596
DECA Initiative Mean (SD)	51.2 (10.9)	53.4 (10.7)	56.7 (12.0)	56.7 (10.5)	Treatment (JS+CS)	−6.5743	1.0586	<0.0001
Missing	70 (23.0%)	91 (29.9%)	119 (32.4%)	196 (53.4%)	Time (Follow-Up vs. Baseline)	0.606	0.8869	0.4945
					Interaction (JS+CS × Follow-Up)	1.9162	1.1374	0.0921
SDQ Total Problems Mean (SD)	7.99 (5.88)	7.79 (5.95)	6.65 (6.18)	5.85 (5.87)	Treatment (JS+CS)	2.0777	0.5232	<0.0001
Missing	74 (24.3%)	88 (28.9%)	101 (27.5%)	181 (49.3%)	Time (Follow-Up vs. Baseline)	−0.4308	0.4098	0.2932
					Interaction (JS+CS × Follow-Up)	−0.0408	0.5574	0.9416
SDQ Externalizing Mean (SD)	5.36 (4.25)	5.18 (4.08)	4.13 (4.07)	3.69 (3.86)	Treatment (JS+CS)	1.6939	0.3659	<0.0001
Missing	74 (24.3%)	88 (28.9%)	101 (27.5%)	181 (49.3%)	Time (Follow-Up vs. Baseline)	−0.1869	0.289	0.5178
					Interaction (JS+CS × Follow-Up)	−0.2006	0.3936	0.6102
SDQ Internalizing Mean (SD)	2.63 (2.57)	2.62 (2.51)	2.53 (2.69)	2.16 (2.60)	Treatment (JS+CS)	0.3805	0.2245	0.0901
Missing	74 (24.3%)	88 (28.9%)	101 (27.5%)	181 (49.3%)	Time (Follow-Up vs. Baseline)	−0.2309	0.1903	0.225
					Interaction (JS+CS × Follow-Up)	0.1561	0.2568	0.5433

Note: DECA = Devereux Early Childhood Assessment; SDQ = Strengths and Difficulties Questionnaire. Higher scores on DECA scales indicate more positive developmental outcomes; higher scores on SDQ scales indicate more problematic behaviors. Statistical effects are derived from mixed-effects models.

No significant treatment X time interaction effects were detected for any outcome measures. This finding suggests that while overall improvements occurred in some child domains (particularly attachment/relationships), the pattern of change over time was similar for both the JS+CS and HC2 groups, with neither group showing differential rates of improvement.

3.2. Mediator Analyses

Seventy mediation models were tested (see Supplementary Table S1). These models were pre-specified based on the JS+CS conceptual framework, and we hypothesized that multiple teacher-level factors (e.g., stress, self-efficacy, and classroom practices) could independently mediate different child social–emotional outcomes. We used a theory-driven approach to examine all plausible intervention mechanisms, rather than exploratory or data-driven analysis. To enhance clarity and support interpretation, Figure 3 provides a consolidated visual summary of the key mediation pathways identified across all models. These pathways illustrate the extent to which teacher perceptions and observed practices explained the relationship between JS+CS and various child outcomes.

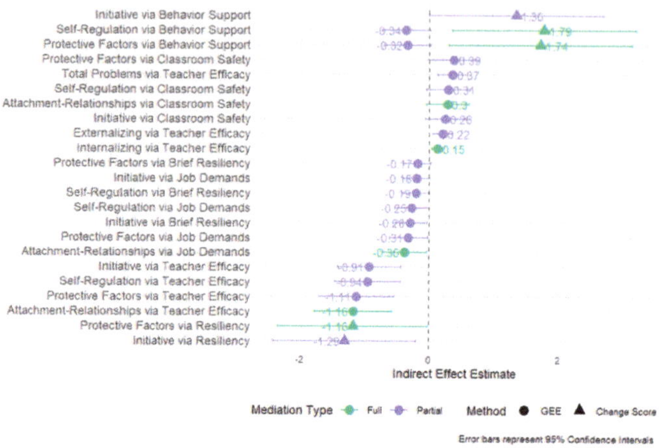

Figure 3. Significant indirect effects of the JS+CS intervention: combined mediation pathways from generalized estimating equations and change score analyses.

Our analyses revealed that observed teacher safety practices within the classroom significantly mediated the relationship between the JS+CS intervention and multiple child outcomes in the intended direction. Teacher safety practices fully mediated the relationship between JS+CS and teacher perceptions of children's attachment/relationships (Z = 1.818). Specifically, JS+CS had a significant positive association with teachers' observed safety practices within classrooms, which in turn increased teachers' ratings of children's attachment/relationships. Teacher safety practices also partially mediated the relationships between JS+CS and teacher perceptions of children's initiative (Z = 1.652) and self-regulation (Z = 1.780). The JS+CS intervention positively influenced safety practices, which subsequently led to improvements in these developmental domains. Similarly, teacher safety practices partially mediated the relationship between JS+CS and teacher perceptions of children's overall resilience as measured by the DECA total protective factors (Z = 1.973). JS+CS significantly improved observed teacher safety practices within classrooms, which in turn enhanced teachers' ratings of children's overall resilience.

Beyond resilience, teacher safety practices partially mediated the relationship between JS+CS and teacher ratings of children's externalizing behaviors (Z = −1.699). The JS+CS intervention had a positive impact on observed teacher practices related to safety environments (e.g., COVID-19 protocols and self-regulation spaces for children), and these improved safety environments reduced teachers' ratings of children's externalizing behavior problems.

Our mediator analyses also revealed several significant mediational pathways between the JS+CS intervention and child outcomes in unintended directions. The mediational effects primarily operated through classroom-level factors, particularly teacher efficacy and job demands.

Teacher efficacy emerged as the most consistent and powerful mediator across multiple outcome domains. The JS+CS intervention was associated with decreased teacher efficacy, which in turn predicted lower scores on all DECA subscales, including attachment/relationships (Z = −3.777), initiative (Z = −3.622), self-regulation (Z = −3.576), and total protective factors (Z = −3.718). Conversely, this reduced teacher efficacy was linked to increased behavioral problems as measured by the SDQ, including externalizing problems (Z = 2.916), internalizing problems (Z = 3.004), and total problems (Z = 3.155).

Childcare worker job demands represented another significant mediational pathway. The JS+CS intervention was associated with increased job demands, which subsequently predicted decreased scores on attachment/relationships (Z = −2.115), initiative (Z = −1.659), self-regulation (Z = −1.902), and total protective factors (Z = −2.005). Additionally, increased job demands were associated with higher levels of externalizing (Z = 1.553) and total behavior problems (Z = 1.605).

Significant partial mediation was observed across several models, including teachers' reported use of adaptive coping strategies or resilience. For child initiative, the indirect effect through teacher resilience was significant, indicating that lower teacher resilience in the JS+CS group partially explained reduced child initiative (Z = −2.086), self-regulation (Z = −1.805), and total protective factors (Z = −1.607).

Teacher-observed behavior management practices (HERS-C) partially mediated the effects between JS+CS and child self-regulation, total protective factors, and externalizing behaviors. The JS+CS intervention was associated with decreased teacher-observed behavior management practices, which subsequently predicted decreased scores on child self-regulation (Z = −1.820) and total protective factors (Z = −1.758) and higher levels of externalizing behavior problems (Z = 1.572).

No other teacher practices, beliefs, or stress mediated the relationship between JS+CS and child outcomes.

3.3. *Mediation Analysis: Change Score Models*

Among the seventy models tested (see Supplementary Table S2), five demonstrated significant mediation, indicating that changes in specific teacher-related factors explained the impact of the intervention on child emotional and behavioral improvements (see Figure 3). Notably, improvements in teachers' perceptions of their own behavioral support fully mediated the intervention's effect on increasing child protective factors (indirect effect = 1.739; SE = 0.725; Z = 2.40; $p = 0.017$), even though the overall treatment effect was not significant. Similarly, teacher ratings of the child's resiliency mediated the impact on protective factors (indirect effect = −1.161; SE = 0.590; Z = −1.97; $p = 0.049$), also with full mediation. For children's social relationship strengths, the indirect pathway through increased teacher behavioral support was again significant (indirect effect = 1.793; SE = 0.728; Z = 2.46; $p = 0.014$), reflecting partial mediation. Likewise, for internalizing behavior (emotional distress), changes in teacher-reported behavior and resiliency explained a portion of the intervention's effect (indirect effects = 1.361 and −1.294, respectively, $p < 0.05$), indicating partial mediation. In contrast, variables such as teacher self-efficacy, teacher stress, and workplace resources or control were not significant mediators in any models.

While most mediators demonstrated consistent effects across both analytic methods, two outcomes, self-regulation and protective factors via behavior support, showed discrepancies between the GEE and change score mediation analyses. Figure 3 serves as a visual synthesis of all 70 mediation models presented in Supplementary Table S1. This figure was designed to highlight the most robust and theoretically meaningful mediation pathways to help readers navigate the complexity of the findings.

In the GEE-based longitudinal models, behavior support was not a statistically significant mediator for either outcome, with indirect effects that were negative and non-significant (self-regulation: indirect effect = −0.345, SE = 0.189, and $p = 0.069$; protective factors: indirect effect = −0.323, SE = 0.184, and $p = 0.078$). In contrast, the change score analyses revealed significant positive mediation for both outcomes (self-regulation: Indirect effect = 1.793, SE = 0.728, and $p = 0.014$; protective factors: indirect effect = 1.739, SE = 0.725, and $p = 0.017$), suggesting that increases in teacher-rated behavior support from baseline until follow-up were associated with improvements in children's developmental outcomes.

These inconsistencies may reflect methodological differences between the approaches, with GEE models capturing population-averaged effects across timepoints, while change score models isolate within-person changes over time. The divergent findings suggest that although population-level effects of behavior support were modest, individual-level improvements in behavior support may play a meaningful role in enhancing child outcomes.

3.4. Moderator Analyses

Teacher-reported problematic child behaviors were evaluated as potential moderators of JS+CS intervention effects on children's protective factors (see Supplementary Table S3 for comprehensive results). Teacher perceptions of children's total problem behaviors (β = 2.59, SE =1.26, p = 0.04; see Figure 4) and children's internalizing behaviors (β = 3.17, SE =1.27, p = 0.01; see Figure 5) significantly moderated the relationship between JS+CS and improvements in children's DECA initiative outcomes. No other teacher-reported problematic child behaviors significantly moderated the relationship between JS+CS and improvements in other DECA outcomes (i.e., attachment/relationships and self-regulation). Additionally, we conducted moderator analyses to explore whether the effects of JS+CS varied by child gender, race/ethnicity, and language proficiency. No statistically significant three-way interactions were observed in these subgroups.

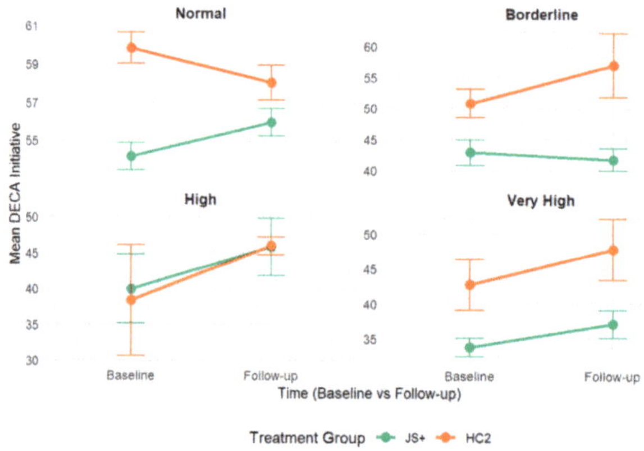

Figure 4. DECA initiative scores by intervention group, stratified by SDQ total problems.

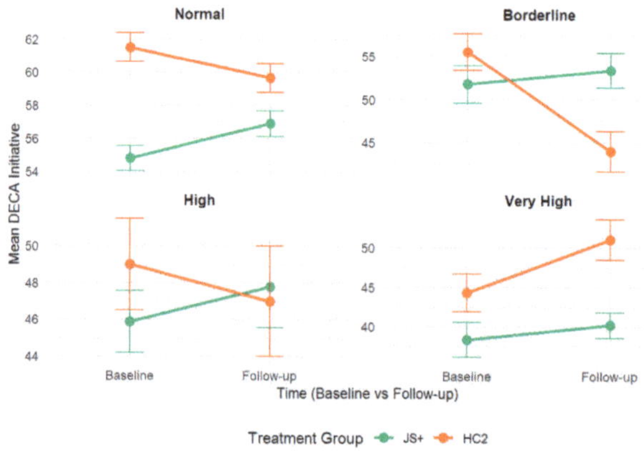

Figure 5. DECA initiative scores by intervention group, stratified by SDQ internalizing problems.

4. Discussion

The purpose of this study was to explore the impact of JS+CS, an IECMHC program adapted for public health crises like COVID-19, on child social–emotional outcomes in ECE settings. Our primary aim was to determine whether JS+CS would improve child protective factors and reduce problem behaviors, as well as to examine whether effects on child outcomes were mediated by teacher stress, self-efficacy, and classroom practices. Additionally, we hypothesized that baseline child behaviors would moderate the relationship between the intervention and outcomes, relative to an active control group. Mediation findings suggested that classroom practices related to safety and behavior support may be critical pathways through which JS+CS influences positive changes in children's social–emotional development. Findings, though modest, indicate that the JS+CS approach—emphasizing reflective consultation and classroom-based support—may contribute to meaningful changes in early learning environments, even amid implementation challenges and the ongoing impact of the COVID-19 pandemic. Although there were limited between-group effects, the results of this study offer several insights into the effectiveness of JS+CS, as well as areas for further refinement.

4.1. Child Protective Factors Mediated by Teacher Stress, Classroom Practices, and Self-Efficacy

Teacher implementation of JS+CS practices had a positive effect on children's protective factors over time, though the magnitude of the effect was modest. Mediation analysis revealed that improvements in teacher practices, particularly those related to classroom safety practices and behavior support, were key mechanisms through which the intervention influenced child protective factors.

However, while these findings suggest that JS+CS has the potential to enhance social–emotional development in children, the main effects on child outcomes of assignment to the JS+CS intervention condition compared to the HC2 active control condition were not observed. The limited between-group effects may be partially explained by the absence of statistically significant group-by-time interaction effects, which suggests that improvements in child outcomes occurred similarly across both JS+CS and HC2 conditions. This may reflect a limitation in statistical power due to attrition and differential dropout at follow-up. Alternatively, it is possible that both interventions, despite their differing emphases, had similar impacts on child social–emotional development. Given that HC2, while focused on physical health, also provided consistent support during a high-stress period, it may have exerted beneficial effects that narrowed observable differences between groups. It is possible that the initial differences in baseline characteristics between the two groups, despite randomization at the center level, may have masked the impact of the intervention. In addition, teachers in the JS+CS centers may have had a heightened awareness of children's behavioral difficulties due to the program's emphasis on mental health consultation, thereby influencing their ratings. The reflective coaching approach employed in JS+CS may have resulted in lower reported teacher self-efficacy, as consultants focused on fostering insight and autonomy rather than providing directive strategies. Research shows that teachers may overestimate their abilities relative to perceptions of their supervisors [75], and therefore, follow-up assessments after reflective supervision may offer a more accurate reflection of teachers' classroom confidence. Additionally, teachers in the JS+CS condition reported higher job demands, likely due to the intervention's more intensive structure and the time commitment required for consultation. In contrast, the HC2 intervention included more structured lesson plans and was easier to implement, which may have contributed to its relatively higher feasibility and lower burden on teachers. Given the limited between-group effects, further refinements to the JS+CS intervention, such as a more structured, versus reflective, approach, may be needed to see more pronounced effects on child outcomes.

4.2. Children's Problematic Behaviors Mediated by Teacher Stress, Classroom Practices, and Self-Efficacy

The study found that JS+CS led to reductions in children's externalizing behaviors over time, which were mediated through changes in classroom safety practices. These mediation results suggest that the JS+CS intervention has the potential to decrease problematic behaviors by improving classroom safety strategies. However, the effect sizes were modest, indicating that while there was a positive trend, the intervention may need to be adapted to provide more continuous access to resources for teachers to achieve more significant reductions in child behavior problems. For example, a mobile application that offers access to ongoing resources with quick accessibility may be more effective in reducing job demands [76].

Another consideration is the differential focus of the two interventions. Even though the JS+CS intervention and HC2 are designed to have differential outcomes, other studies have found that pediatric nutrition and physical wellness interventions for young children can also have a benefit on children's psychosocial outcomes [77]. While JS+CS centered on social–emotional learning and mental health consultation, HC2 targeted physical health behaviors, such as nutrition and physical activity, which have also been linked to cognitive and behavioral benefits [69].

Timing may have also played a role. The JS+CS and HC2 interventions were delivered during the COVID-19 pandemic, a period in which any form of professional support may have been perceived as particularly valuable. The HC2 model may have been equally effective as JS+CS in supporting teacher behaviors during the pandemic, and this indirectly benefited children's socio-emotional outcomes, regardless of its primary nutrition and wellness focus.

4.3. Children's Protective Factors Moderated by Children's Externalizing and Internalizing Behaviors

Some child baseline problem behaviors moderated the relationship between JS+CS implementation and improvements in child social–emotional protective factors. For children exhibiting higher levels of internalizing behaviors at baseline, assignment to the JS+CS intervention condition increased scores on initiative compared to children with similar levels of problem behaviors in the HC2 control group. For children who exhibited lower levels of total problem scores, JS+CS increased children's initiative compared to children with similar levels of total problem scores in the HC2 control condition. Teachers in JS+CS, compared to teachers in HC2, were able to more effectively utilize the intervention strategies to improve social–emotional outcomes in children who started with higher levels of internalizing problem behaviors. This suggests that JS+CS may be particularly beneficial for children who are at greater risk for developmental delays in social–emotional skills. However, even in these cases, the effect sizes remained modest, suggesting that while the intervention holds promise for children with more pronounced behavioral challenges, additional support or intensified interventions may be necessary for larger and more consistent outcomes. It is also important to note that baseline levels of behavior problems were relatively low across the sample, possibly limiting the potential for observable improvements. In addition, the DECA measure may show natural improvement over time as children mature and adapt to classroom environments, and it therefore may not be reflective of the intervention outcomes.

4.4. Limitations

Several limitations should be considered when interpreting these findings. While childcare sites were randomized, teachers in the JS+CS condition rated children as exhibiting more behavioral challenges and fewer protective factors at baseline, which may have influenced the results despite rigorous analytic controls. Future studies should examine additional baseline characteristics to determine potential confounding factors. Additionally, missing data was relatively high—a common issue in community-based effectiveness trials—but intent-to-treat analyses were used to retain as much data as possible. It is also important to acknowledge that teacher-reported measures may pose potential biases, as reflected in the literature [78]. We would also use caution in generalizing the findings outside of Miami-Dade County.

Another important consideration is the potency of the active control condition. HC2 may have been more effective than anticipated, especially during the COVID-19 pandemic, providing meaningful support that narrowed the gap between groups. Consultant turnover was also more pronounced in JS+CS, potentially impacting the consistency and quality of intervention delivery. Finally, long-term follow-ups are needed to assess whether JS+CS may yield delayed benefits that were not captured within this study's timeframe.

4.5. Future Directions

Despite these challenges, JS+CS still demonstrated value in specific domains, and the findings offer direction for future iterations of research. As the field moves into the post-pandemic era, future work should explore how to deliver JS+CS in a way that reduces teacher burden and maintains implementation fidelity, potentially through more streamlined or app-based models. Examining center-level outcomes may also help elucidate how contextual factors influence teacher–child dynamics. Additionally, future studies should explore subgroup effects in greater depth to determine whether specific populations, such as children of different racial/ethnic backgrounds, gender identities, or baseline symptom levels, benefit differentially from the JS+CS intervention. It will also be critical to investigate whether JS+CS yields stronger outcomes in non-pandemic conditions, as earlier studies [79] suggested more promising results. Finally, future studies should examine how fidelity moderates program impact and assess whether observed trends persist or evolve over longer-term follow-ups. Given multiple significant relationships between teacher factors and child outcomes, these outcomes can inform state and federal policies by reinforcing the need to fund and scale ECMHC services within childcare center licensing regulations. Policymakers could leverage JS+CS as a model to support legislation that requires or incentivizes access to mental health consultation in childcare centers, particularly in under-resourced and high-risk communities, as a means to promote equity and reduce disproportionality in early childhood disciplines.

5. Conclusions

These findings highlight the complexity of implementing mental health interventions in ECE settings, particularly in the aftermath of a public health crisis. Despite the modest effect sizes, the mediation results provide a promising indication that teacher practices, particularly safety and behavior supports, are key pathways through which the JS+CS intervention positively impacted child social–emotional development. Both JS+CS and HC2 resulted in some improvements in certain social–emotional outcomes, underscoring the potential of these interventions in enhancing children's well-being. Future research should explore hybrid approaches that integrate both social–emotional learning and physical health promotion to create more comprehensive support systems for young children. Providing more robust professional development, ongoing coaching, and continuous access to resources may help educators manage their own well-being while fostering positive child outcomes. The promising mediation results suggest that with continued refinement and support, interventions like JS+CS have the potential to create lasting improvements in both teacher practices and child social–emotional development.

Supplementary Materials: The following supporting information can be downloaded at https://www.mdpi.com/article/10.3390/children12070812/s1: Table S1: Complete mediation analysis of JS+CS intervention effects on child outcomes via classroom- and teacher-level factors (GEE methods); Table S2: Mediation analysis of JS+CS intervention effects on child outcomes via classroom- and teacher-level factors (change score methods); Table S3: Generalized estimating equation (GEE) models examining the moderating role of SDQ risk categories on intervention effects for DECA outcomes.

Author Contributions: Conceptualization, R.N., T.K.L., E.H. and J.F.J.; methodology, R.N., Y.P., Y.A. and J.F.J.; acquisition of data: E.H., Y.A. and C.V.; formal analysis, R.N., Y.P., R.J.B.-S. and J.F.J.; interpretation of data, T.K.L., Y.A., S.M.S.G., T.R. and C.V.; writing—original draft, R.N., T.K.L., Y.P., E.H., Y.A. and J.F.J.; writing—review and editing, R.N., T.K.L., Y.P., R.J.B.-S., E.H., S.M.S.G., Y.A., T.R., C.V. and J.F.J. All authors have read and agreed to the published version of the manuscript.

Funding: This research was made possible by funding from the Eunice Kennedy Shriver National Institute of Child Health and Human Development [grant number R01HD105474].

Institutional Review Board Statement: This study was conducted in accordance with the Declaration of Helsinki and approved by the University of Miami Institutional Review Board on 6 June 2022 (20220115).

Informed Consent Statement: Informed consent was obtained from all subjects involved in the study.

Data Availability Statement: Requests for data can be sent to the corresponding author.

Acknowledgments: We would like to thank the childcare center staff in Miami-Dade and Broward counties who participated in this study.

Conflicts of Interest: The authors declare no conflicts of interest.

Abbreviations

The following abbreviations are used in this manuscript:

CDC	Centers for Disease Control and Prevention
DECA	Devereux Early Childhood Assessment
ECE	Early care and education
GEE	Generalized estimating equation
HC2	Healthy Caregivers–Healthy Children
HERS-C	Health Environment Rating Scale-Classroom
IECMHC	Infant and early childhood mental health consultation
IRB	Institutional Review Board
JS+CS	Jump Start Plus COVID Support
SDQ	Strengths and Difficulties Questionnaire

References

1. Institute of Medicine; National Research Council. *From Neurons to Neighborhoods: The Science of Early Childhood Development*; The National Academies Press: Washington, DC, USA, 2000; p. 608.
2. Lloyd, C.M.; Carlson, J.; Alvira-Hammond, M. *Federal Policies can Address the Impact of Structural Racism on Black Families' Access to Early Care and Education*; ED614026; Institute of Educational Sciences: Bethesda, MD, USA, 2021; p. 19.
3. Bocknek, E.L.; Iruka, I.U.; Brophy-Herb, H.E.; Stokes, K.; Johnson, A.L. *Belongingness as the Foundation of Social and Emotional Development: Focus on Black Infants, Toddlers, and Young Children*; Springer International Publishing: Cham, Switzerland, 2024; pp. 11–30.

4. Darling-Churchill, K.E.; Lippman, L. Early childhood social and emotional development: Advancing the field of measurement. *J. Appl. Dev. Psychol.* **2016**, *45*, 1–7. [CrossRef]
5. Jones, S.M.; Zaslow, M.; Darling-Churchill, K.E.; Halle, T.G. Assessing early childhood social and emotional development: Key conceptual and measurement issues. *J. Appl. Dev. Psychol.* **2016**, *45*, 42–48. [CrossRef]
6. Phillips, D.A.; Lowenstein, A.E. Early Care, Education, and Child Development. *Annu. Rev. Psychol.* **2011**, *62*, 483–500. [CrossRef] [PubMed]
7. Johnson-Staub, C. *Equity Starts Early: Addressing Racial Inequities in Child Care and Early Education Policy*; Center for Law and Social Policy (CLASP): Washington, DC, USA, 2017.
8. Capizzano, J.A.; Main, R. *Many Young Children Spend Long Hours in Child Care*; No. 22; Urban Institute: Washington, DC, USA, 2005.
9. Hoffman, T.K.; Kuvalanka, K.A. Behavior problems in child care classrooms: Insights from child care teachers. *Prev. Sch. Fail. Altern. Educ. Child. Youth* **2019**, *63*, 259–268. [CrossRef]
10. Mondi, C.F.; Rihal, T.K.; Magro, S.W.; Kerber, S.; Carlson, E.A. Childcare providers' views of challenging child behaviors, suspension, and expulsion: A qualitative analysis. *Infant Ment. Health J.* **2022**, *43*, 695–713. [CrossRef]
11. Gilliam, W.S.; Shahar, G. Preschool and Child Care Expulsion and Suspension: Rates and Predictors in One State. *Infants Young Child.* **2006**, *19*, 228–245. [CrossRef]
12. Sanders-Phillips, K.; Settles-Reaves, B.; Walker, D.; Brownlow, J. Social inequality and racial discrimination: Risk factors for health disparities in children of color. *Pediatrics* **2009**, *124*, S176–S186. [CrossRef]
13. U.S. Department of Education. *2013–2014 Civil Rights Data Collection: A First Look*; Office for Civil Rights: Washington, DC, USA, 2016.
14. Zeng, S.; Corr, C.P.; O'Grady, C.; Guan, Y. Adverse childhood experiences and preschool suspension expulsion: A population study. *Child Abus. Negl.* **2019**, *97*, 104149. [CrossRef]
15. Lamont, J.H.; Devore, C.D.; Allison, M.; Ancona, R.; Barnett, S.E.; Gunther, R.; Holmes, B.; Lamont, J.H.; Minier, M.; Okamoto, J.K.; et al. Out-of-School Suspension and Expulsion. *Pediatrics* **2013**, *131*, e1000–e1007. [CrossRef]
16. Mathis, E.; Hartz, K.; Berkowitz, M.; Carlson, A.; Kimport, R.; Brown, C.; Biel, M.G.; Domitrovich, C.E. Using early childhood mental health consultation to facilitate the social–emotional competence and school readiness of preschool children in marginalized communities. *Sch. Ment. Health* **2022**, *14*, 608–623. [CrossRef]
17. Natale, R.; Kolomeyer, E.; Futterer, J.; Mahmoud, F.D.; Schenker, M.; Robleto, A.; Horen, N.; Spector, R. Infant and early childhood mental health consultation in a diverse metropolitan area. *Infant Ment. Health J.* **2022**, *43*, 440–454. [CrossRef] [PubMed]
18. Iruka, I.U.; Harper, K.; Lloyd, C.M.; Boddicker-Young, P.; De Marco, A.; Jarvis, B. *Anti-Racist Policymaking to Protect, Promote, and Preserve Black Families and Babies*; Equity Research Action Coalition; Frank Porter Graham Child Development Institute, The University of North Carolina at Chapel Hill: Chapel Hill, NC, USA, 2021.
19. Bingham, G.E.; Phelps, C.; Dean, M.P. Examining The Preschool to First-Grade Literacy and Language Outcomes of Black Children Experiencing a High-Quality Early Childhood Program. *Elem. Sch. J.* **2023**, *123*, 367–395. [CrossRef]
20. Panchal, U.; Salazar De Pablo, G.; Franco, M.; Moreno, C.; Parellada, M.; Arango, C.; Fusar-Poli, P. The impact of COVID-19 lockdown on child and adolescent mental health: Systematic review. *Eur. Child Adolesc. Psychiatry* **2023**, *32*, 1151–1177. [CrossRef] [PubMed]
21. Penna, A.L.; de Aquino, C.M.; Pinheiro, M.S.N.; do Nascimento, R.L.F.; Farias-Antúnez, S.; Araújo, D.A.B.S.; Mita, C.; Machado, M.M.T.; Castro, M.C. Impact of the COVID-19 pandemic on maternal mental health, early childhood development, and parental practices: A global scoping review. *BMC Public Health* **2023**, *23*, 388. [CrossRef]
22. Office of the Surgeon General (OSG). *Protecting Youth Mental Health: The U.S. Surgeon General's Advisory*; US Department of Health and Human Services: Washington, DC, USA, 2021.
23. Centers for Disease Control and Prevention. *Youth Risk Behavior Survey Data Summary & Trends Report: 2013–2023*; CDC: Atlanta, GA, USA, 2024.
24. Fox, L.; Hemmeter, M.L. A programwide model for supporting social emotional development and addressing challenging behavior in early childhood settings. In *Handbook of Positive Behavior Support*; Sailor, W., Dunlap, G., Sugai, G., Horner, R., Eds.; Springer: New York, NY, USA, 2009; pp. 177–202.
25. Gilliam, W.S.; Maupin, A.N.; Reyes, C.R. Early childhood mental health consultation: Results of a statewide random-controlled evaluation. *J. Am. Acad. Child Adolesc. Psychiatry* **2016**, *55*, 754–761. [CrossRef]
26. Harvard Global Health Institute. The Path to Zero: Key Metrics for COVID Suppression–Pandemics Explain. Available online: https://globalepidemics.org/key-metrics-for-covid-suppression/ (accessed on 21 April 2024).
27. Lopez, Y. 'Like Paying for a Luxury Car': Childcare Costs in Miami Are Holding Families Back. *Miami Herald*. Available online: https://www.miamiherald.com/news/business/article248956749.html (accessed on 28 March 2021).

28. Lingras, K.A.; Mrozinski, K.; Clavin, A.; Handevidt, A.; Moberg, L.; Michaels, C.; Mischke, M.; Schreifels, T.; Fallon, M. Guidelines for 0–3 Childcare During COVID-19: Balancing Physical Health and Safety with Social Emotional Development. Available online: https://perspectives.waimh.org/2021/03/19/guidelines-for-0-3-childcare-during-covid-19-balancing-physical-health-and-safety-with-social-emotional-development/ (accessed on 27 May 2025).
29. Gilliam, W.S.; Malik, A.A.; Shafiq, M.; Klotz, M.; Reyes, C.; Humphries, J.E.; Murray, T.; Elharake, J.A.; Wilkinson, D.; Omer, S.B. COVID-19 Transmission in US Child Care Programs. *Pediatrics* **2021**, *147*, e2020031971. [CrossRef]
30. Edmondson, A.C.; Higgins, M.; Singer, S.; Weiner, J. Understanding Psychological Safety in Health Care and Education Organizations: A Comparative Perspective. *Res. Hum. Dev.* **2016**, *13*, 65–83. [CrossRef]
31. Souto-Manning, M.; Melvin, S.A. Early Childhood Teachers of Color in New York City: Heightened stress, lower quality of life, declining health, and compromised sleep amidst COVID-19. *Early Child. Res. Q.* **2022**, *60*, 34–48. [CrossRef]
32. Wilinski, B.; Morley, A.; Wu, J.H.-C. From "Survival Mode" to "#winning": Michigan Pre-K Teachers' Experiences During the First Year of COVID-19. *Early Child. Educ. J.* **2025**. [CrossRef]
33. Grant, K. Young children's behaviour and contextual risk factors in the UK. *Educ. Psychol.* **2017**, *39*, 1230–1246. [CrossRef]
34. Whitaker, R.C.; Dearth-Wesley, T.; Gooze, R.A. Workplace stress and the quality of teacher–children relationships in Head Start. *Early Child. Res. Q.* **2015**, *30*, 57–69. [CrossRef]
35. Zinsser, K.M.; Silver, H.C.; Shenberger, E.R.; Jackson, V. A Systematic Review of Early Childhood Exclusionary Discipline. *Rev. Educ. Res.* **2022**, *92*, 743–785. [CrossRef]
36. Natale, R.; Agosto, Y.; Shearer, R.J.B.; George, S.M.S.; Jent, J. Designing a virtual mental health consultation program to support and strengthen childcare centers impacted by COVID-19: A randomized controlled trial protocol. *Contemp. Clin. Trials* **2023**, *124*, 107022. [CrossRef] [PubMed]
37. Davis, A.E.; Perry, D.F. *Healthy Futures: Evaluation of Early Childhood Mental Health Consultation by the District of Columbia Department of Behavioral Health*; Georgetown Univer Center for Child and Human Development: Washington, DC, USA, 2015.
38. Hunter, A.; Davis, A.; Perry, D.F.; Jones, W. *The Georgetown Model of Early Childhood Mental Health Consultation: For School-Based Settings*; Georgetown University Center for Child and Human Development: Washington, DC, USA, 2016.
39. Bronfenbrenner, U. *The Ecology of Human Development*; Harvard University Press: Cambridge, MA, USA, 1979.
40. Bronfenbrenner, U. Ecological models of human development. In *Readings on the Development of Children*, 2nd ed.; Gauvain, M., Cole, M., Eds.; Freeman: New York, NY, USA, 1994; Volume 1, pp. 37–43.
41. Silver, H.C.; Davis Schoch, A.E.; Loomis, A.M.; Park, C.E.; Zinsser, K.M. Updating the evidence: A systematic review of a decade of Infant and Early Childhood Mental Health Consultation (IECMHC) research. *Infant Ment. Health J.* **2023**, *44*, 5–26. [CrossRef]
42. Vuyk, M.A.; Sprague-Jones, J.; Reed, C. Early Childhood Mental Health Consultation: An Evaluation of Effectiveness in a Rural Community. *Infant Ment. Health J.* **2016**, *37*, 66–79. [CrossRef]
43. Center of Excellence for Infant and Early Childhood Mental Health Consultation. The Evidence Base for Infant and Early Childhood Mental Health Consultation (IECMHC). Available online: http://www.iecmhc.org/documents/CoE-Evidence-Synthesis.pdf (accessed on 15 April 2025).
44. Mondi, C.F. Supporting social and emotional learning through infant and early childhood mental health consultation. *Soc. Emot. Learn. Res. Pract. Policy* **2025**, *5*, 100084. [CrossRef]
45. Bailey, C.S.; Denham, S.A.; Curby, T.W.; Bassett, H.H. Emotional and organizational supports for preschoolers' emotion regulation: Relations with school adjustment. *Emotion* **2016**, *16*, 263–279. [CrossRef]
46. Bulotsky-Shearer, R.J.; Fernandez, V.A.; Bichay-Awadalla, K.; Bailey, J.; Futterer, J.; Qi, C.H. Teacher-child interaction quality moderates social risks associated with problem behavior in preschool classroom contexts. *J. Appl. Dev. Psychol.* **2020**, *67*, 101103. [CrossRef]
47. Curby, T.W.; Rudasill, K.M.; Edwards, T.; Pérez-Edgar, K. The role of classroom quality in ameliorating the academic and social risks associated with difficult temperament. *Sch. Psychol. Q.* **2011**, *26*, 175–188. [CrossRef]
48. Perry, D.F.; Allen, M.D.; Brennan, E.M.; Bradley, J.R. The evidence base for mental health consultation in early childhood settings: A research synthesis addressing children's behavioral outcomes. *Early Educ. Dev.* **2010**, *21*, 795–824.
49. Duran, F.B.; Hepburn, K.S.; Kaufmann, R.K.; Le, L.T.; Allen, M.D.; Brennan, E.M.; Green, B.L. *Early Childhood Mental Health Consultation*; Center on the Social and Emotional Foundations for Early Learning: Nashville, TN, USA, 2010.
50. Mackrain, M.; LeBuffe, P.; Powell, G. *Devereux Early Childhood Assessment for Infants and Toddlers*; Kaplan Early Learning Company: Lewisville, NC, USA, 2007.
51. LeBuffe, P.A.; Naglieri, J.A. *The Devereux Early Childhood Assessment for Preschoolers, Second Edition (DECA-P2) Assessment, Technical Manual, and User's Guide*; Kaplan: Lewisville, NC, USA, 2012.
52. LeBuffe, P.A.; Naglieri, J.A. The Devereux Early Childhood Assessment (DECA): A measure of within-child protective factors in preschool children. *NHSA Dialog* **1999**, *3*, 75–80. [CrossRef]
53. Naglieri, J.A.; LeBuffe, P.A.; Shapiro, V.B. Assessment of social-emotional competencies related to resilience. In *Handbook of Resilience in Children*; Goldstein, S.B.R., Ed.; Springer: Cham, Switzerland, 2013; pp. 215–225.

54. Crane, J.; Mincic, M.; Winsler, A. Parent–teacher agreement and the reliability of the Devereux Early Childhood Assessment (DECA) for English- and Spanish-speaking, ethnically diverse children living in poverty. In *Self-Regulation and Early School Success*, 1st ed.; Routledge: London, UK, 2013; pp. 115–129.
55. Patel, S.; Sanders, L.M.; Uhlhorn, S.; Natale, R. Health Promotion in Child-Care Centers: A Randomized, Controlled Trial. In Proceedings of the Pediatric Academic Societies 2011 Annual Meeting, Platform Presentation (CTSA Student Research Award), Denver, CO, USA, 30 April–3 May 2011.
56. Goodman, R. The Strengths and Difficulties Questionnaire: A research note. *J. Child Psychol. Psychiatry* **1997**, *38*, 581–586. [CrossRef] [PubMed]
57. American Academy of Pediatrics. *Caring for Our Children, National Health and Safety Performance Standards*; American Academy of Pediatrics: Itasca, IL, USA, 2019.
58. Gellar, S.; Lynch, K. *Teacher Opinion Survey Revised*, Unpublished manuscript; Virginia Commonwealth University Intellectual Property Foundation: Richmond, VA, USA, 1999.
59. Sinclair, V.G.; Wallston, K.A. The development and psychometric evaluation of the Brief Resilient Coping Scale. *Assessment* **2004**, *11*, 94–101. [CrossRef] [PubMed]
60. Hall, L.A.; Gurley, D.N.; Sachs, B.; Kryscio, R.J. Psychosocial predictors of maternal depressive symptoms, parenting attitudes, and child behavior in single-parent families. *Nurs. Res.* **1991**, *40*, 214–220.
61. Gómez, M.L.; Ashford, K.; Linares, A.M.; Hall, L.A. A pilot test of the Everyday Stressors Index–Spanish version in a sample of Hispanic women attending prenatal care. *J. Nurs. Meas.* **2015**, *23*, 519–531. [CrossRef]
62. Curbow, B.; Spratt, K.; Ungaretti, A.; McDonnell, K.; Breckler, S. Development of the child care worker job stress inventory. *Early Child. Res. Q.* **2000**, *15*, 515–536. [CrossRef]
63. Jent, J.F.; St. George, S.M.; Agosto, Y.; Rothenberg, W.A.; Howe, E.; Velasquez, C.; Mansoor, E.; Garcia, E.G.; Bulotsky-Shearer, R.J.; Natale, R. Virtual robotic telepresence early childhood mental health consultation to childcare centers in the aftermath of COVID-19: Training approaches and perceived acceptability and usefulness. *Front. Psychol.* **2024**, *15*, 1339230. [CrossRef]
64. Harris, P.A.; Taylor, R.; Thielke, R.; Payne, J.; Gonzalez, N.; Conde, J.G. Research electronic data capture (REDCap): A metadata-driven methodology and workflow process for providing translational research informatics support. *J. Biomed. Inform.* **2009**, *42*, 377–381. [CrossRef]
65. Centers for Disease Control and Prevention. Schools and Childcare Programs Guidance for COVID-19 Prevention. Available online: https://www.cdc.gov/covid/index.html (accessed on 10 November 2023).
66. Hemmeter, M.L.; Barton, E.; Fox, L.; Vatland, C.; Henry, G.; Pham, L.; Veguilla, M. Program-wide implementation of the Pyramid Model: Supporting fidelity at the program and classroom levels. *Early Child. Res. Q.* **2022**, *59*, 56–73. [CrossRef]
67. Natale, R.A.; Lopez-Mitnik, G.; Uhlhorn, S.B.; Asfour, L.; Messiah, S.E. Effect of a child care center-based obesity prevention program on body mass index and nutrition practices among preschool-aged children. *Health Promot. Pract.* **2014**, *15*, 695–705. [CrossRef]
68. Natale, R.A.; Messiah, S.E.; Asfour, L.; Uhlhorn, S.B.; Delamater, A.; Arheart, K.L. Role modeling as an early childhood obesity prevention strategy: Effect of parents and teachers on preschool children's healthy lifestyle habits. *J. Dev. Behav. Pediatr.* **2014**, *35*, 378–387. [CrossRef] [PubMed]
69. Natale, R.A.; Messiah, S.E.; Asfour, L.S.; Uhlhorn, S.B.; Englebert, N.E.; Arheart, K.L. Obesity prevention program in childcare centers: Two-year follow-up. *Am. J. Health Promot.* **2017**, *31*, 502–510. [CrossRef] [PubMed]
70. R Core Team. *R: A Language and Environment for Statistical Computing*; R Foundation for Statistical Computing: Vienna, Austria, 2024.
71. Wickham, H. Tidyverse: Easily Install and Load the Tidyverse. Available online: https://tidyverse.tidyverse.org (accessed on 27 May 2025).
72. Wickham, H.; Averick, M.; Bryan, J.; Chang, W.; McGowan, L.D.; François, R.; Grolemund, G.; Hayes, A.; Henry, L.; Hester, J.; et al. Welcome to the Tidyverse. *J. Open Source Softw.* **2019**, *4*, 1686. [CrossRef]
73. Balise, R.; Odom, G.; Grealis, K.; Cardozo, F. rUM: R Templates from the University of Miami. Available online: https://raymondbalise.github.io/rUM/ (accessed on 15 April 2025).
74. Rich, B. Table1: Tables of Descriptive Statistics in HTML. Available online: https://github.com/benjaminrich/table1 (accessed on 15 April 2025).
75. Dassa, L.; Nichols, B. Policy implications of infant mental health. *Infant Ment. Health J.* **2019**, *40*, 123–132. [CrossRef]
76. Natale, R.; Howe, B.; Valesquez, C.; Guzman Garcia, E.; Granja, K.; Caceres, B.; Erban, E.; Ramirez, T.; Jent, J. Co-Designing an Infant Early Childhood Mental Health Mobile App for Early Care and Education Teachers Professional Development: A Community-Based Participatory Research Approach. *JMIR Form. Res.* **2025**, *in press*.
77. Carson, V.; Lee, E.-Y.; Hewitt, L.; Jennings, C.; Hunter, S.; Kuzik, N.; Stearns, J.A.; Unrau, S.P.; Poitras, V.J.; Gray, C.; et al. Systematic review of the relationships between physical activity and health indicators in the early years (0–4 years). *BMC Public Health* **2017**, *17*, 33–63. [CrossRef]

78. Accavitti, M.R.; Williford, A.P. Teacher perceptions of externalizing behaviour subtypes in preschool: Considering racial factors. *Early Child Dev. Care* **2022**, *192*, 932–946. [CrossRef]
79. Natale, R.A.; Kolomeyer, E.; Robleto, A.; Jaffery, Z.; Spector, R. Utilizing the RE-AIM framework to determine effectiveness of a preschool intervention program on social-emotional outcomes. *Eval. Program Plan.* **2020**, *79*, 101773. [CrossRef]

children

MDPI

Article

Efficacy, Feasibility, and Utility of a Mental Health Consultation Mobile Application in Early Care and Education Programs

Ruby Natale [1,*], Yue Pan [2], Yaray Agosto [1], Carolina Velasquez [1], Karen Granja [1], Emperatriz Guzmán Garcia [1] and Jason Jent [1]

1 Mailman Center for Child Development, University of Miami Miller School of Medicine, Miami, FL 33136, USA; yagosto@med.miami.edu (Y.A.); cxv308@med.miami.edu (C.V.); kxg495@med.miami.edu (K.G.); eguzmangarcia@med.miami.edu (E.G.G.); jjent@med.miami.edu (J.J.)

2 Department of Public Health Sciences, University of Miami Miller School of Medicine, Miami, FL 33136, USA; panyue@med.miami.edu

* Correspondence: rnatale@med.miami.edu

Abstract: Background/Objectives: Preschool children from low-income, ethnically diverse communities face disproportionate rates of behavioral challenges and early expulsion from early care and education (ECE) programs. This study evaluated the efficacy, feasibility, and utility of Jump Start on the Go (JS Go), a bilingual, AI-enabled mobile application. JS Go is designed to deliver a 14-week early childhood mental health consultation model in under-resourced ECE settings. **Methods**: This mixed-methods study compared JS Go to the standard in-person Jump Start (JS) program. Participants included 28 teachers and 114 children from six centers (three JS Go, three JS). Quantitative measures assessed teacher classroom practices and child psychosocial outcomes at baseline and post-intervention. App usability and acceptability were only evaluated post-intervention. Seven semi-structured interviews were conducted post-intervention with JS Go directors/teachers to assess the app's feasibility for implementing the four program pillars: safety, behavior support, self-care, and communication. **Results**: JS Go was more effective than JS in promoting teacher classroom practices related to behavior support and resiliency. Both programs were similar in improving children's protective factors and reducing internalizing behaviors, with consistent effects across English and Spanish-speaking children. Teachers rated the JS Go app with high acceptability, though predicted future usage showed greater variability. Rapid qualitative analysis showed that participants found the app easy to use, frequently accessed its resources, and considered it helpful for reinforcing key strategies across the four program pillars. **Conclusions**: JS Go is a novel approach to providing mental health consultation. It represents a promising mobile adaptation of the established JS consultation model, with important implications for future practice and research.

Keywords: childcare; mental health consultation; mobile health; artificial intelligence; young children; classroom practices; mobile childcare app

1. Introduction

Early care and education (ECE) programs play a vital role in the health and development of young children [1,2]. Children living in low-income communities are more likely to exhibit behavioral challenges within ECE programs [3]. Preschool children who exhibit challenging behaviors are suspended and expelled from ECE programs at three times the rate of children in K-12 schools [4], and rates are disproportionately higher for males who are ethnic minorities [5]. Research suggests that Infant and Early Childhood Mental Health

Consultation (IECMHC) is one way to address challenging behaviors before they get to the point where children are expelled from preschool [6]. Yet, there are limited resources and a lack of a mental health consultation infrastructure within ECE centers to support this need [7].

To address challenging behaviors, ECE teachers need tools and skills that support the development of prosocial behaviors. Skilled teachers, working in partnership with families, play a central role in building children's social-emotional competencies and shaping long-term developmental outcomes. IECMHC provides ECE teachers with consultation geared towards helping them identify attitudes, beliefs, practices, and conditions that promote a quality classroom environment that supports prosocial skills. The Jump Start (JS) Early Childhood Consultation is a program that uses IECMHC [8]. The program emphasizes collaboration and equal partnership with early learning program directors, recognizing their expertise and leadership in supporting young children. The JS program aims to increase the capacity of all ECE providers (i.e., family childcare homes and childcare centers) to address young children's needs, reduce challenging behaviors that increase risk for preschool expulsion, and alleviate teachers' job-related stress, ultimately creating a positive impact for young children [7]. Traditionally, the program uses a toolkit to provide centers with psychosocial coping strategies to boost resilience. The toolkit is organized around four program pillars: two are psychosocial (Self-Care, Trauma-Informed Behavior Support) and two are safety-related (Safety, Communication). All materials are in English and Spanish to support the linguistic needs of Miami-Dade County. Despite the existence of effective resources such as JS IECMHC, teachers often struggle to access or implement them due to staffing shortages, time constraints, or lack of awareness of available services [9–11]. A scalable, multi-level strategy that is easily accessible is urgently needed to support teachers in addressing child behavior challenges.

Mobile app technology has become very prevalent over the years and may increase the uptake of IECMHC practices by offering just-in-time, on-demand learning [12]. Most existing child development apps target K-12 populations, prioritize behavioral treatment over preventive efforts, and focus on a single level of intervention, such as the caregiver [13–15]. However, mobile apps are also becoming an increasingly common mechanism for providing support to teachers and staff in ECE programs [16]. For example, one study reviewed 43 apps designed for children's health across iOS and Google Play. Researchers found that these apps often aimed to support chronic illness management, foster age-appropriate engagement, and ensure digital health safety. Their study highlighted the importance of designing apps for dual use by children and caregivers, aligning with the broader goals of empowering families and improving access to health interventions [17]. Another study investigated the use of a functional behavior support app with teachers who work with children exhibiting challenging behaviors by helping them develop a behavior support plan. At baseline, teachers showed infrequent use of support strategies with both their target students and the broader classroom. Following the development of behavior support plans via the app, results showed some teachers demonstrated immediate increases in strategy use, while others showed more variable implementation patterns [18].

Despite the promise of digital tools, no existing apps provide real-time, culturally responsive mental health consultation tailored to the daily realities of ECE teachers, particularly in under-resourced, linguistically diverse settings. To address this gap, this project represents the first known effort to translate a gold-standard, community-based IECMHC program into a bilingual, AI-enabled mobile app tailored for ECE teachers [19,20]. Building on the success of the in-person JS model and in response to an urgent need for accessible, low-burden support tools, Jump Start on the Go (JS Go) was developed. The JS Go app extends the program's reach by delivering evidence-based content in a digital format with an Artificial Intelligence (AI) chatbot feature. While traditional IECMHC models are limited by consultant availability, JS Go offers 24/7 access to dynamic, evidence-based content through an integrated platform combining AI, videos, and infographics. AI serves as a digital assistant, delivering real-time, tailored guidance to teachers based on classroom dynamics, reducing intervention delays from days to seconds. JS Go reimagines public-health approaches to mental health consultation by creating a scalable, sustainable model that could transform national access to critical child mental health supports with reduced staffing of traditional approaches.

The purpose of this study was to assess the efficacy, feasibility, and utility of the JS Go mental health intervention delivered via a mobile application as compared to the control group, Jump Start traditional in-person delivery. It was hypothesized that JS Go would be as effective as the traditional Jump Start program. Specifically, the evaluation aimed to answer the following questions: Does the JS Go mobile application improve child psychosocial outcomes, reduce child challenging behaviors, and enhance teacher well-being and classroom practices, in line with the traditional Jump Start in-person consultation model? Does JS Go enhance teacher well-being and classroom practices, in line with the traditional Jump Start in-person consultation model? Was JS Go a useful and acceptable consultation mechanism, and how well was the platform received by teachers? Feasibility was examined through qualitative interviews with directors and teachers to identify implementation barriers and facilitators in real-world ECE settings. JS Go efficacy was evaluated by comparing teacher and child outcomes between the intervention and the standard Jump Start center. Together, these research questions provide a comprehensive examination of a novel mobile application approach to delivering early childhood mental health consultation in real-world ECE settings.

2. Materials and Methods

2.1. Participants

The University of Miami's Institutional Review Board approved this study (IRB study number 20231026), and it is currently registered with ClinicalTrials.gov (NCT06374550). Participants were recruited through the ECE programs, and this included ECE directors and teachers, and parent-child dyads. Six ECEs were randomly selected from a pool of 28 ECEs that met the following criteria: (1) have >30 children ages 2-to-5; (2) serve low-income families; (2) reflect the ethnic diversity of the Miami-Dade County Public School System (60% Hispanic, 20% Non-Hispanic Black, 20% Non-Hispanic White); and (3) have teachers who agree to participate. Parents, teachers, and directors were recruited within the ECEs that were enrolled in this study. To be included, parents, teachers, and directors had to meet the following criteria: (1) must speak English, Spanish, or Creole; (2) must have a child enrolled in the ECE that is participating in this study; and (3) children ages 2–5. The exclusion criteria consisted of any participants who did not speak English, Spanish, or Creole. Participants who agreed to participate completed the informed consent process, whereas the parents/legal guardians completed the informed consent for children enrolled in this study. In accordance with ethical research practices and as per the University of Miami (UM) Institutional Review Board (IRB) requirements, study participation required caregivers to provide written consent. No children were included who would require assent, given that they were of preschool age.

2.2. Procedures

This was a mixed-methods, quasi-experimental matched-controlled study to assess the efficacy of the AI-enhanced digital IECMHC plus human consultation model, JS Go, relative to the traditional JS model (human consultation only). The consultation model was assigned at the childcare center level. Therefore, teachers and children either received the JS Go or the JS intervention at their childcare center. Participants were assessed at pre-intervention/baseline and at post-intervention. Participants received $20 for the baseline assessments and $30 for the post assessments. Teachers completed assessments about themselves and their children, while parents completed assessments about the sociodemographic characteristics of their children. Teachers completed the measures via the JS Go application, which has an applied programming interface with Research Electronic Data Capture (REDCap) [21]. Parents completed the measures via REDCap through email and public hyperlinks. All data were stored in the REDCap system, a secure, web-based application designed exclusively to support data capture for research studies.

Matching for the current study occurred at the child level. Children enrolled in JS Go were matched with children in a previously conducted JS research trial [22]. Children in the JS group (n = 87) were first excluded from the matching process if they were missing both baseline teacher-reported assessments: (1) the Devereux Early Childhood Assessment (DECA) and (2) the Strengths and Difficulties Questionnaire (SDQ) (n = 14). Of the remaining children, an additional 16 were excluded for missing either the teacher-reported DECA or SDQ at baseline. This resulted in a final JS sample of 57 children, which aligned with the JS Go sample (n = 57).

Beyond quantitative measures, directors (n = 3) and teachers (n = 4) within the JS Go intervention completed semi-structured interviews immediately following the JS Go intervention. An interview guide was developed (see Table 1) based on four domains of the RE-AIM framework (effectiveness, adoption, implementation, and maintenance) to explore the center staff's experience with the JS Go app [23]. The same interview guide was used with both directors and teachers. Examples of questions included, "Tell me about your experience with the JS Go program," and "What do you need to maintain the JS Go program, specifically using the app on a regular basis, and use of the strategies in your center?" The bilingual mental health consultant (MHC) who implemented the intervention and was previously trained on rapid qualitative analysis (RQA) conducted interviews in participants' preferred language using the Zoom videoconferencing platform. Interviews lasted on average M = 31.9 min, SD = 11.6 min. All interviews were recorded via Zoom and securely transferred to a HIPAA-compliant university cloud storage system. The MHC downloaded and reviewed the audio files generated by Zoom to ensure accuracy. All interviews were conducted in Spanish and transcribed by the MHC using Microsoft Word Online's transcription feature. All transcripts were analyzed in their original language.

Table 1. Qualitative Interview Guide for JS Go Directors and Teachers.

Q1: **[Effectiveness and Implementation]** Tell me about your experience with the JS Go program? a. How did the program help, if at all, you adopt JS Go practices? b. How are things different for you as a result of the program? c. How confident do you feel about using reflective practices with teachers in your program? d. What are some of the things that you have done, or will do, to use reflective practices with your teachers?
Q2: **[Effectiveness]** How do you think parents can use the JS Go information? a. Was information shared with parents? b. What, if anything, did the parents learn?
Q3: **[Effectiveness]** Tell me how confident you feel in your role as the JS Go director/teacher?

Table 1. *Cont.*

Q4: **[Effectiveness and Adoption]** Tell me about your experience working with your consultant around a. Using self-care strategies, such as creating a resiliency plan? b. Communicating with staff and families, such as having multiple modes of communication? c. Addressing racial equity topics such as not discriminating against someone by race and/or including all races and cultures in the program/classroom?
Q5: **[Implementation]** Tell me about your experience implementing a. Safety practices such as emergency procedures and policies? b. Behavioral supports to prevent challenging behavior and promote social emotional development, such as peer social skills?
Q6: **[Maintenance]** What do you need to maintain the JS Go program, specifically using the app on a regular basis, and use of the strategies in your center? a. What other resources for yourself and your staff? b. What other training for yourself and your staff?
Q7: **[Maintenance]** After reviewing the app's gaming feature screenshots, a. What feedback do you have regarding the gaming screenshots? b. What additional features or changes would you suggest for the gaming feature? c. How helpful can this app be for helping teachers sustain their use of JS Go practices? d. How helpful can this app be for helping new teachers learn to use JS Go practices? e. What can facilitate the continuous usage of the app by the childcare center staff? f. Any other comments, questions, or concerns you would like to share about the app?
Q8: **[Adoption]** How interested would other staff in your center be in being a part of the JS Go program/working with the mental health consultant and using the app on a regular basis?
Q9: **[Implementation]** How well do you think your center is addressing the following: a. Safety b. Behavior Supports c. Self-Care d. Communication
Q10: **[Implementation]** What strategies do you think you can use to continue making improvements in a. Safety b. Behavior Supports c. Self-Care d. Communication

2.2.1. JS Go Intervention

JS Go is an early childhood mental health consultation program that utilizes a hybrid model combining an AI-enhanced mobile application with live mental health consultation. The program is similarly built upon Georgetown University's evidence-based Infant/Early Childhood Mental Health Consultation (I/ECMHC) framework and encompasses the same four fundamental pillars as the traditional JS model: (1) Safety, (2) Behavior Support, (3) Self-Care, and (4) Communication [7,24].

The JS Go model implements a multi-level, multi-modal intervention that provides (1) simplified multilingual video content in English and Spanish within an app, (2) personalized AI-driven guidance aligned with the JS Go curriculum, and (3) secure two-way communication between teachers and consultants. The program was designed through a community-based participatory research approach, ensuring cultural and linguistic relevance for diverse childcare center settings [20].

The JS Go intervention was implemented over 14 weeks, to match the duration of the JS intervention. Participants received weekly one-hour live consultation sessions with mental health consultants focusing on the four core pillars. In addition, the consultant modeled how the teacher could utilize the JS Go app for ongoing support, education, and AI-driven guidance between consultation sessions. The JS Go app includes three key components: multimedia modules demonstrating implementation strategies, AI-augmented support providing on-demand personalized guidance with safety protocols that escalate complex needs to human consultants, and connected communication allowing secure messaging between teachers and consultants with responses within one business day. The AI augmented support chatbot of JS Go was developed and trained as a retrieval-based model in which teachers input questions or describe situations, the system matches these inputs against a database of pre-approved responses, examples, and guidance from the Jump Start curriculum. The AI system implements programmed boundaries that prevent responses outside of the JS Go scope, particularly for crisis-level situations, and withholds responses when confidence thresholds for accuracy are not met. Specifically, the AI includes safety mechanisms that automatically escalate complex cases to human consultants, maintaining expert oversight for critical situations.

This study consisted of implementing a toolkit which included (1) infographics with key points, a reflective question, and applicable tips that pertain to intervention pillars (Self-Care, Behavior Support, Safety, and Communication); and (2) how-to videos demonstrating strategies for each pillar, such as resiliency-based coping ideas for teachers and directors. Structure: The Action Plan is a standardized implementation protocol used by the MHC in each consultation to (1) set the goal based on the pillar for the week, (2) provide strategies for achieving the goals using infographics and "how to" videos located on the JS Go app, (3) have teachers practice strategies while the consultant provides real-time feedback. Approximately three weeks are devoted to each pillar before moving on to the next. The order of pillar discussion was based on a tailored approach considering the areas of need/weaknesses from each participant's Health Environment Rating Scale (HERS) self-assessment (measure discussed later) as well as a conversation with each participant on their agreement with the proposed plan. Dose: the MHC provided 14 weeks of in-person consultations for 1.5 h weekly per center. Classroom-level consultations occurred individually and/or in a small group (two teachers) for 30 min per week, during nap time at the center, to provide teachers with goals/strategies to adopt pillars into their daily lives and manage challenging behaviors of specific children in the classroom. Examples of goals/strategies include helping teachers develop a self-care plan to build resiliency (beliefs) and use coping strategies (self-efficacy). Reflective consultation was facilitated with the use of infographics and videos during the live sessions. For example, reflective questions were asked about the infographics, and both videos and infographics were used to start discussions about pillars and goals. Teachers were shown examples of how to access and utilize the app and were assigned homework between consultations to utilize the chat, review infographics, and watch videos.

The JS Go app served as the primary platform for accessing all toolkit components, including infographics, videos, and an AI-powered chatbot called Avatar Buddy (see Figure 1). The app is a multilingual tool (available in English, Spanish, and Creole) designed to provide IECMHC resources and evidence-based strategies aimed at reducing suspensions and expulsions in early childhood education programs. Key app sections include (a) the **Home** page for central navigation; (b) the **Resources** page, which houses 16 infographics on IECMHC topics such as expulsions and suspensions, discipline, emergency planning, etc.

App users can apply specific filters to access content based on their preferred ECE setting level (program/center, classroom, or child) and/or the JS pillars (safety, behavior support, self-care, and communication); (c) the **Videos** page, which contains brief educational videos aligned with infographic topics and filtered using the same logic; (d) the **Journey** page, which serves as the secure login hub for survey completion; (e) the **Providers** page, offering information about JS community partners; and (f) the **Support** page, which features the AI chatbot equipped to answer questions related to IECMHC topics in both English and Spanish.

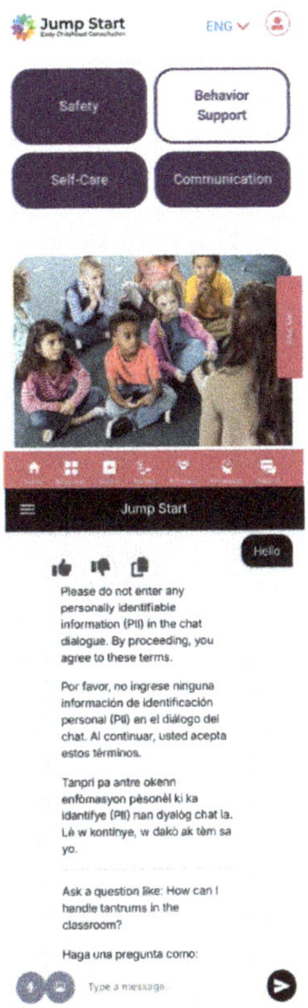

Figure 1. JS Go User Interface.

2.2.2. Matched–Control. Traditional Jump Start

The JS program is an early childhood mental health consultation initiative modeled after Georgetown University's evidence-based I/ECMHC framework. This model encompasses four fundamental pillars: (1) Safety, (2) Behavior Support, (3) Self-Care, and (4) Communication [7,24]. JS is grounded in the Caring for Our Children-National-Health and Safety Standards [25], complemented by CDC COVID-19 guidelines for childcare centers [26], and evidence-based practices for enhancing children's social competence [27].

The consultation model was implemented through weekly one-hour sessions over a 14-week period, delivered by consultants utilizing telepresence robots. JS aimed to (1) enhance children's social, emotional, and behavioral development, and (2) prevent and/or address behavioral challenges by strengthening the capacity of all caregivers (directors, teachers, parents/families), thereby reducing and preventing preschool suspensions and expulsions.

Each pillar of the JS model features a collection of 24 infographics (six per pillar) tailored for classroom teachers. These infographics follow a standardized format with three sections: (1) Reflect, (2) Inform, and (3) Practice. They serve as guides through the consultative process, enabling childcare staff to reflect on their practices and collaboratively develop personalized professional goals.

2.2.3. Consultant Training

The JS and JS Go consultants were clinically trained early childhood mental health professionals with supervision, many holding endorsements from a state infant mental health association. Each consultant underwent extensive training in implementing the JS program, including six virtual onboarding sessions: (1) introduction to Georgetown University's I/ECMHC/Jump Start model and its four pillars, (2) program-level observation training, (3) classroom-level observation training, (4) curriculum infographic review, and (5) exemplar consultation video analysis. JS Go consultants received additional training in how to integrate the use of the JS Go app within consultation services with teachers.

2.3. *Measures*

2.3.1. Sociodemographic Characteristics

Teacher demographic characteristics (e.g., age, gender, race, ethnicity, preferred language, level of education, and years of experience in the ECE setting) were collected via the JS demographic survey at pre-intervention only. Family characteristics (i.e., age, gender, race, ethnicity, primary language spoken in the home, English proficiency) were measured by the JS demographic survey at pre-intervention only.

2.3.2. Teacher Measures

The Health Environment Rating Scale-Classroom (HERS-C) is a 30-min observational assessment developed by our study investigators and used to evaluate classroom implementation across four domains: safety, behavioral supports, communication, and resiliency coping. These domains correspond to both national health and safety standards for early childhood education programs and the four JS Go pillars [8,25]. HERS-C items assess core classroom practices, such as "Classroom has safety guidelines and procedures for responding to crisis situations and adheres to CDC/DCF guidelines" and "Teacher shares behavior expectations and classroom rules using positive language, praise, and redirection when needed". Observers rated implementation on a 7-point Likert scale ranging from "little or no implementation" (1) to "excellent implementation" (7). The measure demonstrated good internal consistency ($\alpha = 0.82$) in this study, and all four domains were examined.

Teachers' beliefs related to their job were measured by the Childcare Worker Job Stress Inventory (CWJSI), which assesses three domains of workplace stress, including job demands, resources, and control [28]. Each subscale is 17 items with responses rated from "very little" (1) to "very much" (5). Sample items include "I feel like I have to be a parent and a teacher to the children" (job demands), "I get praise from the parents for the work that I do" (job resources), and "How much control do you have over the number of children you care for?" (job control). Higher scores indicate greater perceived control, resources, and job-related demands. The domains have strong internal consistency and constructive validity and have been used effectively in prior JS research studies with low-income children [29].

The Teacher Opinion Survey assessed teachers' confidence in managing challenging child behaviors [30]. This 12-item self-report measure uses a 5-point Likert scale from "strongly disagree" (1) to "strongly agree" (5), with higher scores indicating greater confidence. Sample items include, "If I keep trying, I can find some way to reach even the most challenging child", and "If a student in my class became disruptive and noisy, I feel pretty sure that I would know how to respond effectively". The total score demonstrated adequate internal consistency (α = 0.79).

The Brief Resilient Coping Scale was employed to measure teachers' tendencies to cope adaptively with stress. This 4-item instrument, which includes items such as "I look for creative ways to alter difficult situations" and "I believe I can grow in positive ways by dealing with difficult situations", has established reliability and validity [31]. It uses a 5-point rating scale from "does not describe me at all" (1) to "describes me very well" (5). Total scores classify respondents as low (4–13 points), medium (14–16 points), or high (17–20 points) resilient copers. The scale showed good internal consistency in this study (α = 0.835).

Consultation dosage was operationalized as the total number of consultation sessions each teacher received during the intervention period.

2.3.3. Teacher Technology Acceptability of JS Go App Measures

The Technology Acceptance Model Instrument-Fast Form (FF-TAM) is a 16-item checklist that evaluates attitudes toward technology use [32]. It can be modified by listing the technology of interest. Within this study, the mobile application was listed as the technology. The FF-TAM uses an 8-point semantic differential scale ranging from −4 (e.g., inefficient) to +4 (e.g., efficient) to rate items, allowing for a broad range of responses. The FF-TAM has three subscales designed to measure different aspects of technology acceptance, including Usefulness (e.g., unhelpful vs. helpful), Ease of Use (e.g., very cumbersome vs. very usable), and Predicted Future Usage (e.g., For future consultation tasks that are totally within my control, I would probably use telepresence robots as a consultation platform.). All three subscales (i.e., usefulness, ease of use, and predicted future usage) were used in this study. Childcare staff only completed this measure immediately post-intervention. Internal consistency for each of the subscales was high for the childcare staff (α = 99 for all scales).

Participants completed the mHealth App Usability Questionnaire (MAUQ) in either English or Spanish [33]. The MAUQ is a short, reliable, and customizable questionnaire designed to assess the usability of mobile apps and gauge teachers' perceptions of the usefulness of the JS Go app, the quality of the user interface, and the perceived usefulness of the app in delivering early childhood mental health consultation content. Data were collected post-intervention, for a total of one time point. The MAUQ has 18-items organized into three subscales: ease of use and satisfaction (e.g., "It was easy for me to learn to use the app"), system interface arrangement (e.g., "The information in the app was well organized, so I could easily find the information I needed"), and usefulness (e.g., "The app has all the functions and capabilities I expected it to have"). Participants rated JS Go using a seven-point Likert scale (1 strongly disagree to 7 strongly agree). The Cronbach's alpha for the MAUQ in this sample was α = 0.90 for the Ease of Use subscale, α = 0.93 for the Interface subscale, and α = 0.92 for the Usefulness subscale.

In addition to the MAUQ, the Mobile Application Rating Scale (MARS) in English and Spanish was used to classify and assess the quality of mobile health apps [34]. This 23-item tool was used to measure app objective quality indicators of engagement, functionality, aesthetics, and information quality, as well as app subjective quality. The app quality scores were clustered within the engagement, functionality, aesthetics, and information quality subscales. Sample items include, "Is the app fun/entertaining to use?" (engagement), "How accurately/fast do the app features (functions) and components (buttons/menus) work?" (functionality), "How good does the app look?" (aesthetics), "Is app content correct, well written, and relevant to the goal/topic of the app?" (information quality), and "Would you recommend this app to people who might benefit from it?" (app subjective quality). Each

MARS item used a 5-point scale (1-Inadequate, 2-Poor, 3-Acceptable, 4-Good, 5-Excellent). In cases where an item may not be applicable for all apps, an option of Not applicable was included. Data were collected post-intervention, for a total of one time point. The Cronbach's alpha for the MARS in this sample was $\alpha = 0.96$ for the functionality subscale, $\alpha = 0.90$ for the aesthetics subscale, and $\alpha = 0.93$ for the information quality subscale.

2.3.4. Child Measures

The Devereux Early Childhood Assessment (DECA) instrument was used to measure protective factors that promote resilience in young children. These included the DECA for Infants and Toddlers (DECA-I/T) [35] and the DECA for Preschoolers, Second Edition (DECA-P2) [36], both validated, reliable, standardized, and norm-referenced teacher-report measures for children from 1 month through 5 years [37,38]. The DECA-I/T consists of 36 items, while the DECA-P2 contains 38 items, each rated on a five-point scale from "never" (0) to "very frequently" (4). Both instruments yield three subscales: Initiative (ability to use independent thoughts and actions to meet needs), Self-Regulation (ability to express emotions and behaviors in healthy ways), and Attachment/Relationships (mutual, strong relationships between children and significant adults), as well as a Total Protective Factors (TPF) score. Each DECA item begins with the prompt "During the past 4 weeks, how often did the toddler/child..." followed by behaviors such as "show affection for familiar adults" and "calm herself/himself down". These measures have demonstrated adequate internal consistency in English and Spanish-speaking, low-income, diverse samples [39]. In the current study, the internal consistency for the DECA total protective factors scale was excellent ($\alpha = 0.975$).

The Strengths and Difficulties Questionnaire (SDQ) was used to assess behavioral problems in children. This 25-item screening measure is designed for youth ages 2–17, with specific versions for 2–4-year-olds and 4–17-year-olds, though it has also shown promising reliability for 12–24-month-old children (with better reliability for externalizing than internalizing subscales). The teacher-report version was utilized in this study, with items rated on a three-point Likert scale: "not true" (0), "somewhat true" (1), and "certainly true" (2). Each item describes a specific child behavior, such as "Considerate of other people's feelings", "Often loses temper", and "Many worries or often seems worried". The SDQ comprises five domains: emotional symptoms, conduct problems, hyperactivity/inattention, peer relationship problems, and prosocial behavior. An externalizing score was calculated by summing the conduct problems and hyperactivity/inattention scales, while an internalizing score combined the emotional and peer problems scales. The SDQ has established validity and reliability [40], and in this study, the internal consistency for the total problems scale was good ($\alpha = 0.860$).

2.4. Data Analysis

2.4.1. Quantitative Analysis

Baseline demographic characteristics of teachers and children were summarized by intervention group (JS Go and JS) using descriptive statistics. Categorical variables were reported as frequencies and percentages, and continuous variables were summarized using means and standard deviations (SD). Between-group comparisons for categorical variables were conducted using Chi-square tests or Fisher's exact tests, as appropriate. For continuous variables, independent sample t-tests or ANOVA were used depending on the distribution of the data.

For the evaluation of teacher outcomes, mean scores and standard errors (SE) at baseline (T0) and follow-up (T1) were calculated for each outcome by treatment group. Change scores (T1–T0) were also calculated to describe within-group changes over time. To formally test intervention effects, analysis of covariance (ANCOVA) models were conducted for each outcome, with T1 scores as the dependent variable, intervention group (JS Go vs. JS) as the independent variable, and T0 scores as covariates to adjust for baseline differences. The JS group was used as the reference group. Models were estimated using PROC SURVEYREG in SAS, specifying the program as the clustering variable to account for nesting of teachers within programs and to produce robust standard errors. Model coefficients (β), standard errors, and *p*-values were reported for the effect of treatment group.

To examine changes in child outcomes over time and between treatment groups, generalized estimating equation (GEE) models with an exchangeable correlation structure were used to account for clustering of repeated measurements within participants and clustering within programs. For each outcome, models included main effects for time (T0 vs. T1), treatment group (JS Go vs. JS), and their interaction (time × treatment), with JS and baseline (T0) as reference categories. The models assumed a normal distribution and identity link function. Least square means (LS-means) were calculated to estimate and compare group means over time. A two-sided *p*-value of <0.05 was considered statistically significant. As a sensitivity analysis, all GEE models were re-estimated with additional adjustment for child primary language (Spanish vs. English) to evaluate whether intervention effects were consistent across language groups. The models included main effects of child language and treatment × time × language interactions. A two-sided *p*-value of <0.05 was considered statistically significant. All analyses were conducted using SAS 9.4 and visualized using R (version 4.4.2) [41,42].

2.4.2. Qualitative Analysis

Rapid Qualitative Analysis (RQA) was used to identify themes from semi-structured interviews with seven JS Go center staff (three directors and four teachers) [43–47]. RQA is a validated, time-efficient method grounded in implementation science and designed to maintain methodological rigor while producing timely findings [46]. To guide interviews, a semi-structured protocol was developed by the research team based on implementation science frameworks and the core components of the Jump Start model. The protocol was reviewed for content validity by two IECMHC experts and piloted with a non-study teacher to ensure clarity and cultural responsiveness.

Interview transcripts were first summarized using a standardized template developed by the research team. These templates captured key points across predefined domains (e.g., app use, challenges, perceptions of impact, and recommendations). The MHC who conducted the interview prepared the initial summaries immediately after each session. A second trained research assistant then extracted salient content from the summaries and transferred it into a structured analytic matrix. This matrix allowed for rapid comparison of key themes across participants.

A third team member conducted thematic analysis using the matrix to identify recurring concepts. These initial themes were refined through iterative discussions with the broader study team, including investigators with qualitative and IECMHC expertise. Inter-coder reliability was supported through team-based triangulation and consensus-building discussions. An audit trail was maintained throughout the analytic process to ensure dependability and confirmability of findings.

3. Results

3.1. Teacher Outcomes

3.1.1. Teacher Characteristics

A total of 28 teachers participated in the matched controlled comparison, including 6 in the JS Go group and 22 in the JS group (See Table 2). Given that groups were matched on child characteristics, there was an unequal distribution of total teachers across groups. All participants identified as female and Hispanic, and reported Spanish as their primary language. There were no significant differences between groups in terms of teacher age, race, education, years of experience, consultation dosage, and/or intervention completion.

Table 2. Demographic Characteristics of Teachers by Intervention Group (JS Go vs. JS).

Variable	JS Go (n = 6)	JS (n = 22)	Test Statistic	p-Value
Age (years)—M (SD)	47.63 (8.52)	51.01 (11.95)	F(1,26) = 0.42	0.524
Gender			N/A	N/A
Female	6 (100.0%)	22 (100.0%)		
Race			$X^2(4) = 3.06$	0.549
White	6 (100.0%)	14 (63.6%)		
Black	0 (0.0%)	4 (18.2%)		
Native American	0 (0.0%)	1 (4.5%)		
Multiracial	0 (0.0%)	1 (4.5%)		
Other	0 (0.0%)	2 (9.1%)		
Ethnicity			N/A	N/A
Hispanic	6 (100.0%)	22 (100.0%)		
Primary Language			N/A	N/A
Spanish	6 (100.0%)	22 (100.0%)		
Education Level			$\chi^2(4) = 8.96$	0.062
High School/GED	4 (66.7%)	2 (10.0%)		
Some College	0 (0.0%)	1 (5.0%)		
Associate Degree	0 (0.0%)	2 (10.0%)		
Bachelor's Degree	2 (33.3%)	11 (55.0%)		
Graduate Degree	0 (0.0%)	4 (20.0%)		
Completed Intervention			$\chi^2(2) = 1.37$	0.505
Yes	5 (83.3%)	14 (63.6%)		
No	0 (0%)	4 (18.2%)		
Withdrew	1 (16.7%)	4 (18.2%)		
Number of Consults for Completers M (SD)	13.50 (1.23)	11.80 (2.15)	F(1,19) = 3.27	0.086
Experience (years)—M (SD)	6.56 (8.64)	9.76 (11.40)	F(1,24) = 0.40	0.533

Note. Missing data for education level (n = 2) in the JS group. Percentages are within the treatment group. χ^2 = Pearson's chi-square; N/A = not applicable as all participants were in the same category.

3.1.2. Teacher Descriptive Outcomes at Baseline and Follow-Up

Descriptive statistics for each outcome at baseline and follow-up are summarized in Table 3 and visually shown in Figure 1. At pre-treatment, scores were generally similar across groups for most outcomes. JS Go teachers showed increases from baseline to follow-up in several domains, including HERS-C Safety (+0.42), HERS-C Behavior (+0.45), HERS-C Communication (+0.30), and HERS-C Resiliency (+1.27). JS participants also demonstrated improvements in HERS-C Safety (+0.31), HERS-C Communication (+0.07), and HERS-C Resiliency (+0.43).

In contrast, JS Go participants had decreases in Brief Resiliency Coping (−1.33) and Teacher Opinion Survey scores (−1.83), while JS participants had smaller changes (−0.19 and +1.03, respectively). For Childcare Worker Job Demands, JS Go showed little change (−0.04), whereas JS participants increased by +0.81 points, indicating higher demands. Patterns for Childcare Worker Job Resources and Childcare Worker Job Control indicated slight declines for both groups over time.

Table 3. Descriptive Statistics of Outcomes at T0 (Baseline) and T1 (Follow-up) by Intervention Group (JS Go vs. JS).

Outcome	JS Go			JS		
	Baseline Mean (SE)	Follow-Up Mean (SE)	Change	Baseline Mean (SE)	Follow-Up Mean (SE)	Change
HERS-C Safety	4.58 (0.20)	5.00 (0.18)	0.42	4.98 (0.27)	5.29 (0.57)	0.31
HERS-C Behavior	4.55 (0.19)	5.00 (0.29)	0.45	4.36 (0.54)	4.50 (0.43)	0.14
HERS-C Communication	4.00 (0.00)	4.30 (0.45)	0.3	4.36 (0.41)	4.43 (0.55)	0.07
HERS-C Resiliency	3.33 (0.52)	4.60 (0.55)	1.27	3.50 (1.16)	3.93 (0.27)	0.43
Brief Resiliency Coping	18.33 (1.86)	17.00 (1.79)	−1.33	18.05 (2.34)	17.86 (2.38)	−0.19
Teacher Opinion Survey	48.00 (5.51)	46.17 (2.93)	−1.83	44.76 (5.51)	45.79 (5.16)	1.03
CW Job Demands	2.78 (0.42)	2.74 (0.34)	−0.04	2.55 (0.99)	3.36 (0.58)	0.81
CW Job Resources	4.69 (0.42)	4.54 (0.34)	−0.15	4.48 (0.99)	4.45 (0.37)	−0.03
CW Job Control	3.63 (0.79)	3.06 (0.39)	−0.57	3.46 (0.89)	3.06 (0.67)	−0.4

Note. HERS-C abbreviated for Health Environment Rating Scale-Classroom. CW abbreviated for Childcare Worker.

3.1.3. Teacher Intervention Effects from ANCOVA Models

Results from ANCOVA models evaluating intervention effects at post-treatment (T1), adjusting for pre-treatment values (T0), revealed significant differences between the JS Go and JS groups for several outcomes (See Table 4). All models were adjusted for clustering by program ($n = 6$), and robust standard errors were estimated with degrees of freedom based on the number of clusters (df = 5), ensuring that variability between programs was appropriately accounted for in the inference. Specifically, JS Go participants had significantly lower scores on Childcare Worker Job Demands ($\beta = -0.60$, SE = 0.12, $p = 0.0041$), indicating lower perceived job demands relative to JS. JS Go participants also had significantly higher scores on HERS-C Behavior ($\beta = 0.33$, SE = 0.13, $p = 0.0474$), suggesting that teachers engaged in a higher rate of effective classroom practices to support adaptive child behavior within the classroom. Trend-level differences were observed for HERS-C Safety ($\beta = -0.39$, SE = 0.15, $p = 0.0506$), HERS-C Communication ($\beta = -0.49$, SE = 0.21, $p = 0.07$), and HERS-C Resiliency ($\beta = 0.68$, SE = 0.32, $p = 0.0876$), with JS Go teachers reporting fewer safety and communication classroom practices but more resiliency practices compared to JS teachers. No significant between-group teacher differences were found for Brief Resiliency Coping, Teacher Opinion Survey, Childcare Worker Job Resources, or Childcare Worker Job Control.

Table 4. Results from ANCOVA Models Evaluating Treatment Group Effects at T1 (adjusting for T0).

Outcome	β (JS Go vs. JS)	SE	*p*-Value
HERS-C Safety	−0.39	0.15	0.0506
HERS-C Behavior	0.33	0.13	**0.0474**
HERS-C Communication	−0.49	0.21	0.07
HERS-C Resiliency	0.68	0.32	0.0876
Brief Resiliency Coping	−0.91	0.65	0.2226
Teacher Opinion Survey	−1.35	2.01	0.5331
CW Job Demands	−0.6	0.12	**0.0041**
CW Job Resources	−0.03	0.15	0.8272
CW Job Control	−0.07	0.24	0.7904

Note. HERS-C abbreviated for Health Environment Rating Scale-Classroom. CW abbreviated for Childcare Worker. Bold indicates statistically significant.

3.2. Child Outcomes

3.2.1. Child Characteristics

Table 5 presents the baseline demographic characteristics of the child sample across groups ($N = 114$). There were no significant differences between treatment groups on age, gender, ethnicity, or English proficiency. However, there was a significant difference in racial composition ($p = 0.023$), with a higher proportion of Black children in the JS group (8%) compared to JS Go (0%). The majority of participants identified as White and Hispanic across both groups.

Table 5. Demographic Characteristics of Children by Intervention Group (JS Go vs. JS).

Characteristic	JS Go ($n = 57$)	JS ($n = 57$)	Total ($N = 114$)	p-Value
Age in years, M (SD)	3.70 (0.73)	3.83 (0.91)	3.76 (0.82)	0.436
Gender, n (%)				0.348
Female	28 (49.1%)	33 (57.9%)	61 (53.5%)	
Male	29 (50.9%)	24 (42.1%)	53 (46.5%)	
Race, n (%)				0.023 *
White	47 (88.7%)	41 (82.0%)	88 (85.4%)	
Black	0 (0.0%)	4 (8.0%)	4 (3.9%)	
Native American	2 (3.8%)	2 (4.0%)	4 (3.9%)	
Multiracial	4 (7.5%)	0 (0.0%)	4 (3.9%)	
Other	0 (0.0%)	3 (6.0%)	3 (2.9%)	
Ethnicity, n (%)				0.378
Hispanic	50 (94.3%)	47 (88.7%)	97 (91.5%)	
Non-Hispanic White	2 (3.8%)	2 (3.8%)	4 (3.8%)	
Haitian	0 (0.0%)	3 (5.7%)	3 (2.8%)	
Other	1 (1.9%)	1 (1.9%)	2 (1.9%)	
English proficient, n (%)				0.616
No	25 (47.2%)	22 (42.3%)	47 (44.8%)	
Yes	28 (52.8%)	30 (57.7%)	58 (55.2%)	

Note. Some categories have missing data, resulting in different sample sizes for analyses. Chi-square tests were used for categorical variables, and one-way ANOVA was used for age comparisons. * $p < 0.05$.

3.2.2. Descriptive Statistics of Child Outcomes

Table 6 presents the means, standard errors, and change scores of child outcomes at baseline and follow-up by treatment group. At baseline, children in the JS Go group had lower scores on DECA subscales, including Attachment (44.04 [SE = 1.39]), Initiative (46.61 [SE = 1.22]), Self-Regulation (50.53 [SE = 1.47]), and Total (46.81 [SE = 1.39]), and higher scores on SDQ subscales, including Externalizing (6.79 [SE = 0.49]), Internalizing (5.30 [SE = 0.54]), and Total (9.54 [SE = 0.76]), relative to JS participants (DECA Attachment: 47.77 [SE = 1.10]; Initiative: 50.98 [SE = 1.33]; Self-Regulation: 52.68 [SE = 1.29]; Total: 50.81 [SE = 1.25]; SDQ Externalizing: 4.53 [SE = 0.60]; Internalizing: 4.14 [SE = 0.58]; Total: 6.93 [SE = 0.89]). These differences suggest that JS Go participants had a less favorable starting point compared to JS in terms of protective factors and behavioral functioning.

Both groups demonstrated improvements from baseline to follow-up (See Figure 2), though the magnitude of change varied across outcomes. For DECA subscales, JS Go participants improved by 3.91 points in Attachment (follow-up M = 47.94 [SE = 1.39]), 3.14 points in Initiative (49.75 [SE = 1.51]), 3.49 points in Self-Regulation (54.02 [SE = 1.42]), and 3.73 points in Total (50.54 [SE = 1.42]). JS participants showed comparable improvements with increases of 2.77, 3.13, 1.52, and 3.12 points in Attachment (50.55 [SE = 0.96]), Initiative (54.11 [SE = 1.18]), Self-Regulation (54.20 [SE = 1.16]), and Total (53.92 [SE = 0.99]), respectively.

Table 6. Descriptive Statistics of Child Outcomes at T0 (Baseline) and T1 (Follow-up), by Intervention Group (JS Go vs. JS).

Outcome Mean (SE)	JS Go			JS		
	Baseline	Follow-Up	Change	Baseline	Follow-Up	Change
DECA Attachment	44.04 (1.39)	47.94 (1.39)	3.91	47.77 (1.10)	50.55 (0.96)	2.77
DECA Initiative	46.61 (1.22)	49.75 (1.51)	3.14	50.98 (1.33)	54.11 (1.18)	3.13
DECA Self-Regulation	50.53 (1.47)	54.02 (1.42)	3.49	52.68 (1.29)	54.20 (1.16)	1.52
DECA Total	46.81 (1.39)	50.54 (1.42)	3.73	50.81 (1.25)	53.92 (0.99)	3.12
SDQ Externalizing	6.79 (0.49)	6.35 (0.52)	−0.44	4.53 (0.60)	3.87 (0.51)	−0.65
SDQ Internalizing	5.30 (0.54)	1.87 (0.25)	−3.43	4.14 (0.58)	2.00 (0.34)	−2.14
SDQ Total	9.54 (0.76)	8.21 (0.64)	−1.33	6.93 (0.89)	5.87 (0.78)	−1.06

Note. DECA is abbreviated for Deveraux Early Childhood Assessment. SDQ is abbreviated for Strengths and Difficulties Questionnaire.

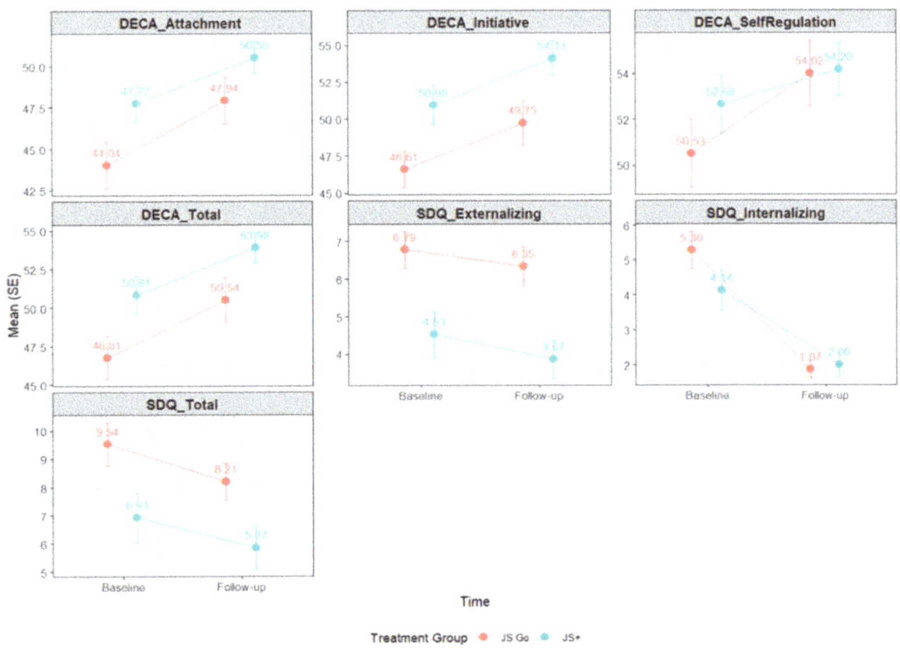

Figure 2. Teacher-reported improvements in child outcomes over time by intervention group.

Similarly, reductions in SDQ scores were observed, reflecting fewer behavioral concerns over time. Among JS Go participants, Externalizing scores decreased by 0.44 points to 6.35 (SE = 0.52), Internalizing decreased by 3.43 points to 1.87 (SE = 0.25), and Total scores decreased by 1.33 points to 8.21 (SE = 0.64). In JS, reductions of 0.65, 2.14, and 1.06 points were observed for child Externalizing (3.87 [SE = 0.51]), Internalizing (2.00 [SE = 0.34]), and Total (5.87 [SE = 0.78]) scores, respectively.

3.2.3. GEE Analysis of Child Outcomes

Results of the updated GEE models are shown in Table 7. Significant main effects of time were observed for DECA Attachment ($\beta = 2.89$, $p = 0.023$), DECA Initiative ($\beta = 3.05$, $p = 0.011$), DECA Total ($\beta = 3.22$, $p = 0.008$), and SDQ Internalizing ($\beta = -2.18$, $p < 0.001$), indicating meaningful within-person changes over time regardless of treatment group.

Table 7. Generalized Estimating Equation (GEE) Results for Child Outcomes.

Outcome	Time Effect (Follow-Up vs. Baseline) β (SE)	p-Value (Time)	Treatment Group (JS Go vs. JS) β (SE)	p-Value (Treatment)	Interaction (Time × Treatment) β (SE)	p-Value (Interaction)
DECA Attachment	2.89 (1.27)	**0.0226**	−3.74 (1.76)	**0.0335**	0.79 (1.78)	0.658
DECA Initiative	3.05 (1.20)	**0.0108**	−4.37 (1.79)	**0.0145**	−0.26 (1.85)	0.8896
DECA Self-Regulation	1.78 (1.29)	0.1666	−2.16 (1.94)	0.2651	1.20 (2.01)	0.5499
DECA Total	3.22 (1.22)	**0.0084**	−4.00 (1.85)	**0.0307**	0.14 (1.88)	0.9421
SDQ Externalizing	−0.74 (0.50)	0.141	2.26 (0.77)	**0.0033**	0.61 (0.67)	0.3642
SDQ Internalizing	−2.18 (0.51)	**<0.0001**	1.16 (0.78)	0.1385	−1.09 (0.71)	0.1253
SDQ Total	−1.16 (0.74)	0.119	2.61 (1.16)	**0.0243**	0.33 (0.98)	0.7369

Note. DECA is abbreviated for Deveraux Early Childhood Assessment. SDQ is abbreviated for Strengths and Difficulties Questionnaire.

Significant main effects of treatment group (JS Go vs. JS) were found for DECA Attachment (β = −3.74, p = 0.034), DECA Initiative (β = −4.37, p = 0.015), DECA Total (β = −4.00, p = 0.031), SDQ Externalizing (β = 2.26, p = 0.003), and SDQ Total (β = 2.61, p = 0.024), indicating that JS Go participants had lower DECA scores and higher SDQ scores compared to JS participants when averaged across time points. No significant time × treatment interactions were detected for any outcomes, indicating that the degree of improvement from baseline to follow-up did not significantly differ by treatment group.

In the sensitivity analysis, adjusting for child primary language, intake of child language (Spanish vs. English) was not significantly associated with any outcomes. Across all models, p-values for language were >0.10, suggesting no meaningful differences in change or post-intervention levels between Spanish-speaking and English-speaking children. No treatment × language interactions were detected, indicating that intervention effects were generally consistent across language groups.

3.3. Teacher Acceptability Ratings of JS Go App

Descriptive statistics for technology acceptability and app quality are presented in Table 8. Overall JS Go teachers reported high levels of perceived usefulness (M = 3.56, SD = 1.01) and ease of use (M = 3.67, SD = 0.82) of the JS Go app on the Technology Fast Form (TFF), though predicted future usage showed greater variability (M = 1.38, SD = 3.63). On the mHealth App Usability Questionnaire (MAUQ), participants rated the app highly across all domains, with average scores near the upper limit of the 7-point scale for ease of use (M = 6.43, SD = 0.59), user interface (M = 6.52, SD = 0.46), and usefulness (M = 6.47, SD = 0.45). Ratings from the Mobile Application Rating Scale (MARS) indicated that teachers found the JS Go app to be of high quality across all subdomains, including engagement (M = 4.73, SD = 0.24), functionality (M = 4.79, SD = 0.51), aesthetics (M = 4.72, SD = 0.53), and information quality (M = 4.67, SD = 0.42). The overall subjective app quality rating was also high (M = 4.73, SD = 0.38), suggesting strong user satisfaction.

Table 8. Descriptive Statistics for JS Go Technology Acceptability and App Quality Measures.

Variable	N	Minimum	Maximum	Mean	Standard Deviation
Technology Fast Form					
Usefulness	6	1	4	3.56	1.01
Ease of Use	6	2	4	3.67	0.82
Predicted Future Usage	6	−4	4	1.38	3.63

Table 8. *Cont.*

Variable	N	Minimum	Maximum	Mean	Standard Deviation
mHealth App Usability Questionnaire					
Ease of Use	6	5	7	6.43	0.59
User Interface	6	6	7	6.52	0.46
Usefulness	6	6	7	6.47	0.45
Mobile App Rating Scale					
Engagement	6	4	5	4.73	0.24
Functionality	6	4	5	4.79	0.51
Aesthetics	6	4	5	4.72	0.53
Information	6	4	5	4.67	0.42
Subjective App Quality	6	4	5	4.73	0.38

3.4. Rapid Qualitative Analysis of Staff Perceptions of JS Go App Feasibility

Interview participants (three directors and four teachers from JS Go centers) identified as White Hispanic females, with a mean age of 50.63 (SD = 9.76) years and 15.0 (SD = 9.58) years of ECE experience. All reported Spanish as their primary language, and 43% had earned a high school diploma or GED as their highest level of education. Semi-structured interviews yielded five primary themes reflecting the center staff's experiences with the JS Go intervention. Specifically, these included (1) the app as a practical and motivating tool with accessibility gaps, (2) the MHC's role in facilitating reflective practices, (3) staff self-efficacy in implementing program pillars, (4) opportunities to strengthen parent engagement, and (5) organizational supports and incentives needed for program sustainability. Themes and translated illustrative quotes are presented in the text below.

Theme 1: JS Go App as a Practical and Motivating Tool with Accessibility Gaps

Staff consistently described the JS Go app as a well-organized and user-friendly resource that supported regular classroom implementation of program pillars. The app's clearly structured content, instructional videos, and AI chat feature were widely praised for offering practical, just-in-time support in reinforcing key strategies and responding to children's challenging behaviors. One teacher noted, "The videos have been a tremendous help in strengthening my experience as a teacher. They have helped me a lot, with routines and with improving how I respond to children's disruptive behaviors". Another, referring to the AI chatbot feature, added, "If you have a direct question, you get an answer along with examples. I like it because it does not just give you the answer, it gives you several examples of how to develop what you are asking about". Participants noted that they frequently revisited the app to access its repository of resources when navigating difficult classroom situations. However, the app's browser-only format was identified as a barrier to consistent access. Participants expressed a strong preference for a downloadable version available through the app store that could function offline, especially in centers with unreliable internet access. As one teacher explained:

> I would like it to be an app that can be downloaded and that offers more resources. Resources that can be taught directly to the children, things we can incorporate into the lesson plan, or in circle time. Having the app be more interactive and easier to have on hand on my phone.

Theme 2: The MHC's Role in Facilitating Reflective Practices

In-person consultation emerged as an essential program component that provided irreplaceable human connection and individualized support. Participants described these interactions as creating reflective spaces where they could process challenges and receive emotional validation. One director noted, "…it is like having a private psychologist. I really enjoyed it because, as I listened to myself, I was self-analyzing my responses and reactions at that moment. That helped me and made me think differently for future occasions". The MHC was consistently viewed as someone who offered both emotional support and practical guidance, particularly in areas such as self-care, racial equity, and communication with families. While participants appreciated the app's streamlined format and usefulness, some emphasized the importance of real dialogue and idea exchange with the consultant. As one teacher explained, "With the app you go straight for the question or you watch a video, but when you are talking, you know, like the communication, it is more. You can share ideas, and sometimes we need to talk". This consultation component, combined with the app's resources, facilitated professional growth by reinforcing existing practices and introducing new strategies. Participants emphasized that the consultant's approach made complex or sensitive topics more approachable and helped build trust and confidence among staff.

Theme 3: Staff Self-Efficacy in Implementing Program Pillars

Participants described increased confidence in applying key components of the JS Go program, particularly in managing classroom behaviors, supporting their own and children's emotional regulation, and promoting a sense of safety. For instance, one director described a shift in her understanding of safety to include not only physical protections but also children's emotional well-being, stating, "It is not just about structure or the physical aspect; it is something more as well".

Additionally, the toolkit materials were frequently cited as helpful for reinforcing strategies introduced in the app and during consultation. Several participants described feeling more capable of responding to challenging behaviors through preventive strategies, positive reinforcement, and relaxation techniques (e.g., verbal reminders, role modeling, "flowers for breathing" method). They noted that these approaches were becoming part of their regular classroom routines, helping them respond more calmly and consistently. One teacher shared, "I feel like I am doing my best and doing things right because I have seen results in the children, and others have told me so too".

Theme 4: Opportunities to Strengthen Parent Involvement

Despite JS Go's emphasis on supporting children's development across settings, parent engagement remained limited throughout implementation. Most participants described minimal communication with families about the program beyond survey distribution or brief, informal updates. While some staff reported mentioning aspects of the program to a few parents, there were no structured strategies or built-in mechanisms for engaging families in the app or reinforcing content at home. Participants acknowledged this as a missed opportunity and expressed interest in strengthening the family engagement component, particularly through more concrete tools or guidance on how to involve parents more intentionally. One director suggested, "That access, and maybe a consultation, or maybe some kind of pages where parents could do the same things, we should definitely incorporate parents more, because they really do need it". Another director noted the potential for the AI chatbot to support families without judgment, stating:

> I think it would be a kind of support for them because they can consult any doubts, and it is like when you consult artificial intelligence. It gives you that immediate response, with a database that is exactly related to what we are looking for with children. So yes, I think it would be a support because sometimes parents might feel like, "Oh, I am not doing a good job as a mom or dad", but they do not want to say it out loud. So, the app feels more private, and they can consult it.

Theme 5: Organizational Supports and Incentives Needed to Sustain JS Go

While participants expressed interest in sustaining the JS Go program, they emphasized that ongoing implementation would depend on both structural supports and staff incentives. Directors and teachers highlighted the importance of leadership involvement, adequate staffing, and time for planning and reflection. Embedding program strategies into existing structures, such as team meetings or onboarding processes for new center staff, was also seen as critical for maintaining continuity. In addition to these structural supports, several participants pointed to the opportunity to earn "training hours" and endorsed the inclusion of interactive components (e.g., "gaming features", "unlocking digital rewards") as factors that could help maintain participation and enthusiasm over time. Regular app updates, including new courses or training announcements, were also viewed as important for sustaining center staff engagement, given the lack of up-to-date content in many programs and teachers' ongoing need to earn in-service hours.

4. Discussion

The current study used a mixed methods approach to examine the feasibility, efficacy, and utility of the JS Go mobile application as a mechanism for delivering IECMHC to early childcare centers. This novel approach integrated traditional in-person consultation with an AI-enhanced mobile platform to address a critical need for accessible mental health support in early childhood settings, particularly those serving diverse, low-income communities. Overall, the findings suggest that JS Go represents a promising digital adaptation of the established Jump Start consultation model, with several important implications for future practice and research.

One objective of this study was to determine if JS Go enhances teacher well-being and classroom practices, in line with the traditional Jump Start in-person consultation model. Teacher outcomes demonstrated some promising trends in favor of the JS Go intervention. Most notably, teachers in the JS Go group reported significantly lower job demands compared to those in the traditional JS group, suggesting that the mobile application may have served to alleviate some of the occupational burden associated with managing challenging behaviors. Further, classroom observation data revealed that JS Go teachers demonstrated significantly higher implementation of effective behavior support practices compared to the traditional JS group. This suggests that the on-demand, accessible nature of the application may have facilitated greater uptake of evidence-based strategies within childcare classrooms. This is especially notable given that 87% of teachers in previous JS research reported feeling overwhelmed by classroom behavioral challenges [48]. The app's multilingual features, infographics, and AI-powered guidance may have provided "just-in-time" learning opportunities that not only reinforced the consultation content between sessions but also may have facilitated more consistent use of behavior support strategies. In terms of other teacher outcomes, JS Go and JS teachers demonstrated similar increases in their observed implementation of the other JS pillars (Safety, Communication, and Resiliency) over time. There were no differences between groups in terms of teacher resilient coping and teacher perceptions of job control and resources. However, it is possible that, given the small sample size for teacher groups (JS Go $n = 6$ teachers; JS $n = 22$ teachers), this study was underpowered to detect significant changes at the teacher level.

Another objective of this study was to determine whether the JS Go mobile application improves child psychosocial outcomes and reduces child challenging behaviors. Children in both the JS Go and JS groups showed significant improvements over time across multiple domains of psychosocial functioning, including teacher perceptions of children's attachment, initiative, and reductions in internalizing behaviors. These positive trajectories align with previous IECMHC research demonstrating benefits for child outcomes [7,49] and provide preliminary evidence that the AI-hybrid digital adaptation of Jump Start maintains effectiveness for child development. If further research confirms equivalent effectiveness, the JS Go digital platform could serve as a scalable and sustainable model for expanding access to early childhood mental health consultation services. Given that fewer than 10% of childcare centers regularly implement IECMHC due to significant workforce and resource constraints [50], JS Go may help extend preventive, multilevel supports to underserved preschool-aged children.

Researchers were also interested in evaluating the utility of JS Go as a consultation mechanism by analyzing teacher ratings of the app's usability and technology acceptability, to assess how well the platform was received and its practical value for teacher end users. The high acceptability ratings from teachers provide compelling evidence for the feasibility of integrating mobile technology and AI support into early childhood mental health consultation. Teachers rated the JS Go app favorably, with particularly strong views of the ease of use, functionality, and information quality. This provides preliminary support that the JS Go app effectively translated the complex content of IECMHC into an accessible digital format that met teachers' needs and expectations. While there was more variability in teachers' perception of their predicted future usage of the app, all other domains were rated highly, suggesting that with appropriate implementation support by mental health consultants, teachers may be more likely to continue to engage with the digital platform over time.

The multilingual design of JS Go appears to have been well-received by this predominantly Spanish-speaking sample, addressing an important gap in culturally and linguistically responsive resources for IECMHC. Of note, there were no differences in child outcomes regardless of whether the child preferred to speak English or Spanish. This feature likely contributed to the high usability ratings and underscores the importance of co-developing with the community, including digital tools that reflect the diversity of the early childhood workforce.

Findings from the RQA illustrate the complementary roles of technology and in-person support and highlight both implementation successes and areas of growth. For future program development, four key recommendations emerge: (1) improve app accessibility through a downloadable version; (2) strengthen the family engagement component with concrete strategies for parent involvement; (3) maintain the dual approach of technology and personal consultation; and (4) develop mechanisms for regular content updates and ongoing training to sustain engagement and implementation over time. The JS Go app emerged as a practical, on-demand resource that helped center directors and teachers reinforce key strategies related to behavior support, self-regulation, and emotional safety. Center staff found the app especially useful for reinforcing practices introduced during consultations, revisiting strategies as needed, accessing resources on their own time, and using the AI chatbot to receive quick, example-based guidance. When paired with individualized consultation, it appeared to facilitate the integration of program pillars into teachers' daily classroom routines, with teachers expressing increased confidence in implementing JS Go practices. To further enhance engagement and implementation sustainability, a token-based gaming feature is being developed that tests users' knowledge of the four program pillars and provides visual tracking of progress. These targeted enhancements are designed to promote staff self-efficacy, implementation fidelity, and program sustainability across diverse ECE settings. Overall, these findings offer practical guidance for the continued development of digital tools that are both scalable and responsive to the realities of ECE programs.

Limitations and Future Directions

Several limitations should be considered when interpreting these findings. The main limitation was the small teacher sample size, with uneven distribution between groups, limited statistical power, and this may have increased the risk of Type II errors. Future studies should aim for larger, more balanced samples to enhance the robustness of findings. Second, although children were matched across intervention groups, significant baseline differences remained, particularly in child behavioral functioning. More stringent matching procedures or randomized designs in future research would strengthen causal inferences about JS intervention effects. Specifically, examining the relative contributions of the digital platform versus human consultation through a randomized controlled design would increase understanding of how to optimize the balance between technology and interpersonal support within IECMHC. Third, the intervention duration of 14 weeks may have been insufficient to detect certain outcomes, particularly those related to teacher well-being and self-efficacy, which may develop over longer timeframes. Longitudinal designs with extended follow-up periods would provide valuable insights into the sustainability of effects and patterns of app usage over time. Fourth, qualitative findings are subject to potential interviewer and coder bias. While double-coding and a structured analytic approach were used to enhance credibility, qualitative interpretations remain context-specific and may not be generalizable. Fifth, this study relied on teacher-reported measures, which introduces potential biases, including social desirability and recall bias. Although these reports offer valuable insight from key informants, future studies should incorporate multi-informant or observational data to strengthen measurement validity.

Lastly, while the technology acceptability measures provided important information about user perceptions, actual app usage data (e.g., frequency, duration, specific content accessed) was not systematically analyzed. Future studies should incorporate detailed app and AI analytics to understand how teachers engage with digital tools and which features most strongly predict implementation and outcomes. Further, refining the AI capabilities of the JS Go AI chatbot based on user interactions could enhance its relevance and effectiveness in addressing teachers' specific needs as they evolve over time and potentially promote ongoing engagement.

Future research should explore the cost-effectiveness of hybrid consultation models compared to traditional approaches, particularly in terms of reach, impact, and sustainability in under-resourced settings. Economic analyses would provide valuable information for policymakers and funders considering investments in digital mental health infrastructure for early childhood mental health consultation systems.

5. Conclusions

Overall, this study provides initial evidence supporting the feasibility, utility, and potential efficacy of JS Go as an innovative approach to delivering IECMHC in early childhood settings. Despite methodological limitations, the findings suggest that integrating mobile technology with traditional consultation may offer a viable strategy for extending the reach of evidence-based mental health support to teachers and children. Children in both groups showed comparable and significant psychosocial gains, indicating that JS Go maintains the effectiveness of traditional IECMHC for child development. High teacher acceptability ratings further support the feasibility of digital platforms in early childhood settings, while qualitative findings highlight the value of pairing technology with interpersonal support. Notably, this study contributes to existing knowledge by demonstrating how hybrid models can deliver culturally responsive, scalable, and just-in-time consultation in an under-resourced, multilingual context. As early childhood programs continue to face significant challenges related to children's behavioral health and teacher well-being, particularly in under-resourced communities, scalable solutions like JS Go represent a promising innovation in the mental health consultation landscape. This technology-enhanced approach not only extends the reach of evidence-based support but also empowers teachers with accessible, culturally and linguistically responsive resources to address challenging child behaviors and emotions in real time. Strengthening the mental health consultation infrastructure through hybrid models such as JS Go has the potential to enhance teacher capacity and improve children's psychosocial outcomes, fostering more nurturing environments in which all young children can thrive. JS Go offers a viable path forward for expanding mental health consultation services in early learning environments. By offering accessible mobile support, this model has the potential to enhance teacher capacity, promote child well-being, and bridge longstanding equity gaps in access to early childhood mental health resources.

Author Contributions: Conceptualization, R.N. and J.J.; methodology, R.N., Y.P., C.V. and J.J.; formal analysis, Y.P., Y.A. and J.J.; data curation, Y.A., C.V., K.G. and E.G.G.; writing—original draft preparation, C.V., Y.A., R.N. and J.J.; writing—reviewing and editing, Y.P., K.G. and E.G.G.; visualization, Y.P. and Y.A.; project administration, R.N., Y.A., C.V. and J.J.; funding acquisition, R.N. and J.J. All authors have read and agreed to the published version of the manuscript.

Funding: This research was funded by the Micah Batchelor Award for Excellence in Children's Health Research [award number BG005747], the Eunice Kennedy Shriver National Institute of Child Health and Human Development [grant number R01HD105474], and The Children's Trust of Miami-Dade County #2212-7574.

Institutional Review Board Statement: The study was conducted in accordance with the Declaration of Helsinki and approved by the Institutional Review Board of the University of Miami (protocol code 20231026 and approved on 4 April 2024).

Informed Consent Statement: Informed consent was obtained from all subjects involved in the study.

Data Availability Statement: Requests for data can be sent to the corresponding author.

Acknowledgments: We would like to thank the childcare center staff, children, and families in Miami-Dade County who participated in this study. We also acknowledge the SpiderBoost and Avatar Buddy development teams for their work in creating and refining the JS Go app.

Conflicts of Interest: The authors declare no conflicts of interest. The funders had no role in the design of the study; in the collection, analyses, or interpretation of data; in the writing of the manuscript; or in the decision to publish the results.

Abbreviations

The following abbreviations are used in this manuscript:

AI	Artificial intelligence
ANCOVA	Analysis of covariance
CWJSI	Childcare Worker Job Stress Inventory
DECA	Devereux Early Childhood Assessment
ECE	Early care and education
FF-TAM	Technology Acceptance Model Instrument-Fast Form
GEE	Generalized estimating equation
HERS-C	Health Environment Rating Scale-Classroom
IECMHC	Infant and early childhood mental health consultation
JS	Jump Start
JS Go	Jump Start on the Go

MARS	Mobile App Rating Scale
MAUQ	mHealth App Usability Questionnaire
MHC	Mental health consultant
REDCap	Research Electronic Data Capture
RQA	Rapid qualitative analysis
SDQ	Strengths and Difficulties Questionnaire
TPF	Total Protective Factors

References

1. Saitadze, I.; Lalayants, M. Mechanisms that mitigate the effects of child poverty and improve children's cognitive and social–emotional development: A systematic review. *Child Fam. Soc. Work.* **2021**, *26*, 289–308. [CrossRef]
2. Harding, J.F.; Paulsell, D. *Improving Access to Early Care and Education: An Equity-Focused Policy Research Agenda*; Mathematica Policy Research: Princeton, NJ, USA, 2018.
3. Hartman, S.; Winsler, A.; Manfra, L. Behavior concerns among low-income, ethnically and linguistically diverse children in child care: Importance for school readiness and kindergarten achievement. *Early Educ. Dev.* **2017**, *28*, 255–273. [CrossRef]
4. Gilliam, W.S.; Shahar, G. Preschool and child care expulsion and suspension: Rates and predictors in one state. *Infants Young Child.* **2006**, *19*, 228–245. [CrossRef]
5. Gilliam, W.S. *Prekindergarteners Left Behind: Expulsion Rates in State Prekindergarten Systems*; Foundation for Child Development: New York, NY, USA, 2005.
6. Albritton, K.; Mathews, R.E.; Anhalt, K. Systematic review of early childhood mental health consultation: Implications for improving preschool discipline disproportionality. *J. Educ. Psychol. Consult.* **2019**, *29*, 444–472. [CrossRef]
7. Natale, R.; Kolomeyer, E.; Futterer, J.; Mahmoud, F.D.; Schenker, M.; Robleto, A.; Horen, N.; Spector, R. Infant and early childhood mental health consultation in a diverse metropolitan area. *Infant Ment. Health J.* **2022**, *43*, 440–454. [CrossRef]
8. Futterer, J.; Mullins, C.; Bulotsky-Shearer, R.J.; Guzmán, E.; Hildago, T.; Kolomeyer, E.; Howe, E.; Horen, N.; Sanders, L.M.; Natale, R. Initial validation of the Health Environment Rating Scale-Early Childhood Consultation-Classroom (HERS-ECC-C). *Infant Ment. Health J.* **2024**, *45*, 449–463. [CrossRef]
9. Natale, R.; Davidson, B.; Woody, M.; Kolomeyer, E.; Mahmoud, F.D.; Valledor, V.; Hidalgo-Ferrer, T.; Schenker, M.; Robleto, A.; Spector, R. A model of care for delivering supports to childcare providers during the COVID-19 pandemic. *Res. Sq.* **2020**. [CrossRef]
10. Collie, R.J. COVID-19 and teachers' somatic burden, stress, and emotional exhaustion: Examining the role of principal leadership and workplace buoyancy. *AERA Open* **2021**, *7*, 1. [CrossRef]
11. Cipriano, C.; Rappolt-Schlichtmann, G.; Brackett, M.A. *Supporting School Community Wellness with Social and Emotional Learning (SEL) During and After a Pandemic*; Edna Bennet Pierce Prevention Research Center, Pennsylvania State University: University Park, PA, USA, 2020.
12. Khaddage, F.; Müller, W.; Flintoff, K. Advancing mobile learning in formal and informal settings via mobile app technology: Where to from here, and how? *J. Educ. Technol. Soc.* **2016**, *19*, 16–26.
13. Cunningham, M.A.; Gorman, C.; McNulty, M.C.; Chavez, C.; Luna-Asturias, C.; Dixon, C.A.; Bull, S.; Berman, S.; Allison, M.A. Engage, develop, learn: A pilot randomized clinical trial to test if a mobile application can enhance home support for early cognitive development among children living in poverty. *mHealth* **2023**, *9*, 4. [CrossRef]
14. Liverpool, S.; Mota, C.P.; Sales, C.M.; Čuš, A.; Carletto, S.; Hancheva, C.; Sousa, S.; Cerón, S.C.; Moreno-Peral, P.; Pietrabissa, G.; et al. Engaging children and young people in digital mental health interventions: Systematic review of modes of delivery, facilitators, and barriers. *J. Med. Internet Res.* **2020**, *22*, e16317. [CrossRef] [PubMed]
15. MacKinnon, A.L.; Silang, K.; Penner, K.; Zalewski, M.; Tomfohr-Madsen, L.; Roos, L.E. Promoting mental health in parents of young children using eHealth interventions: A systematic review and meta-analysis. *Clin. Child Fam. Psychol. Rev.* **2022**, *25*, 413–434. [CrossRef] [PubMed]
16. Hatzigianni, M.; Stephenson, T.; Harrison, L.J.; Waniganayake, M.; Li, P.; Barblett, L.; Hadley, F.; Andrews, R.; Davis, B.; Irvine, S. The role of digital technologies in supporting quality improvement in Australian early childhood education and care settings. *Int. J. Child Care Educ. Policy* **2023**, *17*, 5. [CrossRef]
17. Lee, J.; Su, Z.; Chen, Y. Mobile apps for children's health and wellbeing: Design features and future opportunities. *AMIA Annu. Symp. Proc.* **2024**, *2023*, 1027–1036.
18. McGuire, S.N.; Folkerts, R.; Richards, C.; Meadan, H.; Alqunaysi, R.; Yoon, C.D. Early childhood teachers' use of an FBA iOS app to support students who engage in challenging behaviour: A pilot study. *Technol. Pedag. Educ.* **2024**, *34*, 105–119. [CrossRef]

19. Natale, R.; Howe, E.; Kenworthy LaMarca, T.; St. George, S.M.; Raphael, J.; Schenker, M.; Velasquez, C.; Agosto, Y.; Guzman-Garcia, E.; Granja, K.; et al. Using the RE-AIM Framework to Understand the Role of Program Champions in Sustaining an Infant and Early Childhood Mental Health Intervention: A Qualitative Analysis. *Int. J. Child Care Educ. Policy* 2024, *under review*.
20. Natale, R.; Howe, E.; Velasquez, C.; Guzman Garcia, E.; Granja, K.; Caceres, B.; Erban, E.; Ramirez, T.; Jent, J. Co-designing an infant early childhood mental health mobile app for early care and education teachers: A community-based participatory approach. *JMIR Form. Res.* **2025**, *9*, e66714. [CrossRef] [PubMed]
21. Harris, P.A.; Taylor, R.; Thielke, R.; Payne, J.; Gonzalez, N.; Conde, J.G. Research electronic data capture (REDCap): A metadata-driven methodology and workflow process for providing translational research informatics support. *J. Biomed. Inform.* **2009**, *42*, 377–381. [CrossRef]
22. Natale, R.; Agosto, Y.; Bulotsky Shearer, R.J.; St. George, S.M.; Jent, J. Designing a virtual mental health consultation program to support and strengthen childcare centers impacted by COVID-19: A randomized controlled trial protocol. *Contemp. Clin. Trials* **2023**, *124*, 107022. [CrossRef]
23. Glasgow, R.E.; Battaglia, C.; McCreight, M.; Ayele, R.; Maw, A.M.; Fort, M.P.; Holtrop, J.S.; Gomes, R.N.; Rabin, B.A. Use of the reach, effectiveness, adoption, implementation, and maintenance (RE-AIM) framework to guide iterative adaptations: Applications, lessons learned, and future directions. *Front. Health Serv.* **2022**, *2*, 959565. [CrossRef]
24. Hunter, A.; Davis, A.; Perry, D.F.; Jones, W. *The Georgetown Model of Early Childhood Mental Health Consultation for School-Based Settings*; Georgetown University Center for Child and Human Development: Washington, DC, USA, 2016.
25. American Academy of Pediatrics; American Public Health Association; National Resource Center for Health and Safety in Child Care and Early Education. *Caring for Our Children: National Health and Safety Performance Standards; Guidelines for Early Care and Education Programs*, 4th ed.; American Academy of Pediatrics: Itasca, IL, USA, 2019.
26. National Center for Immunization and Respiratory Diseases (U.S.), Division of Viral Diseases. Guidance for Operating Child Care Programs During COVID-19. Centers for Disease Control and Prevention. 2021. Available online: https://stacks.cdc.gov/view/cdc/107006 (accessed on 16 May 2025).
27. Hemmeter, M.L.; Barton, E.; Fox, L.; Vatland, C.; Henry, G.; Pham, L.; Horth, K.; Taylor, A.; Binder, D.P.; von der Embse, M.; et al. Program-wide implementation of the Pyramid Model: Supporting fidelity at the program and classroom levels. *Early Child. Res. Q.* **2022**, *59*, 56–73. [CrossRef]
28. Curbow, B.; Spratt, K.; Ungaretti, A.; McDonnell, K.; Breckler, S. Development of the child care worker job stress inventory. *Early Child. Res. Q.* **2000**, *15*, 515–536. [CrossRef]
29. Natale, R.; Kenworthy LaMarca, T.; Pan, Y.; Howe, E.; Agosto, Y.; Bulotsky-Shearer, R.J.; St. George, S.M.; Rahman, T.; Velasquez, C.; Jent, J. Strengthening early childhood protective factors through safe and supportive classrooms: Findings from Jump Start+COVID Support. *Children* **2025**, *12*. [CrossRef]
30. Gellar, S.; Lynch, K. *Teacher Opinion Survey Revised*; Virginia Commonwealth University Intellectual Property Foundation and Wingspan, LLC.: Richmond, VA, USA, 1999.
31. Sinclair, V.G.; Wallston, K.A. The development and psychometric evaluation of the Brief Resilient Coping Scale. *Assessment* **2004**, *11*, 94–101. [CrossRef]
32. Chin, W.W.; Johnson, N.; Schwarz, A. A fast form approach to measuring technology acceptance and other constructs. *MIS Q.* **2008**, *32*, 687–703. [CrossRef]
33. Zhou, L.; Bao, J.; Setiawan, I.M.A.; Saptono, A.; Parmanto, B. The mHealth App Usability Questionnaire (MAUQ): Development and validation study. *JMIR mHealth uHealth* **2019**, *7*, e11500. [CrossRef]
34. Stoyanov, S.R.; Hides, L.; Kavanagh, D.J.; Zelenko, O.; Tjondronegoro, D.; Mani, M. Mobile app rating scale: A new tool for assessing the quality of health mobile apps. *JMIR mHealth uHealth* **2015**, *3*, e27. [CrossRef] [PubMed]
35. Mackrain, M.; LeBuffe, P.; Powell, G. *Devereux Early Childhood Assessment for Infants and Toddlers*; Kaplan Early Learning Company: Lewisville, NC, USA, 2007.
36. LeBuffe, P.A.; Naglieri, J.A. *The Devereux Early Childhood Assessment for Preschoolers, Second Edition (DECA-P2) Assessment, Technical Manual and User's Guide*; Kaplan: Lewisville, NC, USA, 2012.
37. LeBuffe, P.A.; Naglieri, J.A. The Devereux Early Childhood Assessment (DECA): A measure of within-child protective factors in preschool children. *NHSA Dialog* **1999**, *3*, 75–80. [CrossRef]
38. Naglieri, J.A.; LeBuffe, P.A.; Shapiro, V.B. Assessment of social-emotional competencies related to resilience. In *Handbook of Resilience in Children*; Goldstein, S., Brooks, R.B., Eds.; Springer: Berlin/Heidelberg, Germany, 2013; pp. 215–225.
39. Crane, J.; Mincic, M.S.; Winsler, A. Parent–teacher agreement and the reliability of the Devereux Early Childhood Assessment (DECA) for English-and Spanish-speaking, ethnically diverse children living in poverty. In *Self-Regulation and Early School Success*, 1st ed.; Routledge: Oxfordshire, UK, 2013; pp. 115–129.
40. Goodman, R. The Strengths and Difficulties Questionnaire: A research note. *J. Child Psychol. Psychiatry* **1997**, *38*, 581–586. [CrossRef]
41. SAS Institute Inc. *SAS/STAT 9.4 User's Guide*; SAS Institute Inc.: Cary, NC, USA, 2013.

42. R Core Team. *R: A Language and Environment for Statistical Computing*; R Foundation for Statistical Computing: Vienna, Austria, 2024.
43. Hamilton, A.B. Qualitative Methods in Rapid Turn-Around Health Services Research. U.S. Department of Veterans Affairs. 2013. Available online: https://www.hsrd.research.va.gov/for_researchers/cyber_seminars/archives/video_archive.cfm?SessionID=780 (accessed on 16 May 2025).
44. Hamilton, A.B.; Finley, E.P. Qualitative methods in implementation research: An introduction. *Psychiatry Res.* **2019**, *280*, 112516. [CrossRef]
45. Hamilton, A.B. Rapid Qualitative Analysis: Updates/Developments. U.S. Department of Veterans Affairs. 2020. Available online: https://www.hsrd.research.va.gov/for_researchers/cyber_seminars/archives/video_archive.cfm?SessionID=3846 (accessed on 16 May 2025).
46. Kowalski, C.P.; Nevedal, A.L.; Finley, E.P.; Young, J.P.; Lewinski, A.A.; Midboe, A.M.; Hamilton, A.B. Planning for and assessing rigor in rapid qualitative analysis (PARRQA): A consensus-based framework for designing, conducting, and reporting. *Implement. Sci.* **2024**, *19*, 71. [CrossRef]
47. St. George, S.M.; Harkness, A.R.; Rodriguez-Diaz, C.E.; Weinstein, E.R.; Pavia, V.; Hamilton, A.B. Applying rapid qualitative analysis for health equity: Lessons learned using "EARS" with Latino communities. *Int. J. Qual. Methods* **2023**, *22*, 16094069231164938. [CrossRef] [PubMed]
48. Natale, R.; Bailey, J.; Kolomeyer, E.; Futterer, J.; Schenker, M.; Bulotsky-Shearer, R. Early childhood teacher workplace stress and classroom practices. *J. Early Child. Teach. Educ.* **2023**, *44*, 897–914. [CrossRef]
49. Gilliam, W.S.; Maupin, A.N.; Reyes, C.R. Early childhood mental health consultation: Results of a statewide random-controlled evaluation. *J. Am. Acad. Child Adolesc. Psychiatry* **2016**, *55*, 754–761. [CrossRef] [PubMed]
50. Williams, P.G.; Yogman, M.; Sells, J.; Alderman, S.; Bauer, N.; Hashikawa, A.; Guevara, J.; Navsaria, D.; Nelson, B.; Peacock, G.; et al. Addressing early education and child care expulsion. *Pediatrics* **2023**, *152*, e2023064049. [CrossRef]

children

MDPI

Article

Promoting Mental Health in Adolescents Through Physical Education: Measuring Life Satisfaction for Comprehensive Development

Santiago Gómez-Paniagua [1], Antonio Castillo-Paredes [2,*], Pedro R. Olivares [3,4] and Jorge Rojo-Ramos [1]

1 Promoting a Healthy Society Research Group (PHeSO), Faculty of Sport Sciences, University of Extremadura, 10003 Cáceres, Spain; sgomezpa@alumnos.unex.es (S.G.-P.); jorgerr@unex.es (J.R.-R.)
2 Grupo AFySE, Investigación en Actividad Física y Salud Escolar, Escuela de Pedagogía en Educación Física, Facultad de Educación, Universidad de Las Américas, Santiago 8370040, Chile
3 Faculty of Education, Psychology and Sport Sciences, University of Huelva, 21007 Huelva, Spain; pedro.olivares@ddi.uhu.es
4 Facultad de Educación, Universidad Autónoma de Chile, Talca 3480094, Chile
* Correspondence: acastillop85@gmail.com

Abstract: Background: Life satisfaction serves as a preventive agent against various emotional, cognitive, and behavioral challenges, making it a crucial cognitive indicator of subjective well-being, particularly during adolescence. Accurately assessing life satisfaction is essential for understanding and promoting adolescent mental health, especially in applied settings such as physical education, which plays a key role in fostering psychological well-being and positive youth development. However, additional investigation is needed to confirm the tools used for this purpose. This study aimed to analyze the psychometric properties, metric invariance, and temporal stability of the Satisfaction with Life Scale (SWLS) in adolescents from a region in southeastern Spain. Thus, the present study sought to answer the following research questions: (1) Does the SWLS demonstrate adequate psychometric properties in an adolescent population? (2) Is the SWLS invariant across gender and residential environments? (3) Does the SWLS show adequate stability over time? **Methods:** A sample of 400 students was assessed using exploratory and confirmatory factor analyses, multigroup comparisons, and test–retest techniques. **Results:** The results showed significant differences in scale scores in the sex and demographic location variables. Also, a robust unifactorial model with five items demonstrated good performance in terms of goodness of fit and internal consistency. Furthermore, full metric invariance was observed across genders, while configural invariance was supported for residential environment. Concurrent validity analyses revealed significant associations with another unidimensional well-being measure, and temporal stability was confirmed through the intraclass correlation coefficient. **Conclusions:** The findings support the SWLS as a potentially valid, reliable, and time-effective tool for assessing adolescent life satisfaction. Its strong psychometric properties make it highly suitable for use in mental health research, longitudinal monitoring, and large-scale studies. Moreover, its ease of administration allows its integration into educational, clinical, community-based, and physical education contexts, offering insightful information for the creation of long-lasting mental health regulations and preventive measures meant to improve the well-being of adolescents. Notwithstanding these encouraging results, some restrictions must be noted. The sample was restricted to a single geographic area, and contextual or cultural factors may have an impact on how satisfied people are with their lives. Furthermore, response biases could have been introduced by using self-report measures.

Children **2025**, *12*, 658

https://doi.org/10.3390/children12050658

Keywords: mental health; adolescents; sex; metric invariance; temporal stability

1. Introduction

The emotional response that each person has to their life and the expectations they have for it, considering their perspectives on work, social life, and personal life, as well as their biological and psychological needs, is what is known as life satisfaction (LS) [1,2]. Both LS and quality of life—more especially, leading a healthy lifestyle—are strongly correlated with health [3]. Accordingly, many studies examining the connection between LS and physical activity (PA) have found that decreased amounts of PA are associated with worse health, which in turn causes LS to decline [4]. Conversely, research has shown that adolescents, irrespective of gender, who engage in more frequent and intense physical exercise have higher LS [5–7]. In addition, due to biological, psychological, cognitive, and social changes that may impact the LS assessment process during adolescence, self-concept may be seen as a sign of how adolescents manage these changes in relation to LS [8]. This has led to the identification of adolescence as a stage of mental health risk in the life cycle. In keeping with this line of reasoning, children's and teenagers' LS appears to be greatly influenced by their educational environment [9]. In other words, higher LS appears to be associated with academic performance, and the most significant mediator for enhancing students' mental health is physical activity (PA) [10].

In a similar vein, many elements have been found to be significant when examining children's and adolescents' SL. In this sense, various variables, such as an individual's gender, can serve as predictors or modify the effect on LS [11]. Research indicates that when focusing on the childhood and adolescent stages, girls typically have lower SV than boys [12]. In addition, living environments also have a significant impact on people's LS levels [13], although there is not much research that repeats these kinds of investigations in children and teenagers [14,15]. However, some research indicates that family functioning and positive youth development are linked, over time, to adolescent SV [16]. Other relationships with SV include family structure, family life cycle stage, and nutrition [17]. In the end, it is anticipated that adolescents with SV will be happier with their lives if they believe they are more capable socially and academically, have the capacity for self-control, and have worthwhile goals to work toward, while adolescents from less affluent families exhibit lower levels of LS [18]. On the other hand, a variety of other pathologies, including cardiovascular illnesses and sleep disorders, are linked to childhood and teenage overweight [19], and these disorders' aftereffects and complications impair children's and teenagers' subjective well-being and lower their LS [20,21].

Because of the evident importance of LS as a protective factor in the normal development of children and adolescents, there are numerous assessment tools available for these populations [22]. Among them, the Satisfaction with Life Scale (SWLS) [23] stands out. It has a five-item single-factor structure, and analyzes the general judgment of adolescents regarding their subjective well-being. Moreover, this scale has been translated over time into different languages [24–26] and validated in different populations [27–29], showing disparate characteristics. The adolescent population has not been an exception, with validations of the scale in different areas around the world, whether in Europe [30,31], Asia [32] or South America [33]. However, as far as Spain is concerned, only Ortuño and colleagues [34] have tested metric invariance in adolescents according to their sociodemographic factors, since other studies that included Spanish adolescents evaluated it by comparing them with their counterparts in other countries [35,36]. Similarly, and to the authors' knowledge, no study has conducted an invariance analysis focused on the area in which the student lives (rural or urban), which has been pointed out as an influential factor in the LS levels of adolescents [13,14], just as no validation study has included data from teenagers living in the region of Extremadura (Spain). Therefore, the current study's objectives were to investigate the SWLS's characteristics and conduct an invariance analysis that takes gender and the environment of a sample of adolescents from a region in southeast Spain under consideration. Similarly, possible differences in the study population according to the variables of analysis will be explored in order to understand the current state of the region. Based on consistent one-factor structures in prior adolescent SWLS validations, we hypothesized that the internal structure would be monofactorial, composed of five items, offer good goodness-of-fit indices, and that the assumption of metric invariance would be met for both the gender variable and the environment. Thus, the present study sought to answer the following research questions:

1. Does the SWLS demonstrate adequate psychometric properties in an adolescent population from Extremadura?
2. Is the SWLS invariant across gender and residential environments?
3. Does the SWLS show adequate stability over time?

2. Materials and Methods

2.1. Participants

Because the goal of this study was to collect as many responses as possible, we used a descriptive cross-sectional design. As per the latest data available on the National Institute of Statistics (www.ine.es), within the Community of Extremadura in Spain, there are 43,043 minors aged 8 to 18. Our study's sample size of 400 participants was greater than the 381 needed to guarantee a 95% confidence level and a ±5% margin of error. The inclusion criteria for participation in the study were regular participation in PE classes and informed consent from parents.

A total of 400 participants comprised the study's sample (Table 1), chosen via convenience sampling in accordance with Salkind's suggested procedures [37], with boys representing the same proportion of the sample (50%, $n = 200$) as girls (50%, $n = 200$). When it came to geographic location, 45% ($n = 180$) of the population lived in rural areas, while the majority (55%, $n = 220$) lived in urban areas. With a mean age of 13.12 years and a standard deviation of 1.94, the group's age variability was deemed to be moderate.

Table 1. Sample characteristics.

Variable	Categories	N	%
Sex	Boy	200	50
	Girl	200	50
Demographic location	Rural	180	45
	Urban	220	55
Variable		**M**	**SD**
Age		13.12	1.94

N: number; %: percentage; SD: standard deviation; M: mean.

In this study, living environments were categorized using the Cáceres Provincial Council's concept. Urban communities were defined as having 20,000 or more inhabitants, whereas rural communities had 20,000 or fewer.

The University of Extremadura's Ethics Committee gave its approval to the study (6/2024), which was carried out in compliance with the Declaration of Helsinki's criteria.

2.2. Procedure

Emails with information on the study, a sample questionnaire, and a request for parental approval were sent to Extremadura's physical education teachers. A list of local public schools offering secondary education was used to choose the teachers. The teachers in question arranged for a member of the study team to visit the center and provide the questionnaires to the pupils after getting the families' signed agreement. A week later, the process would be repeated.

Every student received a tablet from the researcher on the scheduled day, along with a link to the Google Forms questionnaire. The researcher read out each question to make sure the participants understood it. To enable effective data collection and storage, it was decided to employ an electronic questionnaire.

The questionnaire took about five minutes to complete, and anonymous data were gathered between January and February of 2023.

2.3. Instruments

Initially, a set of three sociodemographic questions about sex, housing environment, and age were included in the questionnaire.

Additionally, the Satisfaction with Life Scale (SWLS) (Appendix A), which Atienza and collaborators validated in Spanish [26], was used to gauge teenagers' subjective levels of LS. This instrument has five items that are intended to gauge young people's values for various elements of their lives. A Likert-type scale, with 1 denoting "strongly disagree" and 5 denoting "strongly agree", is used to collect responses. The scale's authors reported a Cronbach's alpha coefficient of 0.84, demonstrating the scale's good reliability when gauging adolescent' LS. This scale gathers items such as "In most aspects, my life is the way I want it to be" or "I am satisfied with my life".

Lastly, the six-level Student's Life Satisfaction Scale (SLSS) in Spanish (Appendix B) was utilized. It was validated by Alfaro et al. [38] and had a Cronbach's alpha score of 0.70. Items 3 and 4 were inverted to make it easier to interpret the results. The scale ranged from "strongly disagree" (1) to "strongly agree" (6).

2.4. Statistical Analysis

The SWLS items and overall scores were analyzed using descriptive statistics. The normality of the data was evaluated using the Kolmogorov–Smirnov test. The Mann–Whitney U test was used to analyze differences by sex and living environment in light of the non-normal distribution. Hedges' g was used to calculate effect sizes.

The Solomon approach was used to randomly split the sample into two subsamples in order to examine the psychometric characteristics of the SWLS. One subsample was subjected to exploratory factor analysis (EFA) using the software FACTOR v.10.10.02, while the other was subjected to confirmatory factor analysis (CFA) using AMOS v.26.0.0. Sample adequacy was evaluated using the Kaiser–Meyer–Olkin (KMO) metric and Bartlett's test of sphericity.

Also, multigroup CFA was used to examine measurement invariance across groups (gender and residential environment). Spearman correlation with a well-being scale that had been validated in Spanish adolescents (SLSS) was used to assess concurrent validity.

Intraclass correlation coefficients (ICCs) with 95% CIs were used to evaluate temporal stability and test–retest reliability. Additionally, the minimal detectable change (MDC) and the standard error of measurement (SEM) were computed.

3. Results

3.1. Descriptive Statistics and Differences

The descriptive statistics and differences for each of the items that make up the SWLS questionnaire by gender and setting are presented in Table 2. In terms of effect size, values below 0.20 are considered to have no effect, a modest influence for coefficients between 0.21 and 0.49, a moderate effect for values between 0.50 and 0.79, and a substantial effect for values above 0.80 [39].

Table 2. Descriptive statistics and differences on SWLS scale.

Item	Total		Men		Women				Rural		Urban			
	Me	IQR	Me	IQR	Me	IQR	*p*	g	Me	IQR	Me	IQR	*p*	g
1	4.00	2.0	4.00	2.0	4.00	1.0	0.01	0.18	4.00	2.0	4.00	2.0	0.93	0.04
2	5.00	1.0	5.00	1.0	4.00	1.0	0.03	0.22	4.00	1.0	5.00	1.0	0.46	0.05
3	5.00	1.0	5.00	1.0	5.00	1.0	<0.01	0.22	5.00	1.0	5.00	1.0	0.53	0.01
4	4.00	1.0	5.00	1.0	4.00	1.0	0.05	0.13	5.00	1.0	4.00	1.0	<0.01	0.23
5	4.00	2.0	4.00	2.0	4.00	2.0	0.01	0.20	4.00	2.0	4.00	2.0	0.23	0.13
SWLS	4.20	1.0	4.40	1.0	4.00	1.0	<0.01	0.26	4.20	1.0	4.20	1.0	0.84	0.01

Note: Me = median value; IQR = interquartile range; g = Hedges' g; SWLS: Satisfaction with Life Scale.

Looking at the gender variable, male students showed statistically significantly higher scores on all items of the questionnaire. However, items 1 and 4 showed insignificant effect sizes, although the rest of the items and the total score showed modest effects. Moreover, some item-level differences were observed by residential environment, with urban students showing higher scores in items one, two and five, although in items three and four, rural students obtained a higher mean score. The sole item that also revealed statistically significant differences favoring students from rural contexts was item 4, indicating a modest effect of these differences.

3.2. EFA and CFA

First, the sample was divided into two equal subsamples using Solomon's method [40], one for the EFA and the other for the CFA. This allows analysis of whether the model explored in one subsample (EFA) is replicated in a second (CFA), establishing a procedure in which all possible sources of common variance are equally represented in each subsample. The RULS method enabled the identification of a unidimensional structure for the questionnaire (Table 3), supported by the amount of variance explained through eigenvalues [41] and the reliability estimates obtained via expected a posteriori (EAP) scores [42].

Table 3. Eigenvalues and variance proportion for the items of the scale.

Items	Eigenvalues	Proportion of Variance
1. In most ways, my life is close to my ideal.	3.37	0.67
2. The conditions of my life are excellent.	0.52	0.10
3. I am satisfied with my life.	0.48	0.09
4. So far, I have gotten the important things I want in life.	0.45	0.09
5. If I could live my life over, I would change almost nothing.	0.18	0.04

Due to the outcome, no rotation mechanism was selected because the structure was one-dimensional. The feasibility of conducting the EFA was confirmed through favorable sample adequacy metrics, with a KMO value of 0.834 and a statistically significant Bartlett's test result ($\chi^2 = 551.3$; df = 10; $p < 0.001$). Table 4 presents the factor loading matrix for a one-factor solution comprising five items.

Table 4. Unrotated loading matrix.

Items	Load	Communality
1. In most ways, my life is close to my ideal.	0.73	0.53
2. The conditions of my life are excellent.	0.79	0.62
3. I am satisfied with my life.	0.92	0.84
4. So far, I have gotten the important things I want in life.	0.70	0.49
5. If I could live my life over, I would change almost nothing.	0.72	0.52

Once the EFA confirmed the structure of the scale, a CFA was conducted using the second subsample to assess the model's characteristics (see Figure 1). All items were retained, as they satisfied the established criteria: absence of cross-loadings above 0.40, communalities exceeding 0.30, and factor loadings equal to or greater than 0.60.

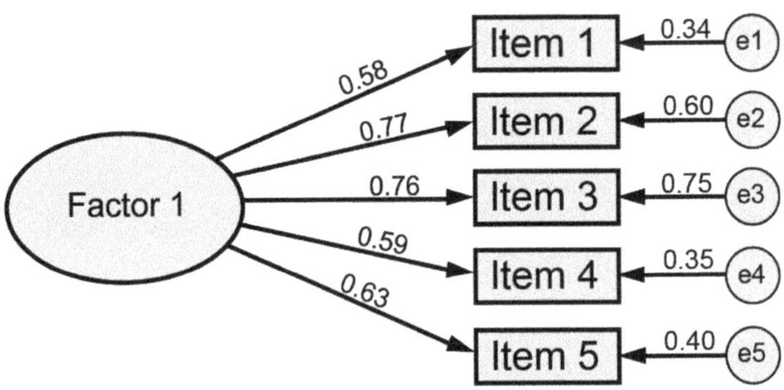

Figure 1. Factorial structure.

The model's goodness-of-fit indices were found to be satisfactory, even though the factorial structure was maintained without introducing correlations between the error terms of items 4 and 5, as suggested in prior studies [25]. To assess model fit, several indicators were considered: the chi-squared-to-degrees of freedom ratio (CMIN/DF) with a threshold below 3 [43]; the root mean square error of approximation (RMSEA) and the root mean square of residuals (RMSR), both expected to be under 0.08 [44,45]; and comparative (CFI) and normed fit indices (NFI), with recommended values above 0.90 [46].

In this analysis, the CMIN/DF reached a value of 2.17 ($\chi^2 = 10.86$, df = 5), while the CFI and NFI were 0.98 and 0.97, respectively. Additionally, the RMSEA and RMSR values were 0.07 and 0.03, indicating an adequate model fit. Table 5 displays the standardized factor loadings by group.

Table 5. Factor loadings of different subgroups.

Item	Men	Women	Rural	Urban	Total
	Loadings (R^2)	Loadings (R^2)	Loadings (R^2)	Loadings (R^2)	Loadings (R^2)
1	0.58 (0.34)	0.59 (0.35)	0.60 (0.36)	0.59 (0.35)	0.58 (0.34)
2	0.74 (0.55)	0.81 (0.65)	0.73 (0.54)	0.81 (0.65)	0.77 (0.60)
3	0.84 (0.70)	0.88 (0.78)	0.81 (0.65)	0.90 (0.81)	0.76 (0.75)
4	0.61 (0.37)	0.59 (0.34)	0.61 (0.38)	0.60 (0.36)	0.59 (0.35)
5	0.58 (0.34)	0.65 (0.43)	0.73 (0.53)	0.56 (0.31)	0.63 (0.40)

Note: All standardized factor loadings estimated were statistically significant ($p < 0.01$).

3.3. Measurement Invariance

Likewise, multiple multigroup confirmatory factor analyses were performed to assess measurement invariance across groups. To determine whether the nested models demonstrated invariance, a change in the comparative fit index (CFI) of less than 0.01 was used as the evaluation criterion [47].

The fit indices obtained from the successive multigroup analyses revealed a variation of less than 0.01 between the unconstrained and constrained models, thereby supporting the presence of measurement invariance across both variables (Table 6).

Table 6. Metric invariance for gender and demographic location.

Model	χ^2	df	CMIN/DF	CFI	NFI	RMSEA	RMSR	ΔCFI
Gender								
Unconstrained	19.35	8	2.42	0.984	0.97	0.06	0.03	
Configural Invariance	23.12	12	1.93	0.984	0.97	0.05	0.04	<0.01
Metric Invariance	30.27	17	1.78	0.982	0.96	0.04	0.04	<0.01
Scalar Invariance	31.51	18	1.75	0.981	0.96	0.04	0.04	<0.01
Demographic Location								
Model	**χ^2**	**df**	**CMIN/DF**	**CFI**	**NFI**	**RMSEA**	**RMSR**	**ΔCFI**
Unconstrained	19.93	8	2.49	0.984	0.97	0.06	0.03	
Configural Invariance	27.79	12	2.32	0.979	0.96	0.06	0.05	<0.01
Metric Invariance	39.91	17	2.35	0.969	0.95	0.06	0.05	>0.01
Scalar Invariance	39.91	18	2.22	0.967	0.95	0.05	0.05	<0.01

3.4. Internal Consistency, Concurrent Validity, and Temporal Stability

Furthermore, as measures of scale reliability, McDonald's omega and Cronbach's alpha were employed [48]. As far as internal consistency is concerned, the scale showed acceptable values in both measurement times: Cronbach's alpha (time 1 = 0.83, time 2 = 0.82) and McDonald's omega (time 1 = 0.83, time 2 = 0.82).

In the same vein, the analysis of the relationship between the SWLS and SLSS scores indicated a statistically significant and direct correlation of moderate magnitude ($\rho = 0.60$, $p < 0.001$).

Finally, in order to assess the temporal stability of the SWLS, test–retest reliability was assessed using the intraclass correlation coefficient (ICC) between the two measurement times with 95% confidence interval. These results were classified by the intervals defined by Cicchetti [49]: poor (<0.40), fair (0.40–0.60), good (0.60–0.75), or excellent (>0.75). In accordance with recommendations for selecting the ICC [50], it was based on two-way random effects, utilizing the mean of multiple measurements and absolute agreement. Furthermore, calculations were made for the minimal detectable change (MDC) and standard error of measurement (SEM) [51,52].

The values related to temporal stability are shown in Table 7. The ICC between 0.6 and 0.75 showed good reliability of the questionnaire in the two data collections.

Table 7. Temporal stability.

SWLS	M (SD)	ICC (95% CI)	SEM	MDC (%)	MDC90 (%)	MDC95 (%)
Time 1 Time 2	4.06 (0.77) 4.24 (0.65)	0.70 (0.62, 0.76)	0.39	0.88 (13.32)	0.91 (21.92)	1.08 (26.12)

Note: M = mean value; SD = standard deviation; ICC = intraclass correlation coefficient; SEM = standard error of measurement; MDC = minimal detectable change.

4. Discussion

The primary objective of this study was to evaluate the psychometric properties of the SWLS in a population of adolescents belonging to a region of southeastern Spain (Extremadura), as well as to confirm its metric invariance according to gender and the environment where they live. Likewise, an update of the current state of LS of adolescents in the region was produced, finding differences in the sex variable and in the area of residence.

As for the differences found in gender, the most current literature exploring SL at the international level in some thirty countries shows that in general terms, female adolescents show lower levels compared to their male peers [53]. In the Spanish context, Aymerich et al. [54] conducted a retrospective study in 600 Spanish adolescents, identifying female students as the most vulnerable, with the most dangerous period being from 10 to 12 years of age. Likewise, in a sample of 2400 adolescents aged 12 to 17 years in southern Spain, Reina Flores et al. [55] found similar results. However, Casas Aznar et al. [56] found positive differences favoring females in a large number of adolescents enrolled in secondary education. As researchers note [57], these discrepancies could be due to females having more social support, but revealing negative emotions more often than men in daily life, causing LS levels to level out over time.

To the best of the authors' knowledge, there is a dearth of scientific research examining how adolescent behavior varies depending on their place of residence. Overall, Márquez and Long [58] assessed LS levels in 15-year-old adolescents from 46 nations and discovered that in spite of the recent reduction, pupils from rural settings had higher levels. Similar findings were reported in an Indian study that examined university students' LS in this setting, which explained why urban students performed worse because of their busy schedules and stress accumulation [59]. However, the latest scientific publications indicate that the trend is towards equality, finding similar scores for students in both contexts, although this varies depending on the society being studied [60]. Numerous psychosocial reasons could be the cause of the lack of notable variances. For instance, adolescents living in urban settings may experience higher levels of academic anxiety, lower feelings of belonging at school, and more exposure to victimization, insecurity, and family conflict, all of which are linked to behavioral problems and poorer psychological well-being [61–66]. Potential urban benefits, including greater access to services or educational opportunities, may be offset by these pressures. According to Jiménez Boraita et al. [67] and Sharma et al. [59], rural youth's reported LS may also be influenced by their greater levels of health-related well-being and longer sleep duration.

In this sense, the results confirmed adequate values in the sample of Spanish-speaking adolescents, as other studies had previously ratified [34,68]. This study established a unifactorial structure composed of five items that yielded good goodness-of-fit indices, like other international studies [69,70], though despite the improvement in these indices, the correlation of items four and five was not necessary to statistically define the model, as recent studies pointed out [32,71]. Likewise, the reliability values obtained are in agreement with previous studies carried out on samples of adolescents in the same country [34,35].

Regarding metric invariance, numerous studies have tested the gender variable. In this sense, Emerson and collaborators have already indicated that gender bias in the questionnaire was not a factor to be taken into account [72]. More recent studies focusing on adolescent populations have confirmed this assertion: in France [73], India [32], and Peru or Portugal [74]. Likewise, Jovanović et al. [71] carried out a study of the scale in 24 countries, asserting the metric invariance of the instrument with respect to gender in 21 of the regions explored. However, they suggested that this invariance should not be taken for granted and needed to be evaluated prior to the application of the questionnaire, mainly due to the complexity of the results obtained.

To the authors' knowledge, the environment in which the adolescent resides has not been the subject of study in terms of metric invariance. Nevertheless, it has been pointed out as an important limitation in previous research, due to the fact that there are many regions in which the population is evenly distributed between urban and rural areas [75].

Moreover, moderate concurrent validity was obtained when compared with another measurement scale of the same construct, as already demonstrated in previous literature [75,76]; however, there are few studies in which it is compared with another unifactorial measure of LS. On the other hand, temporal stability remains a parameter little analyzed in the different SWLS validations. The vast majority of studies use bivariate correlations to assess the temporal stability of the instrument [32,77], although the statistical literature has pointed out that the ICC is more appropriate for assessing the temporal stability of measures associated with health-related quality of life because the measures to be compared at both instants are randomly selected [78]. In this context, Silva et al. [30] found very similar test–retest results to those of this study.

Limitations and Future Lines

This research presents a series of limitations like any other. First, no data were collected from students at baccalaureate level (from 16 to 18 years old), so LS levels in late adolescence cannot be contrasted. Also, the results of this study should be regarded cautiously primarily because of its design, which makes it impossible to establish case–effect correlations. Furthermore, because it was limited to the community of Extremadura, sociocultural factors could have affected the outcomes, in addition to the convenience sampling technique used to choose the participants. Finally, there are few examples in the scientific literature that explore the temporal stability of the questionnaire and the metric invariance of the selected sample, the main reason for the study, so the results cannot be verified.

Future studies should try to include teenagers from different regions of Spain in the sample, going beyond the current regional setting. This would improve the findings' generalizability and provide a more thorough comprehension of life happiness in many sociocultural contexts. Furthermore, adding further waves of data collection would make it easier to create longitudinal research on adolescent well-being and enable the assessment of long-term temporal stability. In addition to expanding the geographic and temporal scope, it would be very beneficial to incorporate other factors like social media use, academic achievement, and socioeconomic position, all of which have been strongly connected to teenage life satisfaction. More in-depth understanding of certain risk and protective factors in the mental health of children and adolescents may be possible by investigating the ways in which these variables interact with subjective well-being.

Moreover, examining metric invariance across further subgroups—such as educational stage or age—may help tailor well-being assessments to different developmental periods, increasing the scale's diagnostic precision. In the long term, validating brief and stable tools like the Satisfaction with Life Scale (SWLS) may support the creation of screening protocols and personalized interventions in educational and community settings. These insights could inform the design of targeted mental health policies and programs that foster comprehensive development and emotional resilience in adolescents, particularly in underrepresented or vulnerable populations.

In practice, schools and educational authorities might use short, validated instruments like the SWLS to conduct periodic LS evaluations in order to identify children who may be at risk of poor well-being and send them to school professionals or mental health specialists. Additionally, preparing educators to analyze and use these findings may facilitate the incorporation of emotional health into lesson planning, particularly in high-stress settings [79,80]. Using brief, dependable measures would enable cost-effective large-scale monitoring in underserved populations or remote schools where access to psychological help is limited.

Moreover, by integrating LS metrics into youth development initiatives, public health authorities might direct funding toward areas or populations with consistently low satisfaction ratings. Using information from LS evaluations to design focused workshops on social belonging, stress management, and emotional regulation would allow for evidence-based interventions centered on the real needs of teenagers.

5. Conclusions

A tool widely validated in other contexts that allows the analysis of LS levels in adolescents was assessed in a sample of students from the Autonomous Community of Extremadura (Spain). The results suggested a monofactorial structure composed of five items, without the need for error correlation and reporting acceptable goodness-of-fit indices. On the other hand, the instrument showed total invariance for gender and configural invariance for the students' place of residence. Likewise, reliability and temporal stability indicators were also satisfactory within the specific sample. Nevertheless, these findings should be interpreted with caution due to the regional nature of the sample, which may limit the generalizability of the results.

Author Contributions: Conceptualization, S.G.-P.; data curation, P.R.O.; formal analysis, S.G.-P.; investigation, P.R.O.; methodology, J.R.-R.; resources, J.R.-R.; software, A.C.-P.; validation, A.C.-P.; writing—original draft, S.G.-P. All authors have read and agreed to the published version of the manuscript.

Funding: The APC was funded by the Open Access Program of the Universidad de Las Américas.

Institutional Review Board Statement: The study was conducted according to the guidelines of the Declaration of Helsinki and approved by the Ethics Committee of the University of Extremadura (6/2024) on 26 November 2024.

Informed Consent Statement: Informed consent was obtained from all subjects involved in the study.

Data Availability Statement: The datasets are available through the corresponding author upon reasonable request. The data are not publicly available due to privacy.

Conflicts of Interest: The authors declare no conflicts of interest.

Appendix A

Table A1. Escala de Satisfacción con la Vida (SWLS).

1.	En la mayoría de los aspectos mi vida es como yo quiero que sea
2.	Las circunstancias de mi vida son muy buenas
3.	Estoy satisfecho con mi vida
4.	Hasta ahora he conseguido de la vida las cosas que considero importantes
5.	Si pudiera vivir mi vida otra vez no cambiaría casi nada

Appendix B

Table A2. Escala de Satisfacción con la Vida para Estudiantes (SLSS).

1.	Mi vida va bien
2.	Mi vida es perfecta
3.	Me gustaría cambiar muchas cosas de mi vida
4.	Te gustaría tener otro tipo de vida
5.	Tengo una buena vida
6.	Tengo lo que quiero en la vida
7.	Mi vida es mejor que la mayoría de los chichos/as de mi edad

References

1. Bear, G.G.; Minke, K.M.; National Association of School Psychologists (Eds.) *Children's Needs III: Development, Prevention, and Intervention*; National Association of School Psychologists: Bethesda, MD, USA, 2006; ISBN 978-0-932955-79-1.
2. Baştuğ, G.; Duman, S. Examining Life Satisfaction Level Depending on Physical Activity in Turkish and German Societies. *Procedia-Soc. Behav. Sci.* **2010**, *2*, 4892–4895. [CrossRef]
3. Anand, M.; Arora, D. Burnout, Life Satisfaction and Quality of Life among Executives of Multi National Companies. *J. Indian Acad. Appl. Psychol.* **2009**, *35*, 159–164.
4. Zullig, K.J.; Valois, R.F.; Huebner, E.S.; Drane, J.W. Adolescent Health-Related Quality of Life and Perceived Satisfaction with Life. *Qual. Life Res.* **2005**, *14*, 1573–1584. [CrossRef]
5. Vaquero-Solís, M.; Gallego, D.I.; Tapia-Serrano, M.Á.; Pulido, J.J.; Sánchez-Miguel, P.A. School-Based Physical Activity Interventions in Children and Adolescents: A Systematic Review. *Int. J. Environ. Res. Public Health* **2020**, *17*, 999. [CrossRef]
6. Chen, S.; Ho, W.K.Y.; Ahmed, M.D. Physical Activity and Its Relationship with Life Satisfaction among Middle School Students: A Cross-Culture Study. *Sustainability* **2020**, *12*, 6932. [CrossRef]
7. Feng, B.; Xu, K.; Zhou, P. Association between Vigorous Physical Activity and Life Satisfaction in Adolescents. *Front. Public Health* **2022**, *10*, 944620. [CrossRef]
8. Vijayakumar, N.; Op De Macks, Z.; Shirtcliff, E.A.; Pfeifer, J.H. Puberty and the Human Brain: Insights into Adolescent Development. *Neurosci. Biobehav. Rev.* **2018**, *92*, 417–436. [CrossRef]
9. Baltacı, H.Ş.; Karataş, Z. Perceived Social Support, Depression and Life Satisfaction as the Predictor of the Resilience of Secondary School Students: The Case of Burdur. *Eurasian J. Educ. Res.* **2015**, *15*, 111–130. [CrossRef]
10. Hughes, C.W.; Barnes, S.; Barnes, C.; DeFina, L.F.; Nakonezny, P.; Emslie, G.J. Depressed Adolescents Treated with Exercise (DATE): A Pilot Randomized Controlled Trial to Test Feasibility and Establish Preliminary Effect Sizes. *Ment. Health Phys. Act.* **2013**, *6*, 119–131. [CrossRef]
11. Slapšinskaitė, A.; Lukoševičiūtė, J.; Šmigelskas, K. Interplay between Adolescent Physical Activity and Life Satisfaction: Gender as Potential Effect Modifier. *Int. J. Public Health* **2020**, *65*, 1355–1363. [CrossRef]

12. Goswami, H. Children's Subjective Well-Being: Socio-Demographic Characteristics and Personality. *Child Ind. Res.* **2014**, *7*, 119–140. [CrossRef]
13. Swami, V.; Todd, J. Rural-Urban Differences in Body Appreciation and Associations with Life Satisfaction in Adults from Sabah, Malaysia. *Body Image* **2022**, *43*, 385–392. [CrossRef]
14. Yeresyan, I.; Lohaus, A. Stress and Wellbeing among Turkish and German Adolescents Living in Rural and Urban Areas. *Rural Remote Health* **2014**, *14*, 2695. [CrossRef]
15. Abreu, D.P.D.; Viñas, F.; Casas, F.; Montserrat, C.; González-Carrasco, M.; Alcantara, S.C.D. Estressores Psicossociais, Senso de Comunidade e Bem-Estar Subjetivo Em Crianças e Adolescentes de Zonas Urbanas e Rurais Do Nordeste Do Brasil. *Cad. Saúde Pública* **2016**, *32*, e00126815. [CrossRef]
16. Shek, D.T.L.; Liu, T.T. Life Satisfaction in Junior Secondary School Students in Hong Kong: A 3-Year Longitudinal Study. *Soc. Indic. Res.* **2014**, *117*, 777–794. [CrossRef]
17. Schnettler, B.; Miranda-Zapata, E.; Grunert, K.G.; Grønhøj, A.; Jiménez, P.; Lobos, G.; Lapo, M.; Orellana, L.; Hueche, C. Satisfaction with Life, Family and Food in Adolescents: Exploring Moderating Roles of Family-Related Factors. *Curr. Psychol.* **2022**, *41*, 802–815. [CrossRef]
18. Calmeiro, L.; Camacho, I.; De Matos, M.G. Life Satisfaction in Adolescents: The Role of Individual and Social Health Assets. *Span. J. Psychol.* **2018**, *21*, E23. [CrossRef]
19. Barlow, S.E.; Dietz, W.H. Management of Child and Adolescent Obesity: Summary and Recommendations Based on Reports From Pediatricians, Pediatric Nurse Practitioners, and Registered Dietitians. *Pediatrics* **2002**, *110*, 236–238. [CrossRef]
20. Hassan, H.; Paulis, W.D.; Bindels, P.J.E.; Koes, B.W.; Van Middelkoop, M. Somatic Complaints as a Mediator in the Association between Body Mass Index and Quality of Life in Children and Adolescents. *BMC Fam. Pract.* **2021**, *22*, 214. [CrossRef]
21. Lebacq, T.; Dujeu, M.; Méroc, E.; Moreau, N.; Pedroni, C.; Godin, I.; Castetbon, K. Perceived Social Support from Teachers and Classmates Does Not Moderate the Inverse Association between Body Mass Index and Health-Related Quality of Life in Adolescents. *Qual. Life Res.* **2019**, *28*, 895–905. [CrossRef]
22. Huebner, E.S. Research on Assessment of Life Satisfaction of Children and Adolescents. *Soc. Indic. Res.* **2004**, *66*, 3–33. [CrossRef]
23. Diener, E.; Emmons, R.A.; Larsen, R.J.; Griffin, S. The Satisfaction with Life Scale. *J. Personal. Assess.* **1985**, *49*, 71–75. [CrossRef] [PubMed]
24. Arrindell, W.A.; Heesink, J.; Feij, J.A. The Satisfaction With Life Scale (SWLS): Appraisal with 1700 Healthy Young Adults in The Netherlands. *Personal. Individ. Differ.* **1999**, *26*, 815–826. [CrossRef]
25. Glaesmer, H.; Grande, G.; Braehler, E.; Roth, M. The German Version of the Satisfaction With Life Scale (SWLS): Psychometric Properties, Validity, and Population-Based Norms. *Eur. J. Psychol. Assess.* **2011**, *27*, 127–132. [CrossRef]
26. Atienza, F.L.; Pons, D.; Balaguer, I.; García-Merita, M. Propiedades Psicométricas de La Escala de Satisfacción Con La Vida En Adolescentes. *Psicothema* **2000**, *12*, 314–319.
27. Pons, D.; Atienza, F.L.; Balaguer, I.; García-Merita, M.L. Satisfaction with Life Scale: Analysis of Factorial Invariance for Adolescents and Elderly Persons. *Percept. Mot. Ski.* **2000**, *91*, 62–68. [CrossRef]
28. Cerezo, M.V.; Soria-Reyes, L.M.; Alarcón, R.; Blanca, M.J. The Satisfaction with Life Scale in Breast Cancer Patients: Psychometric Properties. *Int. J. Clin. Health Psychol.* **2022**, *22*, 100274. [CrossRef]
29. López-Ortega, M.; Torres-Castro, S.; Rosas-Carrasco, O. Psychometric Properties of the Satisfaction with Life Scale (SWLS): Secondary Analysis of the Mexican Health and Aging Study. *Health Qual. Life Outcomes* **2016**, *14*, 170. [CrossRef]
30. Silva, A.D.; Taveira, M.D.C.; Marques, C.; Gouveia, V.V. Satisfaction with Life Scale Among Adolescents and Young Adults in Portugal: Extending Evidence of Construct Validity. *Soc. Indic. Res.* **2015**, *120*, 309–318. [CrossRef]
31. Di Fabio, A.; Gori, A. Measuring Adolescent Life Satisfaction: Psychometric Properties of the Satisfaction With Life Scale in a Sample of Italian Adolescents and Young Adults. *J. Psychoeduc. Assess.* **2016**, *34*, 501–506. [CrossRef]
32. Areepattamannil, S.; Bano, S. Psychometric Properties of the Satisfaction with Life Scale (SWLS) Among Middle Adolescents in a Collectivist Cultural Setting. *Psychol. Stud.* **2020**, *65*, 497–503. [CrossRef]
33. Arias Gallegos, W.L.; Huamani Cahua, J.C.; Caycho-Rodríguez, T. Satisfacción Con La Vida En Escolares de La Ciudad de Arequipa. *Propós. Represent.* **2018**, *6*, 351–379. [CrossRef]
34. Ortuño-Sierra, J.; Aritio-Solana, R.; Chocarro De Luis, E.; Nalda, F.N.; Fonseca-Pedrero, E. Subjective Well-Being in Adolescence: New Psychometric Evidences on the Satisfaction with Life Scale. *Eur. J. Dev. Psychol.* **2019**, *16*, 236–244. [CrossRef]
35. Atienza, F.L.; Balaguer, I.; Corte-Real, N. Factorial Invariance of the Satisfaction with Life Scale in Adolescents from Spain and Portugal. *Psicothema* **2016**, *3*, 353–358. [CrossRef]
36. Esnaola, I.; Benito, M.; Antonio-Agirre, I. Measurement Invariance of the Satisfaction With Life Scale (SWLS) by Country, Gender and Age. *Psicothema* **2017**, *4*, 596–601. [CrossRef]
37. Salkind, N.J.; Escalona, R.L.; Valdés Salmerón, V. *Métodos de Investigación*; Prentice-Hall: Hoboken, NJ, USA, 1999; ISBN 978-970-17-0234-5.

38. Alfaro, J.; Guzman, J.; Sirlopu, D.; Garcia, C.; Reyes, F.; Gaudlitz, L. Propiedades Psicométricas de La Escala de Satisfacción Con La Vida En Los Estudiantes (SLSS) de Huebner En Niños y Niñas de 10 a 12 Años de Chile. *Ann. Psychol.* **2016**, *32*, 383. [CrossRef]
39. Cohen, J. *Statistical Power Analysis for the Behavioral Sciences*, 2nd ed.; Routledge: New York, NY, USA, 2013; ISBN 978-1-134-74270-7.
40. Lorenzo-Seva, U. SOLOMON: A Method for Splitting a Sample into Equivalent Subsamples in Factor Analysis. *Behav. Res.* **2022**, *54*, 2665–2677. [CrossRef]
41. Larsen, R.; Warne, R.T. Estimating Confidence Intervals for Eigenvalues in Exploratory Factor Analysis. *Behav. Res. Methods* **2010**, *42*, 871–876. [CrossRef]
42. Ferrando Piera, P.J.; Lorenzo Seva, U. A Note on Improving EAP Trait Estimation in Oblique Factor-Analytic and Item Response Theory Models. *Psicológica* **2016**, *37*, 235–247.
43. Yaşlioğlu, M.; Toplu Yaşlioğlu, D. How and When to Use Which Fit Indices? A Practical and Critical Review of the Methodology. *Istanb. Manag. J.* **2020**, *88*, 1–20. [CrossRef]
44. Kenny, D.A.; Kaniskan, B.; McCoach, D.B. The Performance of RMSEA in Models with Small Degrees of Freedom. *Sociol. Methods Res.* **2015**, *44*, 486–507. [CrossRef]
45. Shi, D.; Maydeu-Olivares, A.; Rosseel, Y. Assessing Fit in Ordinal Factor Analysis Models: SRMR vs. RMSEA. *Struct. Equ. Model. Multidiscip. J.* **2020**, *27*, 1–15. [CrossRef]
46. Bentler, P.M. Comparative Fit Indexes in Structural Models. *Psychol. Bull.* **1990**, *107*, 238–246. [CrossRef]
47. Cheung, G.W.; Rensvold, R.B. Evaluating Goodness-of-Fit Indexes for Testing Measurement Invariance. *Struct. Equ. Model. Multidiscip. J.* **2002**, *9*, 233–255. [CrossRef]
48. Dunn, T.J.; Baguley, T.; Brunsden, V. From Alpha to Omega: A Practical Solution to the Pervasive Problem of Internal Consistency Estimation. *Br. J. Psychol.* **2014**, *105*, 399–412. [CrossRef]
49. Cicchetti, D.V. Guidelines, Criteria, and Rules of Thumb for Evaluating Normed and Standardized Assessment Instruments in Psychology. *Psychol. Assess.* **1994**, *6*, 284–290. [CrossRef]
50. Koo, T.K.; Li, M.Y. A Guideline of Selecting and Reporting Intraclass Correlation Coefficients for Reliability Research. *J. Chiropr. Med.* **2016**, *15*, 155–163. [CrossRef]
51. De Vet, H.C.; Terwee, C.B.; Ostelo, R.W.; Beckerman, H.; Knol, D.L.; Bouter, L.M. Minimal Changes in Health Status Questionnaires: Distinction between Minimally Detectable Change and Minimally Important Change. *Health Qual. Life Outcomes* **2006**, *4*, 54. [CrossRef]
52. Wyrwich, K.W.; Tierney, W.M.; Wolinsky, F.D. Using the Standard Error of Measurement to Identify Important Changes on the Asthma Quality of Life Questionnaire. *Qual. Life Res.* **2002**, *11*, 1–7. [CrossRef]
53. Marquez, J. Gender Differences in School Effects on Adolescent Life Satisfaction: Exploring Cross-National Variation. *Child Youth Care Forum* **2024**, *53*, 389–409. [CrossRef]
54. Aymerich, M.; Cladellas, R.; Castelló, A.; Casas, F.; Cunill, M. The Evolution of Life Satisfaction Throughout Childhood and Adolescence: Differences in Young People's Evaluations According to Age and Gender. *Child Ind. Res.* **2021**, *14*, 2347–2369. [CrossRef]
55. Reina, M.D.C. Percepciones de Autoevaluación: Autoestima, Autoeficacia y Satisfacción Vital En La Adolescencia. *Psychol. Soc. Educ.* **2017**, *2*, 55. [CrossRef]
56. Casas Aznar, F.; Buxarrais Estrada, M.R.; González Carrasco, M.; Tey, A.; Noguera i Pigem, E.; Rodríguez Rodríguez, J.M.; Figuer Ramírez, C. Los valores y su influencia en la satisfacción vital de los adolescentes entre los 12 y los 16 años: Estudio de algunos correlatos. *Apunt. Psicol.* **2004**, *22*, 3–23.
57. Chui, W.H.; Wong, M.Y.H. Gender Differences in Happiness and Life Satisfaction Among Adolescents in Hong Kong: Relationships and Self-Concept. *Soc. Indic. Res.* **2016**, *125*, 1035–1051. [CrossRef]
58. Marquez, J.; Long, E. A Global Decline in Adolescents' Subjective Well-Being: A Comparative Study Exploring Patterns of Change in the Life Satisfaction of 15-Year-Old Students in 46 Countries. *Child Ind. Res.* **2021**, *14*, 1251–1292. [CrossRef]
59. Sharma, R.; Sarita; Kumar, D. Life Satisfaction of Youth Residing in Rural and Urban Areas: A Comparative Study. *Indian J. Posit. Psychol.* **2023**, *14*, 35–38.
60. Marquez, J.; Main, G. Can Schools and Education Policy Make Children Happier? A Comparative Study in 33 Countries. *Child Ind. Res.* **2021**, *14*, 283–339. [CrossRef]
61. Kohli, S.; Malik, A. Academic Anxiety and Wellbeing amongst Rural and Urban Adolescents. *Indian J. Posit. Psychol.* **2013**, *4*, 148.
62. Anderman, E.M. School Effects on Psychological Outcomes during Adolescence. *J. Educ. Psychol.* **2002**, *94*, 795–809. [CrossRef]
63. Anderman, E.M.; Kimweli, D.M.S. Victimization and Safety in Schools Serving Early Adolescents. *J. Early Adolesc.* **1997**, *17*, 408–438. [CrossRef]
64. Stanley, L.R.; Comello, M.L.G.; Edwards, R.W.; Marquart, B.S. School Adjustment in Rural and Urban Communities: Do Students from "Timbuktu" Differ from Their "City Slicker" Peers? *J Youth Adolesc.* **2008**, *37*, 225–238. [CrossRef]
65. Zhang, W.; Fuligni, A.J. Authority, Autonomy, and Family Relationships Among Adolescents in Urban and Rural China. *J. Res. Adolesc.* **2006**, *16*, 527–537. [CrossRef]

66. Oldfield, J.; Humphrey, N.; Hebron, J. The Role of Parental and Peer Attachment Relationships and School Connectedness in Predicting Adolescent Mental Health Outcomes. *Child Adoles. Ment. Health* **2016**, *21*, 21–29. [CrossRef]
67. Jiménez Boraita, R.; Arriscado Alsina, D.; Gargallo Ibort, E.; Dalmau Torres, J.M. Hábitos y Calidad de Vida Relacionada Con La Salud: Diferencias Entre Adolescentes de Entornos Rurales y Urbanos. *An. Pediatría* **2022**, *96*, 196–202. [CrossRef]
68. Álvarez, C.A.; Briceño, A.M.; Álvarez, K.; Abufhele, M.; Delgado, I. Estudio de Adaptación y Validación Transcultural de Una Escala de Satisfacción Con La Vida Para Adolescentes. *Rev. Chil. Pediatr.* **2018**, *89*, 51–58. [CrossRef]
69. Bai, X.; Wu, C.; Zheng, R.; Ren, X. The Psychometric Evaluation of the Satisfaction with Life Scale Using a Nationally Representative Sample of China. *J. Happiness Stud.* **2011**, *12*, 183–197. [CrossRef]
70. Clench-Aas, J.; Nes, R.B.; Dalgard, O.S.; Aarø, L.E. Dimensionality and Measurement Invariance in the Satisfaction with Life Scale in Norway. *Qual. Life Res.* **2011**, *20*, 1307–1317. [CrossRef]
71. Jovanović, V.; Rudnev, M.; Arslan, G.; Buzea, C.; Dimitrova, R.; Góngora, V.; Guse, T.; Ho, R.T.H.; Iqbal, N.; Jámbori, S.; et al. The Satisfaction with Life Scale in Adolescent Samples: Measurement Invariance across 24 Countries and Regions, Age, and Gender. *Appl. Res. Qual. Life* **2022**, *17*, 2139–2161. [CrossRef]
72. Emerson, S.D.; Guhn, M.; Gadermann, A.M. Measurement Invariance of the Satisfaction with Life Scale: Reviewing Three Decades of Research. *Qual. Life Res.* **2017**, *26*, 2251–2264. [CrossRef]
73. Bacro, F.; Coudronnière, C.; Gaudonville, T.; Galharret, J.-M.; Ferrière, S.; Florin, A.; Guimard, P. The French Adaptation of the Satisfaction with Life Scale (SWLS): Factorial Structure, Age, Gender and Time-Related Invariance in Children and Adolescents. *Eur. J. Dev. Psychol.* **2020**, *17*, 307–316. [CrossRef]
74. Caycho-Rodríguez, T.; Neto, F.; Reyes-Bossio, M.; Vilca, L.W.; García Cadena, C.H.; Pinto Da Costa, M.; Neto, J.; White, M. Factorial Invariance of Satisfaction with Family Life Scale in Adolescents from Peru and Portugal. *J. Gen. Psychol.* **2022**, *149*, 421–442. [CrossRef] [PubMed]
75. Espejo, B.; Martín-Carbonell, M.; Checa, I.; Paternina, Y.; Fernández-Daza, M.; Higuita, J.D.; Albarracín, A.; Cerquera, A. Psychometric Properties of the Diener Satisfaction with Life Scale with Five Response Options Applied to the Colombian Population. *Front. Public Health* **2022**, *9*, 767534. [CrossRef] [PubMed]
76. Appiah, R.; Schutte, L.; Wilson Fadiji, A.; Wissing, M.P.; Cromhout, A. Factorial Validity of the Twi Versions of Five Measures of Mental Health and Well-Being in Ghana. *PLoS ONE* **2020**, *15*, e0236707. [CrossRef] [PubMed]
77. Sovet, L.; Atitsogbe, K.A.; Pari, P.; Park, M.S.A.; Villieux, A. Psychometric Evaluation of the Satisfaction with Life Scale in Togo: A Three-Step Approach. *Eur. Rev. Appl. Psychol.* **2016**, *66*, 243–250. [CrossRef]
78. Vilagut, G. Test-Retest Reliability. In *Encyclopedia of Quality of Life and Well-Being Research*; Michalos, A.C., Ed.; Springer: Dordrecht, The Netherlands, 2014; pp. 6622–6625, ISBN 978-94-007-0752-8.
79. Wu, S.; Zhu, X.; Tian, G.; Kang, X. Exploring the Relationships between Pre-Service Preparation and Student Teachers' Social-Emotional Competence in Teacher Education: Evidence from China. *Sustainability* **2023**, *15*, 2172. [CrossRef]
80. State, T.M.; Kern, L.; Starosta, K.M.; Mukherjee, A.D. Elementary Pre-Service Teacher Preparation in the Area of Social, Emotional, and Behavioral Problems. *Sch. Ment. Health* **2011**, *3*, 13–23. [CrossRef]

children

MDPI

Article

Problematic Internet Use and Its Relationship with Cyberbullying, Anxiety, and Executive Functions in Adolescence

Marta Real-Fernández, Ignasi Navarro-Soria *, Megan Rosales-Gómez and Beatriz Delgado

Department of Developmental Psychology and Didactics, Faculty of Education, University of Alicante, 03690 Alicante, Spain; marta.real.fernandez@gmail.com (M.R.-F.); meganrosales37@gmail.com (M.R.-G.); beatriz.delgado@ua.es (B.D.)

* Correspondence: ignasi.navarro@ua.es

Abstract: Introduction/objectives: Brain development changes during adolescence are directly linked to various cognitive and behavioral challenges characteristic of this stage. The main objective of this study is to investigate the risks associated with Internet use and its relationship with Executive Functions (EFs) and anxiety in a representative sample of Spanish secondary school students. **Methods:** The sample consisted of 1164 participants (48% males) aged 12 to 17 years (M age = 14.86; SD = 1.41) from five selected academic centers. Executive Functions were assessed using the Adolescent and Adult Executive Functioning Questionnaire (ADEXI), anxiety was measured with the Depression, Anxiety and Stress Scale (DASS-21), and Problematic Internet Use (PIU) was evaluated with the Internet Addiction Test (IAT). **Results:** Significant positive correlations were found between the PIU, EF, anxiety, and cyberbullying variables. Predictive models were developed to explain the different variables. **Conclusions:** The results emphasize the need to increase awareness of these issues and to develop effective intervention strategies. Programs that promote responsible Internet use, along with classroom activities addressing anxiety and Executive Functions, could provide clear benefits.

Keywords: Executive Functions; anxiety; cyberbullying; cybervictimization; Problematic Internet Use; adolescence

1. Introduction

Adolescence is a stage characterized by numerous changes, including psychological and emotional changes [1]. During this period, a social shift occurs in which peer relationships gain greater significance [2]. Although this phenomenon has always been present, its manifestation has varied across generations.

Currently, adolescence is accompanied by increasing use of Information and Communication Technologies (ICTs). About 92% of young people aged 10 to 15 are frequent Internet users [3]. While its use is widespread and brings numerous benefits, the literature indicates that inappropriate or excessive use may have significant psychological and behavioral consequences [4]. Although it occurs across all groups and sectors, its greater prevalence among adolescents raises more concerns about the potential negative consequences for this population. Problematic Internet Use (PIU) is at the core of these concerns, and it refers to a behavioral pattern characterized by a loss of control over Internet use, which leads to negative consequences in daily life, such as academic difficulties, physical and mental health problems, and conflicts in social and family relationships. This problematic use differs from normal use of social media or the Internet in that the former significantly interferes with an individual's daily functioning, whereas the latter comprises use through balanced integration in adolescents' lives without causing adverse effects [5]. As previously mentioned, adolescence is one of the most sensitive developmental periods [6]. With age, Internet use tends to normalize, becoming a tool used more frequently in professional settings and less for recreational purposes; adults are generally more aware of the problem and the negative effects of excessive use, and they tend to show greater self-regulation [7,8].

Another risk factor in PIU, in addition to age, is gender. Various authors have pointed out that although boys tend to spend more time on the Internet [9], it is girls who show more problematic patterns of use [4,10]. Although these findings remain controversial, given the many variables that must be considered, they are nonetheless consistent with the fact that girls are more prone to seeking approval and engaging in social comparison [11]. As a result, they experience a stronger emotional impact (such as anxiety and/or depression and damage to self-esteem and self-image) when using social media and messaging platforms. Boys, in contrast, tend to seek out challenge and competition, often through video games and using them as a means of social connection [11]. In this way, we observe that this phenomenon has led to a range of issues, among which cyberbullying can be found. In Spain, cyberbullying has been identified as one of the most prevalent forms of bullying, particularly among youth [12], and, in recent years, reports of cyber-related offences against minors, including cyberbullying, have shown a steady increase. This phenomenon has reached up to a 72% rate of prevalence [13]. Moreover, this growing concern is supported by recent evidence showing that Problematic Internet Use (PIU) is a significant predictor of changes in emotional well-being, externalizing behaviors, and Internet-related risky behaviors, including cyberbullying. One study [14] found that high levels of PIU predicted increases in both proactive and reactive aggressive behaviors, a decrease in positive emotions, and, consequently, a rise in cyberbullying, both in terms of cybervictimization and cyberaggression. These findings are consistent with previous research [15,16], suggesting that adolescents who spend more time online and use the Internet in maladaptive ways are more exposed to its risks, which can increase their involvement in cyberbullying dynamics.

This inappropriate use of ICT and its associated consequences are closely linked to brain development changes characteristic of this stage. One of the most affected elements is Executive Functions (EFs) [17], which enable intentional and deliberate interactions with the world. They include, but are not limited to, attention and concentration, impulse control, decision making, task monitoring, and working memory [18]. These functions serve as essential tools in daily activities that form the foundation of cognitive, psychological, and social development. They emerge from the development of the prefrontal cortex and its connections with other brain regions, beginning in infancy and continuing through adolescence and early adulthood. They are shaped by environmental factors, such as stress, sleep, physical health, and brain plasticity [19]. A study [20] assessed whether there are differences between inhibitory control and cognitive flexibility among victims, perpetrators, bully victims, and witnesses of bullying, and their findings revealed differences in cognitive flexibility, which was lower in victims, but no significant differences in inhibitory control.

Similarly, several studies have investigated the relationship between EFs and psychological symptoms in adolescence, given that, as mentioned earlier, this stage is typically marked by an increased prevalence of emotional difficulties [21,22] It has been found that good use of EFs is associated with a better ability to process emotional information, thereby enabling the capacity to confront personal and social situations with better resilience and coping skills [23]. Consequently, these cognitive abilities also help reduce anxious and depressive symptoms, as they allow individuals to identify and regulate self-destructive thoughts on an emotional level [24]. Regarding externalizing behaviors, research has shown [25] that aggression in children is negatively associated with executive functioning; thus, young people with a prosocial attitude are better able to recall and apply assertive strategies in situations involving anger. These individuals, possessing stronger EFs, may be more capable of inhibiting aggressive responses [26]. The authors also found a bidirectional relationship between peer conflict and EFs in childhood and adolescence, as children and adolescents involved in more interpersonal conflicts tended to exhibit poor functioning.

Considering these findings, deficits in EFs, particularly poor working memory, planning, and inhibitory control, can be understood as potential individual risk factors that could predict and explain the mechanisms underlying aggressive behaviors during this developmental stage [27,28]. The literature extensively reports an inverse relationship between EFs and aggressive behavior [29–32]. For instance, a study conducted with preschool children demonstrated that higher scores related to behavioral problems coincided with lower performance on EF assessments [33]. Furthermore, a systematic review [34] analyzed multiple studies proposing that Executive Functions should be considered key factors for understanding the individual characteristics underlying aggressive behavior, which consequently sustain bullying dynamics. Among the reviewed studies, those of [25,34–40] stood out, determining that EFs (working memory, shifting, and inhibition) correlated significantly with various forms of aggression and played a crucial role in regulating this type of behavior. Inhibitory control is fundamental because it allows individuals to regulate inappropriate behaviors in specific contexts and respond appropriately to complex situations, thereby facilitating effective adaptation to constantly changing environments and contributing to the prevention of behavioral problems [41]. Likewise, working memory, along with cognitive flexibility, also represents one of the core processes and plays a critical role in resolving social conflicts [42].

Furthermore, using the brief EF questionnaire Webexec with adolescents from Spain, one study [43] aimed to analyze whether Webexec correlated with internalizing symptoms, such as anxiety and aggressive behavior. Their findings indicated a positive correlation between EFs and these symptoms. Another study obtained similar results, particularly highlighting a greater difference in the state of anxiety [44]. Furthermore, in another study, the findings not only reinforced the relationship between EFs and manifestations of anxiety and/or depression but also emphasized its importance in the educational context [45]. Consistent with this evidence, other studies have linked anxiety to different EF components, such as inhibition, cognitive flexibility, working memory, organization, categorizing, planning, attention, verbal fluency, decision making, initiative, and emotional regulation, among others. According to [46], there is an inverse correlation between anxiety and inhibitory capacity. However, they found no significant relationship between anxiety and other EF components. In contrast, another study [47] aimed to determine whether anxiety symptoms were associated with dysexecutive symptomatology and found a significant positive correlation between the two. A different study analyzed the relationship between levels of anxiety in adults and their capacity for problem resolution, concluding that the subjects with higher levels of anxiety exhibited more difficulties in problem resolution tasks compared to those with lower anxiety levels [48].

On the other hand, given the strong relationship between these psychological processes, their impact on social media and Internet use can be easily understood. A conducted study [49] analyzed the relationship between PIU and Executive Functions, specifically inhibitory control, planning, and goal achievement. The results showed that lower inhibitory control was associated with PIU and was more frequent in the older age group. Likewise, its relationship to psychopathological mechanisms has been described [50]. A study reviewed the psychological and physical variables that could be associated with PIU and found that anxiety was among them [51]. Similarly, [52] confirmed a significant and direct correlation between PIU and social anxiety, as well as obsessive–compulsive responses. As previously mentioned, one of the consequences of PIU is the emergence of issues like cyberbullying.

Some authors, such as Yudes-Gómez et al. [53], have identified PIU as a strong predictor of both cyberbullying and cybervictimization. Through a study of a large sample of primary and secondary school students, an 8% prevalence of cyberbullying was found, along with high levels of anxiety, aggressiveness, and shifts in interests related to problematic ICT use among both perpetrators and victims compared to non-involved individuals [54].

Based on the review of the current literature, the objectives of this study are defined as focusing on exploring the relationships between various psychological and behavioral factors relevant to adolescence. The main objective is to investigate the risks associated with Internet use and its relationship with Executive Functions and anxiety in a representative sample of secondary school students (aged 12 to 17). The specific objectives include examining the relationship between three of these phenomena, PIU, cybervictimization, and cyberbullying, and the previously mentioned variables. It is expected that greater difficulties in EFs and higher levels of anxiety may be linked to increased vulnerability to these factors. Accordingly, the hypotheses proposed are as follows. (H1) There will be a higher likelihood of PIU among students with EF difficulties, high anxiety levels, and a history of experiencing or perpetrating cyberbullying. (H2) Students will be more likely to suffer cybervictimization when they present EF deficits and high anxiety levels and engage in PIU. (H3) A higher likelihood of committing cyberbullying will be associated with EF deficits, high anxiety levels, and PIU.

2. Materials and Methods

2.1. Participants

The sample consisted of 1164 participants (560 males and 604 females). A convenience sampling method was used, as access was readily available to students in the 7th to 11th grades (*Educación Secundaria Obligatoria* and *1° de bachillerato* in Spain) in the province of Alicante (Spain). According to official data from the *Instituto Nacional de Estadística* (INE), the total population of adolescents aged 12 to 17 in the province of Alicante as of 1 January 2023 was 128,312. Therefore, the sample represents approximately 0.91% of the target population in this region. In addition, although a convenience sampling method was used, both private (1) and public (4) schools from the province were included to increase the heterogeneity of the recruited population in terms of school type. Among the participants, 11.2% were in 7th grade, 25.9% were in 8th grade, 28.6% were in 9th grade, 21.5% were in 10th grade, and 12.9% were in 11th grade. Thus, the age range was 12 to 17 years (M = 14.86; DT = 1.41). Table 1 presents the distribution of the sample by sex and age.

The chi-square test for homogeneity showed no statistically significant differences based on gender or school grade ($\chi^2 = 9.79$; $p = 0.28$). Cramer's V was 0.06, indicating a small effect size or a weak association.

Table 1. Sample distribution by sex and school grade.

			School Grade					Total
			7th	8th	9th	10th	11th	
Sex	Male	N	58	141	164	130	67	560
		%	5.0	12.1	14.1	11.2	5.8	48.1
	Female	N	72	160	169	120	83	604
		%	6.2	13.7	14.5	10.3	7.1	51.9
Total		N	130	301	333	250	150	1164
		%	11.2	25.9	28.6	21.5	12.9	100.0

Note: 7th to 10th grades correspond to *Educación Secundaria Obligatoria* (ESO) and 11th grade corresponds to *1st of Bachillerato* in the Spanish educational system.

2.2. Instruments

To assess Executive Function (EF), the Executive Function Questionnaire for Adolescents and Adults was used [55]. This questionnaire is specifically designed for adolescents and adults and consists of 14 items evaluated on a 5-point Likert scale, where 1 corresponds to "definitely not true" and 5 corresponds to "definitely true". Higher scores indicate greater difficulties in the use of EFs. The questionnaire encompasses two subscales: working memory and inhibitory control. The working memory subscale includes 9 items (e.g., "I have difficulty remembering lengthy instructions"), while the inhibitory control subscale consists of 5 items (e.g., "I sometimes have difficulty stopping an activity I like"). This instrument has demonstrated strong reliability and internal consistency across all of its subscales (working memory $\alpha = 0.87$; inhibition $\alpha = 0.72$), as well as for the total score ($\alpha = 0.90$).

To assess the variable anxiety, the short version of the Depression, Anxiety and Stress Scale (DASS-21) [56] was used. This is a self-reported measure divided into three subscales that evaluate the presence and severity of depression, anxiety, and stress. It employs a Likert-type response scale ranging from 0 to 3 points. Each subscale consists of 7 items, and the total score (ranging from 0 to 21 points) is obtained by summing up the scores of the three subscales. The instrument has demonstrated high reliability and strong internal consistency across all of its subscales ($\alpha = 0.86$). For this study, only the anxiety subscale was used.

To assess PIU, the Internet Addiction Test (IAT) Spanish version [57] was used. This assessment tool consisting of 20 items rated on a 5-point Likert scale (1 = rarely to 5 = always) evaluates symptoms of Internet addiction through 3 factors: loss of control (inability to control use and neglect of duties), emotional need (satisfaction of emotional needs), and dependence. For Spain, the three factors accounted for 46.68% of the variance. Factor 1 (7 items) explained 18.16% of the variance and measured social and occupational dysfunctions, as well as difficulties with time management. Factor 2 (8 items) explained 15.55% of the variance and measured psychological conflicts related to Internet use. Factor 3 (4 items) explained 13.14% of the variance and measured affective reactions. Item 14 did not load significantly onto any factor. This model demonstrated excellent fit (CFI = 0.989; TLI = 0.987; RMSEA = 0.023; SRMR = 0.040). The total score of the 20 items ranges from 20 to 100, where 20 to 39 suggests controlled Internet use, 40 to 69 represents frequent problems due to Internet use, and scores from 70 to 100 correspond to significant problems related to Internet use. It demonstrates good internal consistency (loss of control $\alpha = 0.81$, emotional need $\alpha = 0.78$, dependence $\alpha = 0.75$, total $\alpha = 0.91$) [58].

In order to evaluate cyberbullying, the Cyberbullying: Screening of Peer Harassment Questionnaire [59] was used. This is a self-reported measure consisting of two sections that assess different forms of harassment: face-to-face bullying and a broad set of digital harassment behaviors (cyberbullying). The present study focuses specifically on the latter. The questionnaire measures 15 types of harassment behaviors through digital means. Among the behaviors assessed are sending offensive and insulting messages, sexual harassment, spreading photos or videos, password theft, social exclusion on social media, threats, and defamation, among others. It includes three roles, victims, perpetrators, and observers, although only the first two were measured in this study. The instrument employs a triangular response system where the respondent indicates whether they have experienced these harassment behaviors as a victim or perpetrated them as an aggressor over the past year. It consists of 30 items rated on a 4-point Likert scale (0 = never to 3 = always). The test demonstrates adequate internal consistency ($\alpha = 0.91$), as reported by the authors, and its structure comprises three factors (victim, aggressor, and observer), which explain 40.15% of the variance [60]. The reliability indices for the cyberbullying subscales in the study sample were satisfactory in terms of victimization ($\alpha = 0.87$) and aggression ($\alpha = 0.89$).

2.3. Procedure

Initial contact was established with the schools to conduct the study, followed by a meeting with the administrative team and the guidance department. During this meeting, the objectives of the study were presented, and both institutional approval and the collaboration of educational staff were requested to facilitate the research process. Subsequently, families (parents, guardians, and legal representatives) were informed about the purpose of the study, and informed consent was obtained for the participation of minors. Of the total recruited sample, only 1.2% (n = 15) of students did not participate in the study because their parents did not provide the signed informed consent form. The questionnaires were administered collectively in the corresponding classrooms, ensuring the anonymity of responses. Throughout this phase, the research team was present at all times to clarify any questions and to ensure that students completed the questionnaires independently and without external influence. This supervision enabled a rigorous and controlled data collection process, ensuring both the reliability of responses and adherence to ethical research standards.

2.4. Statistical Analysis

To analyze the relationships between the different variables, the non-parametric Spearman's correlation coefficient test was used. The interpretation of the results follows these criteria: values between 0.10 and 0.30 indicate a small effect size, values between 0.30 and 0.50 represent a moderate effect size, and values greater than 0.50 indicate a large effect size [61].

To assess the predictive capacity of anxiety, Executive Functions, and cyberbullying with regard to PIU, a binary logistic regression analysis was performed, following a stepwise forward regression procedure based on the Wald statistic. This type of logistic modeling allows for the estimation of the probability of an event occurring (in this case, PIU) in the presence of one or more predictors (the other variables). For this purpose, the odds ratio (OR) statistic was used. All outcome variables were transformed into dichotomous variables based on the cutoff points established by the original authors. For the cyberbullying variables, the cutoff point was 16; thus, a score equal to or greater than 16 was coded as "cybervictimization/cyberbullying", and any score below 16 was coded as "no cybervictimization/no cyberbullying". The same procedure was applied to the PIU variable, with a cutoff point of 40.

All analyses were conducted using the statistical software SPSS version 26.0.

3. Results

3.1. Correlations

First, a correlation analysis was conducted among the variables using Spearman's correlation coefficient.

The results show that the relationship between the variables is significant and positive in all cases.

Regarding PIU, a moderate relationship was observed with Executive Functions (0.30–0.33) and anxiety (0.31, 0.33), while the correlation with cyberbullying variables was small (0.19–0.26). Concerning cybervictimization, a moderate relationship was found with Executive Functions (0.31–0.37) and anxiety (0.36), whereas its correlation with PIU was small (0.24–0.30). Cyberbullying showed a small relationship with inhibitory control (0.22) and PIU components (0.19–0.23), while its correlation with working memory and anxiety was low (Table 2).

Table 2. Correlation between different variables.

	1	2	3	4	5	6	7	8	9
1. EFwm	1								
2. EFic	0.73 **	1							
4. Anx	0.44 **	0.36 **	0.44 **	1					
5. Cv	0.31 **	0.37 **	0.36 **	0.36 **	1				
6. Cb	0.09 *	0.22 **	0.15 **	0.09 *	0.46 **	1			
7. PIUlc	0.26 **	0.30 **	0.30 **	0.31 **	0.24 **	0.20 **	1		
8. PIUen	0.33 **	0.33 **	0.35 **	0.33 **	0.30 **	0.23 **	0.67 **	1	
9. PIUdep	0.30 **	0.30 **	0.32 **	0.26 **	0.26 **	0.19 **	0.69 **	0.70 **	1

Note. EFwm = Executive Function (working memory), EFic = Executive Function (inhibitory control), Anx = anxiety, Cv = cybervictimization, Cb = cyberbullying, PIUlc = Problematic Internet Use (loss of control), PIUen = Problematic Internet Use (emotional need), PIUdep = Problematic Internet Use (dependence), * correlation is significant at the 0.05 level (two-tailed), ** correlation is significant at the 0.01 level (two-tailed).

3.2. Logistic Regression

3.2.1. Problematic Internet Use Based on Executive Functions, Anxiety, Cyberbullying, and Cybervictimization

From the data analysis, it was possible to create five predictive models for the explanation of PIU. The logistic regression analyses indicate that PIU is explained by Executive Functions (EFs), anxiety, cyberbullying, and cybervictimization among students. The two models in which Executive Functions (working memory and inhibition) are the predictor variables correctly classify 67.6% of cases ($\chi^2 = 27.07$; $p < 0.001$) and 68.4% of cases ($\chi^2 = 38.89$; $p < 0.001$), with Nagelkerke's R^2 values of 0.078 and 0.111, respectively. The anxiety-based model correctly classifies 63.8% of cases ($\chi^2 = 42.16$; $p < 0.001$), with a goodness-of-fit value (Nagelkerke's R^2) of 0.07. Finally, the PIU models based on cybervictimization and cyberbullying correctly classify 60.1% of cases ($\chi^2 = 56.72$; $p < 0.001$) and 60.1% of cases ($\chi^2 = 31.62$; $p < 0.001$), with Nagelkerke's R^2 values of 0.07 and 0.04, respectively.

The odds ratios (ORs) of the models indicate that students are 1.07 and 1.15 times more likely to exhibit PIU for each one-unit increase in their working memory and inhibition, respectively. Additionally, adolescents have a 1.11 times higher probability of PIU for each one-unit increase in anxiety levels. Likewise, students are 1.14 and 1.20 times more likely to present PIU as their cybervictimization and cyberbullying scores increase by one unit, respectively (see Table 3).

Table 3. Binary logistic regression of the probability of presenting PIU based on EFs, anxiety, cyberbullying, and cybervictimization.

	B	S.E.	Wald	*p*	OR	C.I. 95%
EF working memory	0.07	0.01	25.51	<0.001	1.07	1.04–1.10
Constant	−2.35	0.32	51.61	<0.001	0.09	
EF inhibition	0.14	0.02	35.03	<0.001	1.15	1.10–1.21
Constant	−2.83	0.36	60.13	<0.001	0.05	
Anxiety	0.10	0.02	39.97	<0.001	1.11	1.07–1.14
Constant	−1.72	0.21	63.92	<0.001	0.17	
Cybervictimization	0.13	0.02	40.97	<0.001	1.14	1.09–1.18
Constant	−0.45	0.07	35.01	<0.001	0.63	
Cyberbullying	0.18	0.04	19.16	<0.001	1.20	1.11–1.30
Constant	−0.29	0.07	18.39	<0.001	0.75	

Note: B = coefficient; S.E. = standard error; *p* = probability; OR = odds ratio; C.I. 95% = confidence interval at 95%.

3.2.2. Cybervictimization Based on EFs, Anxiety, and PIU

From the data analysis, it was possible to generate six predictive models that explain cybervictimization. The logistic regression analysis shows that cybervictimization is explained by Executive Functions (EFs), anxiety, and PIU in students. The two models with EFs (working memory and inhibition) as predictor variables correctly classified 63.2% of the cases (χ^2 = 31.89; p < 0.001) and 63.4% of the cases (χ^2 = 45; p < 0.001), with goodness-of-fit values (Nagelkerke R^2) of 0.08 and 0.12, respectively. The explanatory model using anxiety correctly classified 64.8% of the cases (χ^2 = 56.78; p < 0.001), with a goodness-of-fit value (Nagelkerke R^2) of 0.10. Finally, the models of cybervictimization using PIU (loss of control, emotional need, and dependence) correctly classified 61.7% (χ^2 = 40.65; p < 0.001), 63.5% (χ^2 = 63.32; p < 0.001), and 63% (χ^2 = 46.34; p < 0.001) of the cases, with goodness-of-fit values of 0.05, 0.08, and 0.06 (Nagelkerke R^2), respectively.

The odds ratios (ORs) of the models indicate that students have 1.07 and 1.16 times higher probability of being cybervictims for each one-unit increase in their working memory and inhibition, respectively. Additionally, adolescents have a 1.14 times higher probability of experiencing cybervictimization for each one-unit increase in their anxiety. PIU also explained cybervictimization. Specifically, students have 1.08, 1.11, and 1.17 times higher probability of experiencing cybervictimization for each one-unit increase in their PIU scores (loss of control, emotional need, and dependence, respectively) (see Table 4).

Table 4. Binary logistic regression of the probability of experiencing cybervictimization based on EFs, anxiety, and PIU.

	B	S.E.	Wald	*p*	*OR*	C.I. 95%
EF working memory	0.07	0.01	28.45	<0.001	1.07	1.05–1.10
Constant	−1.14	0.30	14.26	<0.001	0.32	
EF inhibition	0.15	0.02	39.16	<0.001	1.16	1.11–1.22
Constant	−1.57	0.33	23.20	<0.001	0.21	
Anxiety	0.13	0.02	47.65	<0.001	1.14	1.09–1.18
Constant	−1.05	0.22	21.84	<0.001	0.35	
PIU loss of control	0.08	0.01	38.02	<0.001	1.08	1.06–1.11
Constant	−0.83	0.21	15.5	<0.001	0.44	
PIU emotional need	0.11	0.01	54.61	<0.001	1.11	1.08–1.14
Constant	−1.03	0.20	26.02	<0.001	0.36	
PIU dependence	0.16	0.03	41.39	<0.001	1.17	1.12–1.23
Constant	−0.71	0.18	15.02	<0.001	0.49	

Note: B = coefficient; S.E. = standard error; *p* = probability; OR = odds ratio; C.I. 95% = confidence interval at 95%.

3.2.3. Cyberbullying Based on EFs, Anxiety, and PIU

From the data analysis, it was possible to create six predictive models for the explanation of cyberbullying. The logistic regression analyses indicate that cyberbullying is explained by Executive Functions (EFs) and PIU among students. No statistically significant results were found for anxiety or working memory. The model with inhibition as the predictor variable correctly classified 62.7% of the cases (χ^2 = 31.89; p < 0.001), with a goodness-of-fit value (Nagelkerke R^2) of 0.04. The models of cyberbullying using PIU (emotional need, loss of control, and dependence) correctly classified 64.9% (χ^2 = 37.05; p < 0.001), 64.2% (χ^2 = 31.75; p < 0.001), and 64.2% (χ^2 = 28.27; p < 0.001) of the cases, with goodness-of-fit values of 0.05, 0.04, and 0.04 (Nagelkerke R^2), respectively.

The odds ratios (ORs) of the models indicate that students are 1.09 times more likely to engage in cyberbullying for each one-unit increase in their inhibition. Additionally, students have 1.07, 1.08, and 1.13 times higher probability of experiencing cybervictimization for each one-unit increase in their PIU scores (loss of control, emotional need, and dependence, respectively) (see Table 5).

Table 5. Binary logistic regression of the probability of perpetrating cyberbullying based on EFs, anxiety, and PIU.

	B	S.E.	Wald	*p*	*OR*	C.I. 95%
EF inhibition	0.08	0.02	14.25	<0.01	1.09	1.04–1.13
Constant	−1.65	0.32	26.98	<0.01	0.19	
PIU loss of control	0.07	0.01	30.88	<0.01	1.07	1.05–1.10
Constant	−1.70	0.21	62,79	<0.01	0.18	
PIU emotional need	0.07	0.01	35.63	<0.01	1.08	1.05–1.10
Constant	−1.64	0.19	73.53	<0.01	0.19	
PIU dependence	0.12	0.02	27.65	<0.01	1.13	1.08–1.18
Constant	−1.48	0.18	65.34	<0.01	1.12	

Note: B = coefficient; S.E. = standard error; *p* = probability; OR = odds ratio; C.I. 95% = confidence interval at 95%.

4. Discussion

The main objective of this research was to analyze the risks associated with Internet use during adolescence and their relationship with Executive Functions (EFs) and anxiety. More specifically, the interaction between three key phenomena was examined—Problematic Internet Use (PIU), cybervictimization, and cyberbullying—and their link to these psychological variables, with the aim of better understanding the factors that may influence the development of risky behaviors in digital environments.

As a preliminary step, the distribution of the sample by sex and age was analyzed, and no statistically significant differences were found. This aligns with findings reported by other researchers [62–64].

The first hypothesis (H1) proposed that Problematic Internet Use (PIU) would be more frequent in adolescents with lower development of Executive Functions, higher levels of anxiety, and a history of cyberbullying and cybervictimization. The results confirmed this hypothesis, both through significant positive correlations and regression analyses, in which five predictive models were developed to explain PIU based on Executive Functions (EFs), anxiety, cyberbullying, and cybervictimization.

The findings align with previous research that has identified an association between deficits in inhibitory control and PIU in adolescents, as demonstrated through multiple linear regression analyses [24]. Similarly, systematic reviews have indicated that certain psychological and physiological variables, including anxiety, may be related to the development of PIU [49]. Furthermore, recent studies have shown a significant relationship between PIU, cyberbullying, and cybervictimization, suggesting that interaction dynamics in digital environments may act as a risk factor for the development of this behavior [50,53].

Difficulties in Executive Functions (EFs) can lead to a pattern of PIU, where a lack of self-control, planning, and emotional regulation fosters greater dependence on online interactions [49]. This tendency is reinforced by impulsivity and difficulties in managing time and priorities, which can lead individuals to neglect their academic, work, or social responsibilities [50].

In this context, anxiety plays a key role, as many individuals turn to the Internet as a maladaptive emotional regulation strategy, seeking temporary relief from their distress through excessive consumption of digital content or interaction on social media [52]. However, this type of coping mechanism can perpetuate Internet dependency, creating a vicious cycle in which avoiding anxiety through excessive use of electronic devices ultimately exacerbates the problem.

Sense of belonging plays a central role during adolescence and is essential for understanding the difficulties related to psychological development and school adjustment. A study [65] examined the relationship between belonging at school and belonging on social media, finding that both variables were negatively correlated with psychological maladjustment and academic performance, with social media addiction acting as a mediating factor. This impact on adolescents' psychological health and school adaptation is crucial for understanding how the phenomenon of cyberbullying emerges. Moreover, disruptions in sense of belonging may also help explain why some adolescents seek refuge in online environments or become involved in harmful digital behaviors, reinforcing the patterns observed in Problematic Internet Use.

Furthermore, the impact of PIU can be observed in both victims and aggressors. Victims, feeling rejected or excluded in face-to-face social environments, may use the Internet as an escape mechanism, seeking refuge in virtual communities or online relationships that provide them with a sense of belonging. On the other hand, aggressors, in addition to using digital platforms to harass their victims, often exhibit higher levels of impulsivity and low inhibitory control, which facilitates the repetition of aggressive behaviors without adequate reflection on the consequences of their actions [20].

These elements collectively reinforce the need for interventions aimed at strengthening Executive Functions, promoting strategies that enable more conscious and adaptive use of the Internet, as well as effective tools for managing anxiety and preventing cyberbullying. Understanding these mechanisms is essential for designing prevention and intervention programs that reduce the negative effects of PIU and promote a healthy balance in the use of digital technologies.

The second hypothesis (H2) proposed that students would have a higher probability of experiencing cybervictimization when they exhibited difficulties in Executive Functions (EFs), high levels of anxiety, and PIU. This relationship is explained by various psychological and behavioral factors that may increase the vulnerability of young people in digital environments.

First, young people with higher anxiety may be more likely to become victims of cyberbullying, as they tend to show signs of emotional insecurity that can be perceived and exploited by aggressors. Additionally, lower competence in social skills may hinder their ability to defend themselves or seek help, increasing their helplessness in the face of online attacks. Furthermore, anxiety can lead to increased time spent in the digital world, thereby raising the likelihood of encountering risky situations [20].

On the other hand, difficulties in Executive Functions (EFs) can also contribute to cybervictimization. Impulsivity and low inhibitory control may lead to more intense reactions to online provocations, which could prolong and escalate conflicts in digital environments. Additionally, poor decision making may result in interactions with strangers or exposure on digital platforms without adequately assessing the potential consequences [50].

These factors reinforce the need for interventions focused on emotional management, the development of social skills, and the strengthening of Executive Functions aiming to reduce young people's vulnerability to cybervictimization and promote safer and more conscious use of the Internet.

The third hypothesis (H3) proposed that the probability of engaging in cyberbullying would be related to difficulties in Executive Functions (EFs), high levels of anxiety, and PIU. The results supported the proposed hypothesis, aligning with previous findings [54]. Likewise, prior research has demonstrated the relationship between Executive Functions

(EFs), inhibition capacity, self-control, and problem-solving skills, which are key factors in participation in cyberbullying dynamics.

Despite these findings, this study has certain limitations that should be considered in future research. Due to its cross-sectional design, it is not possible to establish causal relationships between the analyzed variables. To address this limitation, it would be advisable to conduct prospective longitudinal studies. Likewise, it would be beneficial to include a random sampling method and to identify the reasons why some parents or legal guardians did not provide consent for their children to participate in the study in order to address these issues in future implementation. It would also be appropriate to apply the study to primary education to gain deeper insight into how the use of new technologies and their associated risks emerge at an early age. In addition, it would be valuable to explore the perspectives and knowledge that teachers and parents have regarding the phenomena studied. Finally, to ensure that the results more accurately reflect the national reality, it would be necessary to carry out the evaluation in a greater number of provinces, including schools located in both urban and rural areas.

Beyond the aspects mentioned, we think it would be of interest for future lines of research to focus on the traumatic aspect of cyberbullying, given that the effect of trauma on the brain has been extensively studied. Various authors have shown that individuals who have undergone traumatic experiences often present alterations in the dorsal prefrontal networks, suggesting deficits in executive control, particularly in response inhibition, working memory, attention regulation, cognitive flexibility, and stimulus response inhibition, which tend to worsen in emotionally charged or trauma-related contexts [66–68]. This line of inquiry could help to better understand the impact of trauma on executive functioning, both in victims and in aggressors.

However, the results obtained have practical implications in the educational, mental health, and even family domains, emphasizing the importance of educating and raising awareness among the various agents who accompany young people at this stage of life about how the virtual world operates.

With regard to adolescents, in the educational context, it is recommended to include strategies for self-regulation and critical thinking, promote group work, and strengthen the early detection of psychological difficulties [45]. In the clinical setting, these findings can refine therapeutic interventions and improve emotional regulation in adolescents.

Families can benefit from awareness campaigns fostering open dialogue about Internet use and promoting healthy digital habits [69–72]. Although it may be difficult for some adults to understand, for young people, technology constitutes a bridge between the real and the virtual world. Building upon emotional context, another critical factor to consider is the fear of missing out (FoMO), which directly affects adolescents' well-being today. A previous study [73] investigated the relationship between peer exclusion from WhatsApp classmate groups, FoMO, and emotional symptoms. The findings showed that exclusion from online classmate groups was positively associated with both FoMO and emotional distress. Importantly, FoMO served as a mediating variable, meaning that adolescents who experienced greater online exclusion reported higher levels of FoMO, which in turn was linked to more emotional symptoms. The study highlights how cyber exclusion, also a form of cyberbullying, can negatively affect emotional well-being during early adolescence by increasing the apprehension of being disconnected from peers. Something as simple as knowing whether a child or student is an active member of WhatsApp groups can provide information about a possible situation of marginalization, serving as a modern equivalent of the sociogram and helping to address cases of cyberbullying, which, due to their invisible nature, often go unnoticed.

It is necessary to raise awareness among parents regarding the permissiveness with which smartphones are currently provided at early ages and the little or no supervision that follows. The importance lies in the fact that these devices provide access to unlimited interaction, something previous generations never experienced. In the past, in our social relationships, we received positive or negative feedback from a small group of peers. Now, however, with any content we share through social networks, we are exposed to the opinions of hundreds of peers. Moreover, the way social media platforms operate allows peers to make statements without being aware of the harm they may cause to the recipient, as they do not see their reaction [74]. This means that greater harm can be inflicted without remorse [75].

In the case of teachers, while they do not have access to supervise students' use of social media, they can be trained to teach their students to identify the different roles adopted by aggressors, victims, and bystanders in situations of abuse and thus help prevent such behaviors [76].

Overall, campaigns and intervention projects aimed at the prevention and management of PIU and its associated risks could bring significant benefits to society.

Author Contributions: Conceptualization, M.R.-F., I.N.-S. and B.D.; methodology and formal analysis, B.D.; investigation, M.R.-F., I.N.-S. and B.D.; resources funding acquisition, B.D. and I.N.-S.; writing—original draft preparation, M.R.-F.; writing—review and editing, I.N.-S., B.D. and M.R.-G.; translation from Spanish to English, M.R.-G.; visualization and supervision, B.D. All authors have read and agreed to the published version of the manuscript.

Funding: This research was funded by the Ministry of Science and Innovation, the Agency, and the European Regional Development Fund (Project PID123118NA-100 funded by MCIN/AEI/10.13039/501 100011033/FEDER, EU).

Institutional Review Board Statement: The present study has been approved by the Ethics Committee of the University of Alicante, UA-2023-02-07, approved on 7 February 2023.

Informed Consent Statement: Informed consent was obtained from all subjects involved in the study.

Data Availability Statement: Due to the explicit prohibition by the ethics committee of the disclosure of minors' data, it is not possible to provide such data.

Conflicts of Interest: The authors declare no conflicts of interest.

References

1. Iglesias Diz, J.L. Desarrollo del adolescente: Aspectos físicos, psicológicos y sociales. *Pediatr. Integral* **2013**, *17*, 88–93.
2. Bukowski, W.M.; Laursen, B.; Hoza, B. The snowball effect: Friendship moderates escalations in depressed affect among avoidant and excluded children. *Dev. Psychopathol.* **2010**, *22*, 749–757. [CrossRef]
3. Instituto Nacional de Estadística [INE]. *Encuesta Sobre Equipamiento y uso de Tecnologías de Información y Comunicación en los Hogares (TICH)*; Instituto Nacional de Estadística: Madrid, Spain, 2014. Available online: http://www.ine.es/prensa/np864.pdf (accessed on 8 October 2024).
4. Rial, A.; Golpe, S.; Gómez, P.; Barreiro, C. Variables asociadas al uso problemático de Internet entre adolescentes. *Health Addict: Salud Drogas* **2015**, *15*, 25–38.
5. López, A.D.; Sánchez, J.J.M.; Ruiz, A.B.M.; Hernández, F.J.R. Perfiles de uso de las TIC en adolescentes: Diferencias y similitudes en cuanto al rendimiento académico, el estrés y la mediación parental. *Rev. Investig. Educ.* **2025**, *43*. [CrossRef]
6. Sánchez-Martínez, M.; Otero, A. Factors associated with cell phone use in adolescents in the community of Madrid (Spain). *CyberPsychology Behav.* **2009**, *12*, 131–137. [CrossRef]
7. Beranuy, M.; Chamarro Lusar, A.; Graner, C.; Carbonell, X. Validación de dos escalas breves para evaluar la adicción a Internet y el abuso de móvil. *Psicothema* **2009**, *21*, 480–485.
8. Labrador, F.J.; Villadangos, S.M. Menores y nuevas tecnologías: Conductas indicadoras de posible problema de adicción. *Psicothema* **2010**, *22*, 180–188.

9. Estévez, L.; Bayón, C.; de la Cruz, J.; Fernández-Uría, A. Uso y abuso de Internet en adolescentes. In *Adicción a las Nuevas Tecnologías en Jóvenes y Adolescentes*; Echeburúa, E., Labrador, F., Becoña, E., Eds.; Pirámide: Madrid, Spain, 2009; pp. 101–130.
10. de la Villa Moral, M.; Suárez, C. Factores de riesgo en el uso problemático de Internet y del teléfono móvil en adolescentes españoles. *Rev. Iberoam. Psicol. Salud* **2016**, *7*, 69–78. [CrossRef]
11. Villanueva Blasco, V.J.; Gómez Martínez, S.; Iranzo Ejarque, B.; Serrano Bernal, S.; Aguilar, J.; Grau Aberola, E.; Alapont, L. ¿Existen diferencias en función del sexo en el uso problemático de Internet en adolescentes? *Inform. Psicol.* **2019**, *117*, 47–57. [CrossRef]
12. Ministerio del Interior de España. *Informe Sobre Cibercriminalidad 2023*; Ministerio del Interior: Madrid, Spain, 2023. Available online: https://www.interior.gob.es/opencms/export/sites/default/.galleries/galeria-de-prensa/documentos-y-multimedia/balances-e-informes/2023/Informe-Cibercriminalidad_2023.pdf (accessed on 8 October 2024).
13. Escortell, R.; Delgado, B.; Martínez-Monteagudo, M.C. Cybervictimization, self-concept, aggressiveness, and school anxiety in school children: A structural equations analysis. *Int. J. Environ. Res. Public Health* **2020**, *17*, 7000. [CrossRef]
14. Alonso, C.; Romero, E. Uso problemático de internet en adolescentes: Factores personales de riesgo y consecuencias emocionales y conductuales. *Rev. Iberoam. Psicol. Salud* **2021**, *12*, 76–89. [CrossRef]
15. Arpaci, I.; Abdeljawad, T.; Baloğlu, M.; Kesici, Ş.; Mahariq, I. Mediating effect of internet addiction on the relationship between individualism and cyberbullying: Cross-Sectional Questionnaire Study. *J. Med. Internet Res.* **2020**, *22*, e16210. [CrossRef]
16. Stodt, B.; Wegmann, E.; Brand, M. Predicting dysfunctional internet use: The role of age, conscientiousness, and internet literacy in internet addiction and cyberbullying. *Int. J. Cyber Behav. Psychol. Learn (IJCBPL)* **2016**, *6*, 28–43. [CrossRef]
17. Herrera, E.Y.; Álvarez, G.C.P.; Alencastro, A.G. Desarrollo de las funciones ejecutivas en la infancia. *Rev. Cognosis* **2020**, *5*, 103–114. [CrossRef]
18. Grissom, N.M.; Reyes, T.M. Let's call the whole thing off: Evaluating gender and sex differences in executive function. *Neuropsychopharmacology* **2019**, *44*, 86–96. [CrossRef] [PubMed]
19. Diamond, A. Executive functions. *Annu. Rev. Psychol.* **2013**, *64*, 135–168. [CrossRef]
20. Hoyos, O.; Olmos, K.; De los Reyes, C. Flexibilidad cognitiva y control inhibitorio: Un acercamiento clínico a la comprensión del maltrato entre iguales por abuso de poder. *Rev. Argent. Clin. Psicol.* **2013**, *22*, 219–227.
21. Avenevoli, S.; Swendsen, J.; He, J.P.; Burstein, M.; Merikangas, K.R. Major depression in the national comorbidity survey–Adolescent supplement: Prevalence, correlates, and treatment. *J. Am. Acad. Child. Adolesc. Psychiatry* **2015**, *54*, 37–44. [CrossRef] [PubMed]
22. Esbjørn, B.H.; Hoeyer, M.; Dyrborg, J.; Leth, I.; Kendall, P.C. Prevalence and co-morbidity among anxiety disorders in a national cohort of psychiatrically referred children and adolescents. *J. Anxiety Disord.* **2010**, *24*, 866–872. [CrossRef]
23. Martel, M.M.; Nigg, J.T.; Wong, M.M.; Fitzgerald, H.E.; Jester, J.M.; Puttler, L.I.; Glass, J.M.; Adams, K.M.; Zucker, R.A. Childhood and adolescent resiliency, regulation, and executive functioning in relation to adolescent problems and competence in a high-risk sample. *Dev. Psychopathol.* **2007**, *19*, 541–563. [CrossRef]
24. Mullin, B.C.; Perks, E.L.; Haraden, D.A.; Snyder, H.R.; Hankin, B.L. Subjective executive function weaknesses are linked to elevated internalizing symptoms among community adolescents. *Assessment* **2020**, *27*, 560–571. [CrossRef] [PubMed]
25. Poland, S.E.; Monks, C.P.; Tsermentseli, S. Cool and hot executive function as predictors of aggression in early childhood: Differentiating between the function and form of aggression. *Br. J. Dev. Psychol.* **2016**, *34*, 181–197. [CrossRef] [PubMed]
26. Holmes, C.; Kim-Spoon, J.; Deater-Deckard, J. Linking executive function and peer problems from early childhood through middle adolescence. *J. Abnorm. Child. Psychol.* **2016**, *44*, 31–42. [CrossRef]
27. Ellis, M.L.; Weiss, B.; Lochman, J.E. Executive functions in children: Associations with aggressive behavior and appraisal processing. *J. Abnorm. Child. Psychol.* **2009**, *37*, 945–956. [CrossRef]
28. Verlinden, M.; Veenstra, R.; Ghassabian, A.; Jansen, P.W.; Hofman, A.; Jaddoe, V.W.; Verhulst, F.C.; Tiemeier, H. Executive functioning and non-verbal intelligence as predictors of bullying in early elementary school. *J. Abnorm. Child. Psychol.* **2014**, *42*, 953–966. [CrossRef] [PubMed]
29. Woltering, S.; Lishak, V.; Hodgson, N.; Granic, I.; Zelazo, P.D. Executive function in children with externalizing and comorbid internalizing behavior problems. *J. Child. Psychol. Psychiatry Allied Discip.* **2015**, *57*, 30–38. [CrossRef]
30. Riccio, C.A.; Hewitt, L.L.; Blake, J.J. Relation of measures of executive function to aggressive behavior in children. *Appl. Neuropsychol.* **2011**, *18*, 1–10. [CrossRef]
31. Schoemaker, K.; Mulder, H.; Dekovic, M.; Matthys, W. Executive functions in preschool children with externalizing behavior problems: A meta-analysis. *J. Abnorm. Child. Psychol.* **2013**, *41*, 457–471. [CrossRef]
32. Seguin, J.R. The frontal lobe and aggression. *Eur. J. Dev. Psychol.* **2008**, *1*, 1–20. [CrossRef]
33. López, M.R.; Nieto, A.B.; Conde, A.B.Q.; Bernardo, G.Á. Problemas de conducta y funciones ejecutivas en niños y niñas de 5 años. *Rev. Infad Psicol.* **2016**, *1*, 57–66. [CrossRef]
34. Mesones, F.H.; Dargent, A.G.; Terrones, M.L. El corazón de las Tinieblas: ¿Son. las (dis) Funciones Ejecutivas un Factor Común en las Conductas de Agresión y el Bullying? *Rev. Psicol. Herediana* **2024**, *17*, 9–23. [CrossRef]
35. Granvald, V.; Marciszko, C. Relations between key executive functions and aggression in childhood. *Child. Neuropsychol.* **2015**, *22*, 537–555. [CrossRef]

36. Spann, C.A.; Gagne, J.R. Aggressive behaviors in young siblings: Associations with executive functions and maternal characteristics. *J. Abnorm. Child. Psychol.* **2016**, *44*, 523–533. [CrossRef]
37. Baker, E.R.; Jensen, C.J.; Tisak, M.S. A closer examination of aggressive subtypes in early childhood: Contributions of executive function and single-parent status. *Early Child. Dev. Care* **2017**, *189*, 733–746. [CrossRef]
38. Vazquez-Miraz, P.; Gutierrez, K.; Fernandez, J.; Ramirez, P.; Espinosa, P.; Dominguez, E. Análisis de la relación entre la conducta de bullying y las funciones ejecutivas en niños y adolescentes escolarizados. *Rev. Complutense Educ.* **2021**, *32*, 477–486. [CrossRef]
39. Rohlf, H.L.; Holl, A.K.; Kirsch, F.; Krahe, B.; Elsner, B. Longitudinal links between executive function, anger, and aggression in middle childhood. *Front. Behav. Neurosci.* **2018**, *12*, 27. [CrossRef] [PubMed]
40. O'Toole, S.E.; Tsermentseli, S.; Humayun, S.; Monks, C.P. Cool and hot executive functions at 5 years old as predictors of physical and relational aggression between 5 and 6 years old. *Int. J. Behav. Dev.* **2019**, *43*, 157–165. [CrossRef]
41. Goldstein, M.; Brendel, G.; Tuescher, O.; Pan, H.; Epstein, J.; Beutel, M.; Yang, Y.; Thomas, K.; Levy, K.; Silverman, M.; et al. Neural substrates of the interaction of emotional stimulus processing and motor inhibitory control: An emotional linguistic go/no-go fMRI study. *NeuroImage* **2007**, *36*, 1026–1040. [CrossRef]
42. Ziermans, T.; Dumontheil, I.; Roggeman, C.; Peyrard-Janvid, M.; Matsson, H.; Kere, J.; Klingberg, T. Working memory brain activity and capacity link MAOA polymorphism to aggressive behavior during development. *Transl. Psychiatry* **2012**, *2*, e85. [CrossRef]
43. Morea, A.; Zumalde, E.C. Validación del Cuestionario Breve de Funciones Ejecutivas Webexec: Pruebas de rendimiento y síntomas psicológicos. *Rev. Psicol. Clín Niños Adolesc.* **2020**, *7*, 56–62. [CrossRef]
44. Lavigne-Cerván, R.; Costa-López, B.; Juárez-Ruiz de Mier, R.; Real-Fernández, M.; Sánchez-Muñoz de León, M.; Navarro-Soria, I. Consequences of COVID-19 confinement on anxiety, sleep and executive functions of children and adolescents in Spain. *Front. Psychol.* **2021**, *12*, 334. [CrossRef] [PubMed]
45. Frutos de Miguel, J. Las funciones ejecutivas y la salud mental en el contexto educativo. *Estud. Educ.* 2025; *early access*. [CrossRef]
46. Valcárcel, S. *Control Ejecutivo y Autorregulación Emocional de la Ansiedad en las Relaciones Interpersonales*; Universidad de Jaén: Jaén, Spain, 2014.
47. Magnoli, J.V. La Ansiedad y las Funciones Ejecutivas en Población Adulta. Bachelor's Thesis, Universidad de Palermo, Buenos Aires, Argentina, 2021.
48. Pacheco, A.; Lupiáñez, J.; Acosta, A. Atención y ansiedad: Relaciones de la alerta y el control cognitivo con la ansiedad rasgo. *Psicológica* **2009**, *30*, 1–25.
49. Albertos, A.; Ibabe, I. Uso problemático de las tecnologías, actividades de ocio y funciones ejecutivas en adolescentes. *Rev. Educ.* **2021**, *394*, 101–127. [CrossRef]
50. Hinojo-Lucena, F.J.; Aznar-Díaz, I.; Trujillo-Torres, J.M.; Romero-Rodríguez, J.M. Uso problemático de Internet y variables psicológicas o físicas en estudiantes universitarios. *Rev. Electr. Investig. Educ.* **2021**, *23*, 1–17. [CrossRef]
51. Domínguez Martín, C.; Geijo Uribe, S.; Sánchez Lorenzo, I.; Imaz Roncero, C.; Cabús Piñol, G. Revisión de los mecanismos implicados en el uso problemático de Internet. *Rev. Asoc. Esp. Neuropsiquiatr.* **2012**, *32*, 691–705. Available online: https://www.redalyc.org/articulo.oa?id=265025475011 (accessed on 8 October 2024).
52. Bernal-Ruiz, C.; Rosa-Alcázar, A.I.; González-Calatayud, V.; Rosa-Alcázar, E. ¿Existe relación entre uso problemático de Internet y las respuestas de ansiedad social, obsesivo-compulsivas y el bienestar psicológico en adolescentes? *An. Psicol.* **2017**, *33*, 269–276. [CrossRef]
53. Yudes-Gómez, C.; Baridon-Chauvie, D.; González-Cabrera, J.M. Ciberacoso y uso problemático de Internet en Colombia, Uruguay y España. *Comun. Rev. Cient. Comun. Educ.* **2018**, *26*, 49–58. [CrossRef]
54. Giménez, A.M.; Maquilón, J.J.; Arnaiz, P. Usos problemáticos y agresivos de las TIC por parte de adolescentes implicados en cyberbullying. *Rev. Investig. Educ.* **2015**, *33*, 335–351. [CrossRef]
55. Holst, Y.; Thorell, L.B. Adult executive functioning inventory (ADEXI): Validity, reliability, and relations to ADHD. *Int. J. Methods Psychiatr. Res.* **2018**, *27*, 567–570. [CrossRef]
56. Lovibond, S.H.; Lovibond, P.F. *Manual for the Depression Anxiety Stress Scales (DASS-21)*; Psychology Foundation: Sydney, Australia, 1995.
57. Young, K.S. *Internet Addiction Test (IAT)*; Center for Internet Addiction Recovery: Bradford, PA, USA, 1998.
58. Panova, T.; Carbonell, X.; Chamarro, A.; Ximena Puerta-Cortés, D. Internet Addiction Test research through a cross-cultural perspective: Spain, USA and Colombia La investigación del Internet Addiction Test desde una perspectiva intercultural: España, Estados Unidos y Colombia. *Adicciones* **2021**, *33*, 307–318. [CrossRef]
59. Garaigordobil, M. *Cyberbullying. Screening de Acoso Entre Iguales*; TEAediciones: Madrid, Spain, 2013.
60. Garaigordobil, M.; Aliri, J.; Maganto, C.; Bernaras, E.; Jaureguizar, J. Cyberbullying: Prevalencia de Víctimas, Agresores y Observadores en Función del Nivel Socio-Económico-Cultural. In Proceedings of the 6th International and 11th National Congress of Clinical Psychology, Santiago de Compostela, Spain, 6–8 June 2013; Buela-Casal, G., Buela-Casal, G., Quevedo-

Blasco, G., Eds.; Asociación Española de Psicología Conductual (AEPC): Granada, Spain, 2014; pp. 42–49. Available online: http://www.aepc.es/psclinica_web/ProceedinsPaper.html (accessed on 8 October 2024).
61. Spearman, C. The proof of association between two variables. *Am. J. Psychol.* **1904**, *15*, 72–101. [CrossRef]
62. Piqueras-Rodríguez, J.A.; García-Oliva, C.; Marzo, J.C. Uso problemático de Internet en adolescentes: Relación con sexo, edad, nivel socioeconómico y frecuencia de uso de internet. *Acción Psicol.* **2019**, *16*, 129–141. [CrossRef]
63. Rial, A.; Gómez-Salgado, P.; Isorna, M.; Araujo, M.; Varela, J. EUPI-a: Escala de uso problemático de Internet en adolescentes. Desarrollo y validación psicométrica [PIUS-a: Problematic Internet Use Scale in Adolescents. Development and Psychometric Validation]. *Adicciones* **2015**, *27*, 47–63. [CrossRef]
64. Golpe, S.; Isorna, M.; Gómez-Salgado, P.; Rial, A. Problematic Internet Use and Adolescents: Sport does Matter. *RETOS-Nuevas Tend. Educ. Física Deporte Recreación* **2017**, *31*, 52–57.
65. Fabris, M.A.; Settanni, M.; Longobardi, C.; Marengo, D. Sense of belonging at school and on social media in adolescence: Associations with educational achievement and psychosocial maladjustment. *Child. Psychiatry Hum. Dev.* **2024**, *55*, 1620–1633. [CrossRef] [PubMed]
66. Aupperle, R.L.; Melrose, A.J.; Stein, M.B.; Paulus, M.P. Executive function and PTSD: Disengaging from trauma. *Neuropharmacology* **2012**, *62*, 686–694. [CrossRef]
67. Polak, A.R.; Witteveen, A.B.; Reitsma, J.B.; Olff, M. The role of executive function in posttraumatic stress disorder: A systematic review. *J. Affect. Disord.* **2012**, *141*, 11–21. [CrossRef]
68. Bremner, J.D. Traumatic stress: Effects on the brain. *Dialogues Clin. Neurosci.* **2006**, *8*, 445–461. [CrossRef]
69. Ortega-Barón, J.; Buelga, S.; Cava, M.J.; Torralba, E. Ajuste psicosocial en cibervíctimas y ciberagresores en Educación Secundaria. *An. De Psicol.* **2017**, *33*, 422–431. [CrossRef]
70. Sánchez Pardo, L.; Crespo Herrador, G.; Aguilar-Moya, R.; Bueno-Cañigral, F.J.; Aleixandre-Benavent, R.; Valderrama-Zurián, J.C. *Los Adolescentes y el Ciberacoso*; Ayuntamiento de Valencia: Valencia, Spain, 2016.
71. Real Fernández, M.; Navarro Soria, I.J.; Collado Valero, J.; Lavigne Cerván, R.; Delgado Domenech, B. Ciberacoso y funciones ejecutivas en niños y adolescentes: Una revisión sistemática. *Rev. Educ.* **2022**, *397*, 69–95. [CrossRef]
72. Rivera, J.P.; Reynoso, T.M.; Vilchis, R.M. Efectos de un programa de ciberconvivencia en la prevención del ciberacoso. *Psychol. Soc. Educ.* **2018**, *10*, 239–250. [CrossRef]
73. Marengo, D.; Settanni, M.; Fabris, M.A.; Longobardi, C. Alone, together: Fear of missing out mediates the link between peer exclusion in WhatsApp classmate groups and psychological adjustment in early-adolescent teens. *J. Soc. Pers. Relat.* **2021**, *38*, 1371–1379. [CrossRef]
74. Yot-Domínguez, C.R.; Cotán Fernández, A. Las familias en la investigación sobre el ciberacoso. *Rev. Elec. Edu.* **2020**, *73*, 140–156. [CrossRef]
75. Franz-Torres, M.R.; López-Cruz, M.A. Smartphones y Tablets, desarrollo psicológico y aprendizaje infantil: Una revisión sistemática. *Rev. Psicol. Educ.* **2023**, *18*, 40.
76. De Luca, L.; Nocentini, A.; Menesini, E. The teacher's role in preventing bullying. *Front. Psychol.* **2019**, *10*, 1830. [CrossRef]

children

MDPI

Article

Risk Factors and Clinical Predictors of Suicidal Behaviors and Non-Suicidal Self-Injury Among Pediatric Psychiatry Emergency Admissions Pre- and Post-Pandemic: A Retrospective Cohort Study

Roxana Șipoș [1], Tudor Văidean [1,2,*] and Elena Predescu [1]

[1] Department of Neuroscience, Psychiatry and Pediatric Psychiatry, "Iuliu Hatieganu" University of Medicine and Pharmacy, 57 Republicii Street, 400489 Cluj-Napoca, Romania
[2] Department of Clinical Psychology and Psychotherapy, Faculty of Psychology and Educational Sciences, Babeş-Bolyai University, 37 Republicii Street, 400015 Cluj-Napoca, Romania
* Correspondence: tudor.vaidean@elearn.umfcluj.ro

Abstract: Background: Suicidal behavior (SB) and non-suicidal self-injury (NSSI) are significant public health concerns among adolescents. The COVID-19 pandemic may have exacerbated these issues. Methods: This retrospective cohort study analyzed data from 341 adolescents (aged 6–18 years) presenting to a Romanian pediatric psychiatry emergency department during the years 2019 (pre-pandemic) and 2022 (post-pandemic). All participants underwent a thorough psychiatric assessment, and, together with their caregivers, were questioned on a wide range of potentially relevant issues, such as family, social, school, and life history factors. Logistic regression and random forest models were used to identify predictors of SB and NSSI. Results: SB was significantly predicted in regression models based on a prior suicidal ideation (OR = 68.410; $p < 0.001$), having a parent living abroad (OR = 11.438; $p = 0.020$), depression (OR = 6.803; $p < 0.001$), and conflicts with peers (OR = 0.325, $p = 0.042$), teachers (OR = 0.119, $p = 0.024$), or both (OR = 0.166, $p = 0.012$). The random forest model featured a slightly different order of the main predictors and highlighted the importance of additional predictors, such as prior suicide attempts, gender, and past non-suicidal self-injury. NSSI was mainly predicted by a history of self-harm (OR = 52.437; $p < 0.001$), the number of comorbid psychiatric disorders (OR = 1.709; $p = 0.003$), and conduct disorder (OR = 0.184; $p < 0.001$), to which are added, according to random forest models, new predictors, such as borderline personality disorder, suicidal ideation, and school performance. Post-pandemic increases were observed in depression, suicidal ideation, and possible psycho-traumatic negative life event exposure. Conclusions: This study underscores the complex interplay of individual, familial, and societal factors influencing adolescent self-harm. Comprehensive interventions are needed, with early intervention crucial for those with a history of self-harm. Further research using prospective designs is recommended.

Keywords: adolescent; suicidal behavior; non-suicidal self-injury; risk factors; COVID-19 pandemic

1. Introduction

Non-suicidal self-injury (NSSI) involves deliberate self-harm without suicidal intent and is often employed as a maladaptive coping mechanism for emotional distress [1,2]. NSSI is most prevalent during adolescence, a developmental stage marked by heightened emotional vulnerability and risk-taking behaviors [3]. Prevalence rates of NSSI range from 15% to 25% in community samples, rising to as high as 60% among adolescents in clinical settings, such as emergency departments [4,5]. Research indicates that children and adolescents with psychiatric disorders frequently engage in NSSI and suicide attempts and experience suicidal ideation, underscoring the severity of these behaviors in clinical samples [6]. Despite its non-suicidal intent, NSSI is a robust predictor of future suicidal behavior (SB), emphasizing the critical need for targeted interventions in high-risk populations [7–9]. However, studies show that empirical support for such interventions for children and adolescents is so far extremely low [10].

Suicidal behavior (SB), encompassing suicidal ideation, attempts, and completed suicide, remains one of the leading causes of mortality among adolescents worldwide [11]. Unlike NSSI, SB is driven by an explicit intent to end one's life, often stemming from a combination of individual vulnerabilities (e.g., depression, hopelessness), familial stressors, and societal pressures [12]. Shared predictors, such as emotional dysregulation and adverse childhood experiences, complicate the distinction between NSSI and SB, yet research underscores critical differences in their etiology. For instance, while both behaviors are associated with depression and trauma, SB uniquely correlates with impulsivity, hopelessness, and a history of previous suicide attempts [13,14]. Understanding the nuanced predictors of SB and its interplay with NSSI is essential for early identification and prevention.

The COVID-19 pandemic has significantly amplified mental health concerns among adolescents. Pandemic-related stressors—including social isolation, disrupted routines, increased family conflict, and limited access to mental health services—have been linked to a surge in psychological distress and maladaptive behaviors, including NSSI and SB [15,16]. Recent studies indicate that adolescents faced heightened emotional dysregulation during this period, reflecting the pandemic's exacerbation of pre-existing vulnerabilities, such as depression, anxiety, and adverse childhood experiences [17,18]. Additionally, alarming trends in hospital admissions related to deliberate self-poisoning and substance use among Romanian adolescents have emerged, reflecting the broader mental health challenges during this time [19]. At the same time, protective factors, such as social support, peer networks, and school-based interventions, were significantly reduced, further elevating the risk of self-harm behaviors [20]. These findings emphasize the need to explore the pandemic's varied impacts on NSSI and SB, particularly within high-risk clinical settings.

Despite the growing body of literature, significant research gaps remain in understanding the specific predictors of NSSI and SB across diverse populations and contexts. Many studies focus on community samples, leaving clinical populations—such as adolescents presenting to emergency departments—underexplored [5,21]. Moreover, much of the research has been conducted in Western countries, limiting the generalizability of findings to other cultural and healthcare contexts. For example, Romania, a country with limited mental health resources for adolescents, remains underrepresented in global studies on self-harm and suicide [22]. Understanding predictors of NSSI and SB within Romanian pediatric psychiatry emergency settings is crucial for tailoring culturally sensitive interventions.

In view of these aspects, the main aim of the present study is to investigate the risk factors and clinical predictors of NSSI and SB among adolescents presenting to a Romanian pediatric psychiatry emergency department before and after the COVID-19 pandemic. More specifically, we aim to identify those factors that determine that only a fraction of patients with mental disorders severe enough to present in emergency conditions resort to such behaviors. To this end, we used a retrospective cohort design in which we applied logistic regression and random forest modeling to identify the potential predictors. The underlying hypothesis is that by combining these two statistical procedures we could identify not only factors that already benefit from empirical support (such as certain psychiatric disorders) but also factors that have not been discussed in the literature so far, such as aspects related to the family, social, school, or life history background of patients. Another assumption is that the COVID-19 pandemic could have influenced the dynamics of the factors influencing NSSI and SB, by changing the weights of certain variables or even by introducing some new elements. By exploring the pandemic's impact on these predictors, this research aims to inform the development of targeted prevention and intervention strategies for high-risk populations, ultimately contributing to a better understanding of the mechanisms linking NSSI and SB.

2. Materials and Methods

2.1. Participant Selection

This retrospective cohort study analyzed data from 341 children and adolescents aged 6 to 18 years who were admitted as emergencies to the Pediatric Psychiatry Clinic in Cluj-Napoca during 2019 and 2022. These years were selected to enable a comparative analysis of psychiatric emergencies before (2019) and after (2022) the COVID-19 pandemic. All patients meeting the inclusion criteria were included, with those who did not engage in non-suicidal self-injury (NSSI) or suicidal behavior (SB) serving as the control group.

Inclusion criteria required participants to be between 6 and 18 years of age, admitted for an emergency psychiatric evaluation or treatment, and to have provided informed consent for the use of their medical data for research purposes. Consent was obtained from patients and from their parents or legal guardians. Patients who exclusively utilized outpatient services, declined consent, or had incomplete medical records were excluded.

Psychiatric diagnoses were assigned according to the International Classification of Diseases, 10th Revision (ICD-10), based on comprehensive clinical evaluations conducted by trained child psychiatrists. The study adhered to the principles of the Declaration of Helsinki and received approval from the Emergency Clinical Hospital for Children Cluj-Napoca Clinical Trials Quality Assurance Commission (Approval No. 80/14.12.2020).

2.2. Data Collection

Data were retrospectively extracted from medical records by two independent raters, with discrepancies resolved through a consensus. The dataset included socio-demographic information, family and personal history, clinical characteristics, school-related variables, and self-harm behaviors.

Socio-demographic and clinical information was primarily based on self-reported or parent-reported data documented during clinical evaluations. Reports included details on the socio-economic status, family structure and dynamics, and school-related factors, such as academic performance, bullying, peer conflicts, and disciplinary issues. Clinician observations during emergency admissions supplemented self- or parent-reported accounts where possible.

Psychiatric diagnoses were classified according to ICD-10 and included affective disorders (e.g., depressive episodes, bipolar disorder), anxiety and stress-related disorders (e.g., generalized anxiety disorder, post-traumatic stress disorder [PTSD]), conduct and emotional disorders (e.g., oppositional defiant disorder, adjustment disorder), neurodevelopmental disorders (e.g., attention deficit hyperactivity disorder [ADHD], autism spectrum disorder), substance use disorders, psychotic disorders, and other categories (e.g., eating disorders or somatoform disorders). Personality disorder traits were also recorded when present.

In addition to establishing the psychiatric diagnosis, the assessment of all participants involved asking predetermined questions investigating their family, school, and life context. Information on chronic somatic illnesses, prior psychiatric treatments (e.g., psychotherapy, pharmacological interventions), and potentially psycho-traumatizing negative life events (i.e., parental absence, death of a close person, school failure, history of suicide in the family, serious interpersonal conflicts, severe illness in the family, a history of accidents, or any other event that the patient may have considered to be psycho-traumatizing) was collected. Family-related variables included the parental age, marital status (married, single, divorced/separated, or widowed), employment status, education level, family conflicts, and family history of psychiatric disorders (e.g., depression, anxiety, schizophrenia, bipolar disorder, or substance use disorders).

Self-harm behaviors, including non-suicidal self-injury (NSSI) and suicidal behavior (SB, encompassing suicidal ideation and attempts), were also primarily reported by participants or their parents during emergency consultations. The frequency, method, and circumstances of these behaviors were documented in the medical records by attending clinicians.

2.3. Statistical Analysis

Statistical analyses were conducted using SPSS software (version 17.0) and R (version 4.3.3 for MacOS) alongside R Studio (version 2023.12.1+402) for advanced statistical modeling. Descriptive statistics summarized continuous variables as means and standard deviations, while categorical variables were presented as frequencies and percentages. Analyses were stratified by year (2019 vs. 2022) and by self-harm category, which included a control group, suicidal behaviors (SBs), and non-suicidal self-injury (NSSI).

Comparative analyses employed independent t-tests for continuous variables (e.g., age) and chi-square tests for categorical variables (e.g., gender, diagnosis, school-related conflicts). Given the large number of variables under consideration, Bonferroni corrections or other procedures to handle multiple comparisons were not performed, since such approaches tend to be particularly conservative in such situations and, in attempting to reduce Type I errors, there would have been a high risk of sacrificing statistically significant findings. Instead, to achieve the predictions of interest, we used two different statistical procedures that effectively control for covariates without, however, overdoing it in terms of stringency, and we reported 95% confidence intervals to provide a clearer understanding of the data without stringent multiple correction adjustments.

First, logistic regression models were developed to predict suicidal behavior and NSSI based on variables, including sex, environment, psychiatric diagnosis, and school/family-related conflicts. Two logistic regression models were created for each outcome variable to assess the predictive power of different sets of predictors. Categorical predictors were dummy-coded, and ordinal predictors (e.g., socioeconomic status) were treated as ordinal variables. Supplementary Table S1 displays the predictor variables used in each of the two regression models.

To address potential multicollinearity among predictor variables and to account for complex, non-linear relationships, random forest (RF) models were employed alongside logistic regression. The RF models comprised 2000 decision trees, with hyperparameters (e.g., mtry, sample.fraction, and min.node.size) optimized through a grid search to minimize the root mean squared error (RMSE). Final models utilized mtry = 8, sample.fraction = 0.80, and min.node.size = 5. Sampling without replacement was applied to avoid selection bias [23]. The random forest algorithm is particularly beneficial for managing health-related data, as it can capture intricate interactions among variables and provide insights into complex relationships, making it a valuable tool in the analysis of health data [24]. Statistical significance was set at $p < 0.05$.

3. Results

3.1. Characteristics of the Sample

The study sample included 341 participants, consisting of 200 females and 141 males, aged between 6 and 17 years, with a mean age of 14.57 years (SD = 2.25). The majority of participants (n = 214) were from urban areas. Most of the participants (n = 190) came from stable family environments, although many reported experiencing socioeconomic challenges (n = 190). A significant portion of the sample (71.85%) indicated a history of familial conflict, while 58.65% reported having at least one family member diagnosed with a psychiatric disorder, with substance use disorders (SUDs), particularly tobacco and alcohol use, being the most common (33.13%). Additionally, 14.95% (n = 51) reported a family history of somatic conditions, whereas only 8 participants (2.35%) indicated a neurological disorder in their family history.

A substantial proportion of participants (55.13%, n = 188) reported having experienced at least one significant potentially traumatic negative life event, with parental separation/divorce being the most frequently reported (n = 64). Regarding educational experiences, while most participants (n = 299) were enrolled in school, many reported challenges, including conflicts (n = 234) and poor academic performance (n = 210). However, only a small proportion (16.1%, n = 55) considered family and/or peer conflicts to be severe enough to be categorized as psycho-traumatic experiences.

In terms of psychiatric diagnoses, the most prevalent conditions included depression (41.93%, n = 143), conduct disorder (CD; n = 135), substance use disorder (SUD; n = 134), and attention-deficit/hyperactivity disorder (ADHD; n = 131). On average, participants had 3.13 comorbid conditions (SD = 1.38), with some individuals having as many as eight distinct diagnoses. At the time of the study, 23.16% of participants were receiving psychotherapy, while 21.99% reported not using any form of psychotropic medication. All characteristics of the whole sample are presented in Supplementary Table S2.

The study also compared data collected before (2019) and after (2022) the COVID-19 pandemic. Of the participants, 39.29% were assigned to the control group, while 164 participants exhibited suicidal behaviors, including suicidal ideation (n = 157) and suicide attempts (n = 81). Additionally, 119 participants had engaged in non-suicidal self-injury (NSSI). In total, 163 participants had a history of suicidal ideation, 74 had attempted suicide, and 158 had engaged in NSSI at some point in their lives. Tables 1 and 2 provide detailed comparisons of these characteristics between the pre-pandemic (2019) and post-pandemic (2022) periods.

Table 1. Main demographic characteristics of the sample and the comparison between the pre-pandemic and post-pandemic periods.

Characteristics	PRE-PANDEMIC (n = 194)	POST-PANDEMIC (n = 147)	p
Female:male distribution (%F)	107:87 (55.15%)	93:54 (63.26%)	0.132 †
Age (M ± SD)	14.289 ± 2.437	14.946 ± 1.922	0.007 *†
Urban:rural provenience (%U)	130:64 (67.01%)	84:63 (57.14%)	0.062 ‡
	Family structure (n, %)		
Organized	112 (57.73%)	78 (53.06%)	0.390 ‡
Divorced	30 (15.46%)	34 (23.13%)	0.073 ‡
Cohabitation	2 (1.03%)	2 (1.36%)	0.738 ‡
Institutionalized	28 (14.43%)	18 (12.24%)	0.558 ‡
Disorganized (death of one parent)	22 (11.34%)	15 (10.20%)	0.738 ‡

Table 1. *Cont.*

Characteristics	PRE-PANDEMIC (*n* = 194)	POST-PANDEMIC (*n* = 147)	*p*
	Socioeconomic status (*n*, %)		
Poor	100 (51.54%)	90 (61.22%)	0.075 ‡
Middle	64 (32.98%)	35 (23.81%)	0.064 ‡
Good	28 (14.43%)	18 (12.24%)	0.558 ‡
Very good	2 (1.03%)	4 (2.72%)	0.240 ‡
Conflicts in family (*n*, %)	130 (67.01%)	115 (78.23%)	0.023 *‡
Psychiatric disorders in family (*n*, %)	121 (62.37%)	79 (53.74%)	0.109 ‡
SUD	68 (35.05%)	45 (30.61%)	0.388 ‡
Depression	20 (10.30%)	12 (8.16%)	0.501 ‡
Schizophrenia	14 (7.21%)	12 (8.16%)	0.744 ‡
Anxiety disorders	1 (0.51%)	1 (0.68%)	0.844 ‡
Other disorders	18 (9.27%)	9 (6.12%)	0.285 ‡
Somatic disorders in family (*n*, %)	32 (16.49%)	19 (12.93%)	0.360 ‡
Neurological disorders in family (*n*, %)	2 (1.03%)	6 (4.08%)	0.065 ‡
	Potentially traumatic negative life events (*n*, %)		
Death of one parent	22 (11.34%)	15 (10.20%)	0.738 ‡
Death of someone close	8 (4.12%)	6 (4.08%)	0.985 ‡
Divorce or separation of parents	30 (15.46%)	34 (23.13%)	0.073 ‡
Parents abroad	4 (2.06%)	7 (4.76%)	0.162 ‡
Suicide in family	1 (0.51%)	0 (0%)	0.383 ‡
School failure	8 (4.12%)	3 (2.04%)	0.281 ‡
Severe conflicts with friends or parents	24 (12.37%)	31 (21.09%)	0.030 *‡
Serious illness in family or friends	5 (2.58%)	4 (2.72%)	0.935 ‡
Accidents	1 (0.51%)	1 (0.68%)	0.844 ‡
School attendance (*n*, %)	171 (88.14%)	128 (87.07%)	0.766 ‡
School conflicts (*n*, %)	149 (76.80%)	85 (57.82%)	<0.001 *‡
Only with colleagues	99 (51.03%)	51 (34.69%)	0.003 *‡
Only with teachers	10 (5.15%)	6 (4.08%)	0.643 ‡
With both	40 (20.61%)	28 (19.05%)	0.719 ‡
School performance (*n*, %)			0.014 *‡
Poor	121 (62.37%)	89 (60.54%)	0.731 ‡
Middle	53 (27.31%)	30 (20.41%)	0.141 ‡
Good	14 (7.21%)	26 (17.69%)	0.003 *‡
Very good	6 (3.09%)	2 (1.36%)	0.295 ‡
Suicidal behavior (*n*, %)	81 (41.75%)	83 (56.46%)	0.007 *‡
Suicidal ideation (*n*, %)	75 (38.65%)	82 (55.78%)	0.002 *‡
Past suicidal ideation (*n*, %)	86 (44.33%)	77 (52.38%)	0.140 ‡
Suicidal attempt (*n*, %)	39 (20.10%)	42 (28.57%)	0.069 ‡
Past suicidal attempts (*n*, %)	47 (24.23%)	27 (18.37%)	0.194 ‡
Past suicidal behavior (*n*, %)	90 (46.39%)	79 (53.74%)	0.179 ‡
Self-harm (*n*, %)	70 (36.08%)	49 (33.33%)	0.598 ‡
Past self-harm (*n*, %)	83 (42.78%)	75 (51.02%)	0.131 ‡

‡—chi-square; †—*t* test; * = statistical significance.

Table 2. Comparison of the distribution of diagnoses and therapeutic interventions between the pre-pandemic and post-pandemic period.

Characteristics	PRE-PANDEMIC (n = 194)	POST-PANDEMIC (n = 147)	p
	Diagnostics (n)		
Depression	71 (36.60%)	76 (51.70%)	0.038 *‡
CD	74 (38.14%)	61 (41.50%)	0.531 ‡
ADHD	68 (35.05%)	63 (42.86%)	0.142 ‡
ODD	13 (6.70%)	2 (1.36%)	0.017 *‡
Anxiety disorders	58 (29.90%)	43 (29.25%)	0.897 ‡
Sleep disorders	24 (12.37%)	4 (2.72%)	0.001 *‡
SUD	69 (35.57%)	65 (44.22%)	0.105 ‡
Bipolar disorder	6 (3.09%)	4 (2.72%)	0.840 ‡
PTSD	7 (3.61%)	7 (4.76%)	0.595 ‡
Borderline personality disorder	38 (19.59%)	28 (19.05%)	0.901 ‡
No. of comorbid diagnostics (M ± SD)	3.077 ± 1.373	3.204 ± 1.385	0.401 †
Psychotherapy (n, %)	43 (22.16%)	36 (24.49%)	0.614 ‡
Psychotropic medication (n, %)	151 (77.84%)	115 (78.23%)	0.930 ‡

‡—chi-square; †—*t* test; * = statistical significance.

Cutting and scratching were the most prevalent self-harm methods, increasing significantly from 62.85% pre-pandemic to 79.59% post-pandemic, χ^2 (1, N = 119) = 3.826, p = 0.050, OR = 0.434, 95% CI [0.186, 1.012]. Table 3 presents these data.

Table 3. Main self-harm behaviors before and after the COVID-19 pandemic.

Characteristics	PRE-PANDEMIC	POST-PANDEMIC	p
Self-harm	n = 70	n = 49	
Cutting, scratching	44 (62.85%)	39 (79.59%)	0.05 *
Self-poisoning	6 (8.57%)	2 (4.08%)	0.121
Other	20 (28.57%)	8 (16.32%)	0.145
Suicide attempt	n = 39	n = 42	
Drug ingestion	27 (69.23%)	30 (71.42%)	0.829
Cutting	4 (10.25%)	3 (7.14%)	0.618
Substance intoxication	0 (0%)	1 (2.38%)	0.332
Hanging	0 (0%)	2 (4.76%)	0.168
Defenestration	6 (15.38%)	5 (11.90%)	0.648
Other	2 (5.128%)	1 (2.38%)	0.513

* = statistical significance.

3.2. Stratification by Assessment Period and Group Comparisons

When stratifying the sample based on the assessment period, several significant differences emerged between the pre- and post-pandemic groups. Participants in the post-pandemic sample had significantly higher mean ages (t(339) = 2.694, p = 0.007), d = −0.295, 95% CI [−0.510, −0.079], higher depression rates (χ^2(1, N = 341) = 4.297, p = 0.038), OR = 1.583, 95% CI [1.024, 2.446], and a greater prevalence of family conflict (χ^2(1, N = 341) = 5.206, p = 0.023), OR = 1.769, 95% CI [1.081, 2.897]. They also reported more severe conflicts with parents and/or friends (χ^2(1, N = 341) = 4.698, p = 0.030), OR = 1.893, 95% CI [1.057, 3.390], higher rates of suicidal ideation (χ^2(1, N = 341) = 9.869, p = 0.002), OR = 2.002, 95% CI [1.295, 3.093], and increased suicidal behavior (χ^2(1, N = 341) = 7.249, p = 0.007), OR = 1.809, 95% CI [1.173, 2.790]. Notably, past suicidal ideation rates and prior reports of suicidal behavior did not significantly differ between the two samples.

Educational outcomes also varied significantly between the pre- and post-pandemic groups (χ^2(3, N = 341) = 10.573, p = 0.014). More students in the post-pandemic period reported good academic performance (χ^2(1, N = 341) = 8.855, p = 0.003), OR = 2.763, 95% CI [1.387, 5.505]. Conversely, post-pandemic participants had significantly lower rates of oppositional defiant disorder (χ^2(1, N = 341) = 5.672, p = 0.017), OR = 0.192, 95% CI [0.043, 0.865], sleep disorders (χ^2(1, N = 341) = 10.333, p = 0.001), OR = 0.198, 95% CI [0.067, 0.584], and academic conflicts (χ^2(1, N = 341) = 13.993, p < 0.001), OR = 0.414, 95% CI [0.260, 0.661].

3.2.1. Suicidal Behavior Group vs. Control Group

When comparing participants in the suicidal behavior group to those in the control group, several significant differences were observed. Participants in the suicidal behavior group were older (t(296) = −2.642, p = 0.009), d = 0.308, 95% CI [0.078, 0.537] and more likely to be female (χ^2(1, N = 298) = 23.640, p < 0.001), OR = 3.264, 95% CI [2.010, 5.299]. They exhibited significantly higher rates of depression (χ^2(1, N = 298) = 77.798, p < 0.001), OR = 10.395, 95% CI [5.958, 18.136], anxiety disorders (χ^2(1, N = 298) = 10.100, p = 0.001), OR = 2.276, 95% CI [1.363, 3.801], post-traumatic stress disorder (PTSD; χ^2(1, N = 298) = 10.216, p = 0.001), OR = 22.049, 95% CI [1.293, 375.954], and borderline personality disorder traits (χ^2(1, N = 298) = 18.642, p < 0.001), OR = 4.547, 95% CI [2.189, 9.445]. They also reported more potentially traumatic negative life events (χ^2(1, N = 298) = 12.046, p < 0.001), OR = 2.271, 95% CI [1.424, 3.622], higher school attendance (χ^2(1, N = 298) = 7.978, p = 0.005), OR = 2.882, 95% CI [1.349, 6.156], and greater participation in regular psychotherapy sessions (χ^2(1, N = 298) = 4.421, p = 0.036), OR = 1.825, 95% CI [1.037, 3.211].

In contrast, conduct disorder (χ^2(1, N = 298) = 10.288, p = 0.001), OR = 0.464, 95% CI [0.290, 0.744], and sleep disorders (χ^2(1, N = 298) = 7.814, p = 0.005), OR = 0.249, 95% CI [0.088, 0.706], were significantly less common in the suicidal behavior group. Participants in this group also had significantly higher frequencies of past suicidal ideation (χ^2(1, N = 298) = 149.222, p < 0.001), OR = 36.931, 95% CI [18.892, 72.193], suicide attempts (χ^2(1, N = 298) = 90.887, p < 0.001), OR = 262.557, 95% CI [16.067, 4290.431], and past non-suicidal self-injury (NSSI; χ^2(1, N = 298) = 71.286, p < 0.001), OR = 10.332, 95% CI [5.740, 18.598].

3.2.2. NSSI Group vs. Control Group

Participants in the NSSI group also exhibited significant differences compared to the control group. They had a higher proportion of females (χ^2(1, N = 253) = 11.101, p < 0.001), OR = 2.364, 95% CI [1.419, 3.937], and a greater number of comorbid conditions (t(251) = 3.512, p < 0.001), d = 0.442, 95% CI [0.192, 0.692]. Depression (χ^2(1, N = 253) = 34.483, p < 0.001), OR = 5.249, 95% CI [2.953, 9.332], PTSD (χ^2(1, N = 253) = 9.303, p = 0.002), OR = 20.507, 95% CI [1.171, 359.224], borderline personality disorder traits (χ^2(1, N = 253) = 25.855, p < 0.001), OR = 6.045, 95% CI [2.857, 12.790], family conflicts (χ^2(1, N = 253) = 9.008, p = 0.003), OR = 2.439, 95% CI [1.351, 4.405], and participation in psychotherapy sessions (χ^2(1, N = 253) = 7.513, p = 0.006), OR = 2.264, 95% CI [1.253, 4.091], were all more common in the NSSI group. However, conduct disorder was significantly less prevalent in this group (χ^2(1, N = 253) = 8.474, p = 0.004), OR = 0.469, 95% CI [0.281, 0.784].

Additionally, participants in the NSSI group reported significantly higher frequencies of past suicidal ideation (χ^2(1, N = 253) = 91.060, p < 0.001), OR = 18.291, 95% CI [9.413, 35.543], past self-harm behaviors (χ^2(1, N = 253) = 150.737, p < 0.001), OR = 63.273, 95% CI [28.585, 140.052], past suicide attempts (χ^2(1, N = 253) = 27.182, p < 0.001), OR = 137.038, 95% CI [8.312, 2259.437], and overall suicidal behavior (χ^2(1, N = 253) = 122.326, p < 0.001), OR = 473.069, 95% CI [28.716, 7793.356].

The mean number of past suicide attempts was 0.640 (SD = 0.798) in the suicidal behavior group, with a maximum of four attempts, compared to 0.504 (SD = 0.780) among participants in the NSSI group. Table 4 summarizes demographic characteristics of the suicidal behavior, NSSI, and control groups, while Table 5 details their primary diagnoses.

Table 4. Characteristics of participants in the main groups.

Characteristics	CONTROL (n = 134)	SUICIDAL BEHAVIOR (n = 164)			NSSI (n = 119)
		Ideation (n = 157)	Attempts (n = 81)	Whole (n = 164)	
Pre-pandemic presentation (n, %)	79 (58.95%)	75 (47.77%)	39 (48.15%)	81 (49.39%) ‡	70 (58.82%) ‡
Female:male distribution (%F)	61:73 (45.52%)	114:43 (72.61%)	65:16 (80.24%)	120:44 (73.17%) *‡	79:40 (66.38%) *‡
Age (M ± SD)	14.231 ± 2.678	14.898 ± 1.645	14.864 ± 1.626	14.902 ± 1.670 *†	14.689 ± 1.986 ‡
Urban:rural provenience (%U)	81:53 (60.44%)	104:53 (66.24%)	48:33 (59.25%)	108:56 (65.85%) ‡	79:40 (66.38%) ‡
Family structure (n, %)					
Organized	83 (61.94%)	82 (52.23%)	43 (53.09%)	87 (53.05%) ‡	60 (50.42%) ‡
Divorced	21 (15.67%)	39 (24.84%)	20 (24.69%)	39 (23.78%) ‡	20 (16.81%) ‡
Cohabitation	2 (1.49%)	2 (1.27%)	2 (2.47%)	2 (1.22%) ‡	1 (0.84%) ‡
Institutionalized	17 (12.69%)	18 (11.46%)	7 (8.64%)	19 (11.59%) ‡	21 (17.65%)‡
Disorganized (death of one parent)	11 (8.21%)	16 (10.19%)	9 (11.11%)	17 (10.37%) ‡	17 (14.29%) ‡
Socioeconomic status (n, %)					
Poor	72 (53.73%)	86 (54.78%)	42 (51.85%)	87 (53.05%) ‡	75 (63.03%) ‡
Middle	40 (29.85%)	45 (28.66%)	24 (29.63%)	49 (29.88%) ‡	29 (24.37%) ‡
Good	21 (15.67%)	21 (13.38%)	12 (14.81%)	23 (14.02%) ‡	11 (9.24%) ‡
Very good	1 (0.75%)	5 (3.18%)	3 (3.70%)	5 (3.05%) ‡	4 (3.36%) ‡
Conflicts in family (n, %)	88 (65.67%)	119 (75.80%)	62 (76.54%)	122 (74.39%) ‡	98 (82.35%) *‡
Psychiatric disorders in family (n, %)	75 (55.97%)	95 (60.51%)	43 (53.09%)	96 (58.54%) ‡	72 (60.50%) ‡
SUD	41 (30.60%)	51 (32.48%)	25 (30.86%)	51 (31.10%) ‡	45 (37.82%) ‡
Depression	9 (6.72%)	21 (13.38%)	10 (12.35%)	21 (12.80%) ‡	8 (6.72%) ‡
Schizophrenia	10 (7.46%)	12 (7.64%)	5 (6.17%)	12 (7.32%) ‡	10 (8.40%) ‡
Anxiety disorders	1 (0.75%)	1 (0.64%)	0 (0%)	1 (0.61%) ‡	1 (0.84%) ‡
Other disorders	14 (10.45%)	10 (6.37%)	3 (3.70%)	11 (6.71%) ‡	8 (6.72%) ‡
Somatic disorders in family (n, %)	20 (14.93%)	22 (14.01%)	13 (16.05%)	24 (14.63%) ‡	20 (16.81%) ‡
Neurological disorders in family (n, %)	1 (0.75%)	6 (3.82%)	3 (3.70%)	6 (3.66%) ‡	4 (3.36%) ‡
Potentially traumatic negative life events (n, %)					
Death of one parent	11 (8.21%)	16 (10.19%)	9 (11.11%)	17 (10.37%)	17 (14.29%)
Death of someone close	4 (2.99%)	8 (5.10%)	6 (7.41%)	9 (5.49%)	3 (2.52%)
Divorce or separation of parents	21 (15.67%)	39 (24.84%)	20 (24.69%)	39 (23.78%)	20 (16.81%)
Parents abroad	3 (2.24%)	7 (4.46%)	5 (6.17%)	7 (4.27%)	2 (1.68%)
Suicide in family	0 (0%)	0 (0%)	0 (0%)	0 (0%)	1 (0.84%)
School failure	4 (2.99%)	5 (3.18%)	1 (1.23%)	5 (3.05%)	4 (3.36%)
Severe conflicts with friends or parents	15 (11.19%)	29 (18.47%)	20 (24.69%)	31 (18.90%)	23 (19.33%)
Serious illness in family or friends	3 (2.24%)	5 (3.18%)	2 (2.47%)	5 (3.05%)	4 (3.36%)
Accidents	1 (0.75%)	0 (0%)	0 (0%)	0 (0%)	1 (0.84%)
School attendance (n, %)	111 (82.84%)	146 (93.00%)	77 (95.06%)	153 (93.29%) *‡	107 (89.92%) ‡
School conflicts (n, %)	93 (69.40%)	99 (63.06%)	47 (58.02%)	91 (55.49%) ‡	93 (78.15%) ‡
Only with colleagues	59 (44.03%)	67 (42.68%)	37 (45.68%)	67 (40.85%) ‡	61 (51.26%) ‡
Only with teachers	4 (2.99%)	8 (5.10%)	3 (3.70%)	9 (5.49%) ‡	7 (5.88%) ‡
With both	30 (22.39%)	24 (15.29%)	7 (8.64%)	25 (15.24%) ‡	25 (21.01%) ‡
School performance (n, %)					
Poor	86 (64.18%)	86 (54.78%)	41 (50.62%)	88 (53.66%) ‡	73 (61.34%) ‡
Middle	29 (21.64%)	46 (29.30%)	21 (25.93%)	49 (29.88%) ‡	34 (28.57%) ‡
Good	15 (11.19%)	22 (14.01%)	16 (19.75%)	24 (14.63%) ‡	9 (7.56%) ‡
Very good	4 (2.99%)	3 (1.91%)	3 (3.70%)	3 (1.83%) ‡	3 (2.52%) ‡
Suicidal behavior (n, %)	0 (0%)	157 (100%)	81 (100%)	164 (100%)	76 (63.87%) ‡
Suicidal ideation	0 (0%)	157 (100%)	74 (91.36%)	157 (95.73%) ‡	75 (63.03%) ‡

Table 4. *Cont.*

Characteristics	CONTROL (n = 134)	SUICIDAL BEHAVIOR (n = 164)			NSSI (n = 119)
		Ideation (n = 157)	Attempts (n = 81)	Whole (n = 164)	
Past suicidal ideation	15 (11.19%)	132 (84.08%)	61 (75.31%)	135 (82.32%) *‡	83 (69.75%) ‡
Suicidal attempt	0 (0%)	74 (47.13%)	81 (100%)	81 (49.39%) ‡	40 (33.61%) ‡
Past suicidal attempts	10 (7.46%)	54 (34.39%)	33 (40.74%)	57 (34.76%) *‡	40 (33.61%) ‡
Past suicidal behavior	16 (11.94%)	132 (84.08%)	63 (77.78%)	137 (83.54%) *‡	86 (72.27%) ‡
Self-harm (n, %)	0 (0%)	75 (47.77%)	40 (49.38%)	76 (46.34%) ‡	119 (100%)
Past self-harm (n, %)	18 (13.43%)	100 (63.69%)	51 (62.96%)	101 (61.59%) *‡	108 (90.76%) ‡

‡—chi-square; †—*t* test; * = statistical significance.

Table 5. Comparison of the distribution of diagnoses and therapeutic interventions between the main groups of participants.

Characteristics	CONTROL (n = 134)	SUICIDAL BEHAVIOR (n = 164)			SELF-HARM (n = 119)
		Ideation (n = 157)	Attempts (n = 81)	Whole (n = 164)	
		Diagnostics (n, %)			
Depression	23 (17.16%)	109 (69.43%)	56 (69.14%)	112 (68.29%) *‡	62 (52.10%) *‡
CD	67 (50.00%)	51 (32.48%)	22 (27.16%)	52 (31.71%) *‡	38 (31.93%) *‡
ADHD	56 (41.79%)	50 (31.85%)	26 (32.10%)	53 (32.32%) ‡	48 (40.34%) ‡
ODD	8 (5.97%)	4 (2.55%)	2 (2.47%)	5 (3.05%) ‡	4 (3.36%) ‡
Anxiety disorders	30 (22.39%)	63 (40.13%)	31 (38.27%)	65 (39.63%) *‡	36 (30.25%) ‡
Sleep disorders	15 (11.19%)	5 (3.18%)	3 (3.70%)	5 (3.05%) *‡	12 (10.08%) ‡
SUD	46 (34.33%)	64 (40.76%)	30 (37.04%)	67 (40.85%) ‡	55 (46.22%) ‡
Bipolar disorder	5 (3.73%)	5 (3.18%)	2 (2.47%)	5 (3.05%) ‡	4 (3.36%) ‡
PTSD	0 (0%)	11 (7.01%)	4 (4.94%)	12 (7.32%) *‡	8 (6.72%) *‡
Borderline personality traits	10 (7.46%)	42 (26.75%)	25 (30.86%)	44 (26.83%) *‡	39 (32.77%) *‡
No. of comorbid diagnostics (M±SD)	2.940 ± 1.255	3.102 ± 1.374	3.111 ± 1.360	3.098 ± 1.376 †	3.546 ± 1.489 *†
Psychotherapy (n, %)	23 (17.16%)	45 (28.66%)	18 (22.22%)	45 (27.43%) *‡	38 (31.93%) *‡
Psychotropic medication (n, %)	99 (73.88%)	130 (82.80%)	61 (75.31%)	134 (81.71%) ‡	98 (82.35%) ‡

‡—chi-square; †—*t* test; * = statistical significance.

3.3. Logistic Regressions

3.3.1. Predicting Suicidal Behavior (SB)

Logistic regression Model 1 significantly predicted suicidal behavior, ($\chi^2(312)$ = 236.661, $p < 0.001$), accounting for 57.1% of the variance in the sample (Tjur $R^2 = 0.571$). Details of the regression coefficients and model fit statistics are provided in Supplementary Table S3. Three variables emerged as significant predictors of suicidal behavior. Depression was associated with an increased risk, with a regression coefficient (β) of 1.740 and an odds ratio (OR) of 5.700 ($p < 0.001$). A history of suicidal ideation was the strongest predictor, β = 3.856, OR = 47.261, $p < 0.001$, indicating that individuals with such a history were approximately 47 times more likely to exhibit suicidal behavior. In contrast, school-related conflicts showed a negative association, β = −1.148, OR = 0.317, $p = 0.023$, suggesting that the presence of school-related conflicts was linked to a reduction in the risk of suicidal behavior by approximately 68%.

Overall, Model 1 demonstrated robust performance, with an accuracy of 84.5%, a sensitivity of 83.5%, a specificity of 85.3%, and an area under the curve (AUC) of 0.928. Multicollinearity, assessed using the Variance Inflation Factor (VIF), was within acceptable limits, with a maximum VIF of 2.297, indicating no significant redundancy among the predictors.

Incorporating additional predictors in Model 2 ($\chi^2(298) = 252.910$, $p < 0.001$) significantly enhanced its predictive power for self-harm behaviors. The explained variance increased to 59.9% (Tjur $R^2 = 0.599$), alongside improvements in the overall accuracy (86.5%), AUC (0.937), sensitivity (86.0%), and specificity (87.0%). Multicollinearity remained moderate, with a maximum Variance Inflation Factor (VIF) below 5, ensuring reliable estimates. Depression ($\beta = 1.917$, OR = 6.803, $p < 0.001$) and prior suicidal ideation ($\beta = 4.226$, OR = 68.410, $p < 0.001$) remained significant predictors, with their effects amplified in this model.

Further analysis of school-related conflicts, which were previously significant in Model 1, revealed additional insights. Conflicts with peers ($\beta = -1.125$, OR = 0.325, $p = 0.042$), teachers ($\beta = -2.130$, OR = 0.119, $p = 0.024$), or both ($\beta = -1.797$, OR = 0.166, $p = 0.012$) were significantly associated with a reduced risk of suicidal behavior. Notably, Model 2 also identified a new significant risk factor, having a parent living abroad ($\beta = 2.437$, OR = 11.438, $p = 0.020$), suggesting that this factor may uniquely contribute to the likelihood of self-harm behaviors. These expanded findings, presented in Supplementary Table S4, underscore the importance of examining diverse contextual factors when predicting suicidal behavior.

3.3.2. Predicting NSSI

The logistic regression Model 1 significantly predicted non-suicidal self-injury (NSSI) behaviors ($\chi^2(312) = 197.244$, $p < 0.001$), explaining 51.0% of the variance (Tjur $R^2 = 0.510$). Several key predictors emerged as significant in the model. Conduct disorder was associated with a significantly reduced risk of NSSI ($\beta = -1.468$, OR = 0.230, $p = 0.001$), indicating a protective effect. Conversely, a higher number of comorbid diagnoses ($\beta = 0.554$, OR = 1.741, $p = 0.001$) and, most notably, a history of self-harm ($\beta = 3.739$, OR = 42.054, $p < 0.001$) were strongly associated with an increased risk. Individuals with a history of self-harm demonstrated a striking 42-fold higher likelihood of engaging in future NSSI.

Model 1 demonstrated strong predictive performance, achieving an accuracy of 84.5%, an AUC of 0.911, sensitivity of 80.7%, and specificity of 86.5%. Multicollinearity was assessed and found to be moderate, indicating stable parameter estimates. Detailed regression coefficients and model fit statistics are presented in Supplementary Table S5.

The addition of predictors in Model 2 ($\chi^2(298) = 207.099$, $p < 0.001$) slightly enhanced the predictive capacity for NSSI, increasing the explained variance to 52.8% (Tjur $R^2 = 0.528$). Model 2 also demonstrated modest gains in accuracy (85.0%), the AUC (0.920), and specificity (87.4%), while maintaining similar sensitivity to Model 1. Consistent with the findings from Model 1, conduct disorder remained a significant negative predictor of NSSI ($\beta = -1.691$, OR = 0.184, $p < 0.001$), reinforcing its protective association. In contrast, higher comorbidity ($\beta = 0.536$, OR = 1.709; $p = 0.003$) and a history of self-harm ($\beta = 3.960$, OR = 52.437; $p < 0.001$) emerged as strong positive predictors, with the latter suggesting a more than 52-fold increase in the likelihood of future NSSI. These results underscore the pivotal role of self-harm history in identifying individuals at a heightened risk. Comprehensive regression coefficients and model fit statistics are provided in Supplementary Table S6.

3.4. Random Forest Regressions

3.4.1. Predicting Suicidal Behavior

The random forest model explained 47.0% of the variance in suicidal behavior ($R^2 = 0.470$), slightly less than the logistic regression models, with a prediction error of 13.26%. Both impurity- and permutation-based importance measures consistently identified prior suicidal ideation (impurity: 16.7; permutation: 0.129) and depression (impurity:

7.66; permutation: 0.039) as the top predictors. These variables had also been significant in the logistic regression models, with their ranking remaining consistent across methods.

Interestingly, prior suicide attempts, which were not statistically significant in the logistic regression models (e.g., Model 2: β = −0.054, OR = 0.947, p = 0.919), ranked as the third most important predictor in the random forest model (permutation importance: 0.00931). Additional influential predictors included female sex (permutation importance: 0.00591) and a history of NSSI (permutation importance: 0.00572), both of which demonstrated relatively stable predictive power.

In contrast, the three facets of school-related conflict—significant in the logistic regression models—contributed minimally to the random forest model's predictive accuracy. Among these, conflicts with both teachers and peers ranked 11th (permutation importance: 0.00179), followed by conflicts with peers alone (23rd; permutation importance: 0.000277), while conflicts with teachers alone ranked near the bottom with a negative permutation importance score (−0.000557).

The timing of assessment, categorized as pre- versus post-pandemic, was the ninth most important variable, with a permutation importance score of 0.00234. This variable demonstrated greater relevance than certain potentially psycho-traumatizing negative life events, such as severe conflict (ranked 10th; 0.00190), parental divorce (ranked 13th; 0.00173), or having a parent residing abroad. Notably, while parental absence had been statistically significant in the second logistic regression model, it ranked 38th in the random forest model, with a negative permutation importance score (−0.000332).

A complete breakdown of variable importance scores is available in Supplementary Table S7 and visually depicted in Figure 1. These findings highlight the strengths of the random forest approach in identifying the nuanced contributions of predictors, offering a complementary perspective to the logistic regression results.

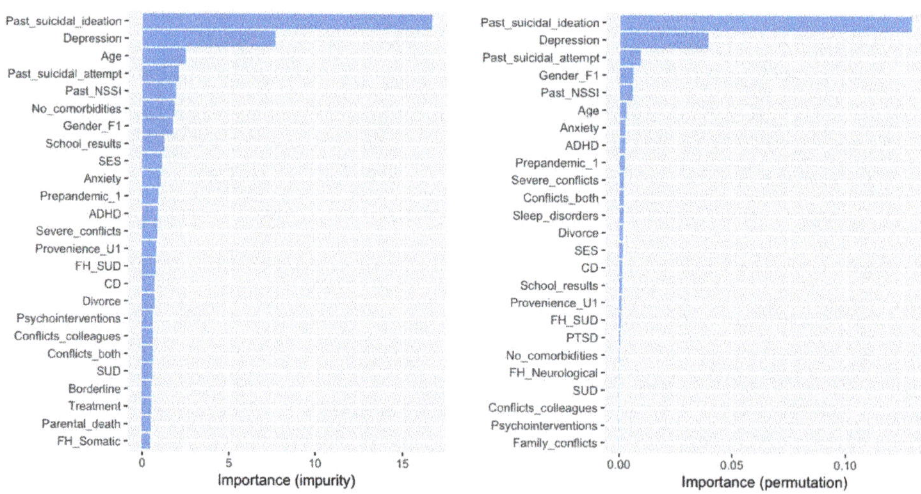

Figure 1. Importance of predictors for suicidal behavior.

3.4.2. Predicting NSSI

The random forest model for predicting non-suicidal self-injury (NSSI) explained 40.3% of the variance (R^2 = 0.403; prediction error = 13.59%), which was lower than the variance explained by the logistic regression models. Consistent with the logistic regression results, a history of NSSI was the most important predictor, with both impurity (16.9) and permutation (0.136) importance scores highlighting its significance. Borderline personality disorder traits, though showing a relatively low permutation importance score (0.0107), emerged as the second most influential predictor in the random forest model. This contrasts the logistic regression models, where borderline personality disorder traits were not significantly associated with NSSI (e.g., Model 2: β = 0.100, OR = 1.105, p = 0.824).

The number of comorbidities, which was a significant predictor in the logistic regression models, showed lower importance in the random forest model (permutation importance: 0.00895), similar to prior suicidal ideation (permutation importance: 0.00877). Other notable predictors in the random forest model included academic performance (0.00569), conduct disorder (0.00544), and anxiety disorders (0.00282).

The timing of presentation, categorized as pre- versus post-pandemic, was ranked eighth in permutation importance (0.00175), surpassing variables, such as past suicide attempts (0.00150; ranked 10th), family conflicts (0.00115; ranked 12th), and other potentially traumatic life events. Among these events, the experience of having a parent living abroad had the lowest permutation importance score (0.000518), ranking 17th.

These results are detailed in Supplementary Table S8 and illustrated in Figure 2.

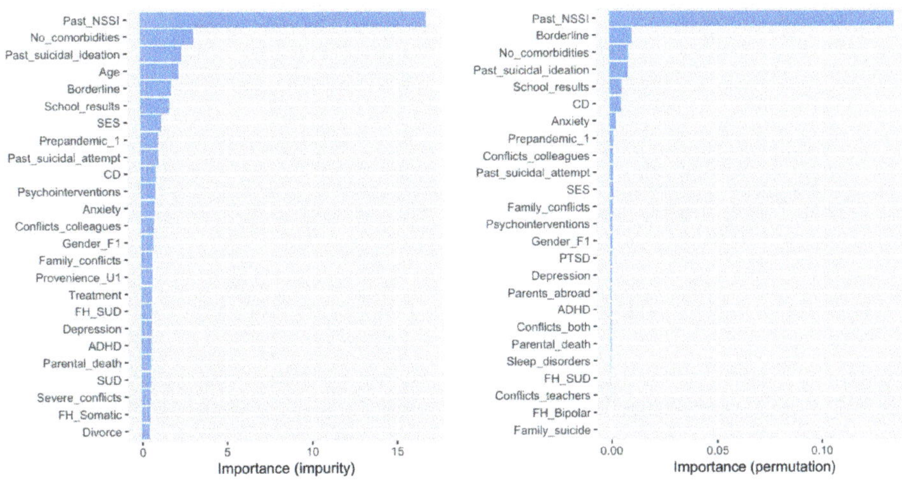

Figure 2. Importance of predictors for NSSI.

4. Discussion

This retrospective cohort study investigated the risk factors and clinical predictors associated with suicidal behavior (SB) and non-suicidal self-injury (NSSI) among pediatric psychiatry emergency admissions, contrasting data from the pre-pandemic year of 2019 with the post-pandemic year of 2022. Our comprehensive analysis elucidates several significant associations that enhance and refine the existing literature surrounding adolescent self-harm in clinical environments.

4.1. Prevalence and Characteristics of Self-Harm

Our sample comprised a notable majority of females (58.65%) with a mean age of 14.57 years (SD = 2.25), mainly hailing from urban settings (62.75%). While many participants came from ostensibly stable family units, a considerable subset (71.85%) reported experiencing familial conflicts. Furthermore, a significant proportion (58.65%) identified at least one family member with a psychiatric disorder, predominantly substance use disorders (33.13%). These findings echo existing research highlighting the familial transmission of psychopathology and the interplay between emotional and behavioral dysfunctions across generations [25–27]. Additionally, we observed that 14.95% of participants reported a family history of somatic conditions, hinting at a possible nexus between mental and physical health vulnerabilities within families. The prevalence of exposure to at least one potentially traumatic negative life event (55.13%), with parental separation or divorce being the most reported ($n = 64$), underscores the importance of considering family dynamics in the assessment and treatment of self-harm behaviors in adolescents [28].

The high prevalence of self-harming behaviors (both SB and NSSI) discovered within our sample aligns with the growing body of evidence documenting the significant burden of these behaviors among adolescents [4,5]. Previous studies have similarly demonstrated elevated rates of self-harm and suicidal ideation among adolescents, particularly in clinical settings [29,30]. Notably, we observed a significant increase in self-harm methods, specifically cutting and scratching, in the post-pandemic period ($\chi^2 = 3.826$, $p = 0.050$). This escalation reflects broader trends reported in the literature, which raised concerns about heightened rates of self-harm during and following the COVID-19 pandemic [15,16,18,31].

The trend of increased self-harm during the pandemic has been substantiated by several studies, indicating that psychological stressors, such as isolation, uncertainty, and changes in routine, contributed to heightened distress among adolescents [20,32]. Pertinently, medication ingestion was identified as the most common method used in suicide attempts among our sample. This finding is consistent with previous research suggesting that adolescents increasingly utilize pharmaceuticals as a method of self-harm [33–35]. Many studies have reported that the accessibility of medications, coupled with emotional distress, contributes to the prevalence of such attempts among youth [36,37].

4.2. Risk and Protective Factors

Our comparative analyses yielded several significant risk factors associated with both suicidal behavior (SB) and non-suicidal self-injury (NSSI) among adolescents admitted to psychiatric emergency services.

Prevalence of Psychiatric Disorders. Individuals within the SB group demonstrated markedly higher rates of depressive disorders, anxiety disorders, post-traumatic stress disorder (PTSD), borderline personality disorder traits (BPDs), and a history of potentially traumatic negative life events, all with statistical significance ($p < 0.05$). This finding corroborates a substantial body of literature that has consistently linked psychiatric disorders with suicidal behaviors. For instance, Barrocas et al. (2015) and Deutz et al. (2016) highlighted the strong association between major depressive disorder and increased suicide risk among adolescents [38,39]. Fang et al. (2024) also concluded that anxiety disorders serve as robust risk factors for both suicidal ideation and attempts, emphasizing the multifaceted nature of these conditions and their impact on youth [40].

Furthermore, PTSD has been recognized as a significant predictor of suicidal behaviors [41]. Adolescents with PTSD often grapple with intrusive memories and heightened emotional distress, which can contribute to self-harm and suicidal ideation [42]. In our analysis, we found that a history of suicidal ideation and attempts, as well as NSSI, were strongly correlated with current suicidal behaviors. This aligns with previous findings by Ribeiro (2016), who pointed out that such a history should be considered a critical indicator of future suicide risk [8].

Gender Differences in Suicidal Behavior. Notably, our study found that females were significantly overrepresented in the SB group ($\chi^2 = 23.640$, $p < 0.001$). This finding is consistent with established gender differences in suicidal behavior, where studies indicate that adolescent girls tend to exhibit higher rates of suicidal ideation and attempts compared to their male counterparts [43]. Researchers have posited that societal norms, emotional expression differences, and coping styles may contribute to these disparities [44].

Academic Conflicts and Reporting Bias. Interestingly, lower rates of academic conflicts were reported in the post-pandemic period, which warrants further investigation [45]. This unexpected finding may reflect a reporting bias, as adolescents may have different thresholds for reporting academic distress after experiencing the unique challenges and disruptions brought on by the pandemic [15]. Alternatively, the complex interplay of factors during this period may have led to changes in academic environments and support systems that reduced reported conflict. Further qualitative research could illuminate these dynamics and help ascertain whether this trend reflects genuine changes in academic pressures or variations in reporting practices among adolescents [46].

NSSI and Associated Risk Factors. The NSSI group exhibited significantly elevated rates of depression, PTSD, borderline personality disorder traits, and family conflicts compared to the control group. The association between NSSI and these psychiatric conditions has been well-documented in the literature. For instance, the link between NSSI and conduct disorder reflects the behavioral problems often seen in adolescents who self-harm [47]. Additionally, family conflicts were prevalent among those exhibiting NSSI, corroborating findings by Tatnell et al. (2014), which indicated that interpersonal relationships, particularly within family settings, significantly impacted self-harming behaviors [48]. Also of interest are the results provided by a recently published systematic umbrella review suggesting the potential usefulness of specific interventions targeting emotional dysregulation as a trans-diagnostic manifestation, such as ER Individual Therapy for Adolescents (ERITA), in reducing NSSI behaviors [49].

A particularly salient finding from our analyses is the strong association between a history of self-harm and current NSSI. This underscores the importance of early intervention and preventive efforts targeting adolescents who have previously engaged in self-injurious behavior. Studies, such as those by Ribeiro et al. (2015), have demonstrated that prior self-harm significantly increases the risk of future episodes, reiterating the necessity for routine screenings and interventions in clinical and educational settings to address these behaviors before they escalate [8].

4.3. *Impact of the COVID-19 Pandemic*

The COVID-19 pandemic has generated unprecedented disruptions globally, particularly affecting mental health across various age groups, with adolescents being particularly vulnerable [20,50]. Our study's comparisons between pre- and post-pandemic periods revealed significant shifts in mental health status and diagnostic profiles among adolescents seeking psychiatric care [51,52]. The findings indicate a complex and multifaceted impact of the pandemic on adolescent mental health, reflecting the interplay of heightened stressors, evolving psychosocial dynamics, and variations in access to mental health services [16,45,53,54].

Changes in Demographics and Depression Rates. One of the most striking contrasts observed was the significant increase in the mean age of adolescents in the post-pandemic sample. This demographic shift may suggest various underlying factors, including changes in the age of onset for mental health issues or alterations in treatment-seeking behavior among older adolescents. Previous research has suggested that older adolescents may experience distinct stressors related to transitions into adulthood, which could exacerbate mental health challenges in the context of a pandemic [55].

Moreover, the post-pandemic sample exhibited substantially higher rates of depression and suicidal ideation, aligning with global trends that have documented a surge in these conditions during the pandemic. A meta-analysis by Wang et al. (2022) reported that depression rates among adolescents increased significantly during COVID-19, driven largely by social isolation, uncertainty, and loss [56]. Furthermore, increased family stress and economic instability during the pandemic have been identified as contributing factors to the decline in adolescent mental health [57]. Our findings, which showed statistically significant differences (all $p < 0.05$), underscore the urgency in addressing mental health needs during and following such crises.

Reports of Potentially Psycho-traumatic Negative Life Events. In addition to higher rates of depression, the increase in reports of potential psycho-traumatic negative life events among adolescents post-pandemic is concerning. The pandemic has exposed youth to a range of traumatic experiences—ranging from the loss of family members to disruptions in daily life—and these experiences can profoundly impact mental health [58]. Studies have indicated that exposure to such traumatic events significantly heightens the risk of developing PTSD and other stress-related disorders [59]. Furthermore, parental stress has emerged as a significant factor influencing child mental health, underscoring the importance of family dynamics in these contexts [60]. Our findings reaffirm the critical need for mental health services to incorporate trauma-informed approaches in their interventions for adolescents, especially in the context of global crises.

Decreased Rates of Oppositional Defiant Disorder and Sleep Disorders. Conversely, we observed lower rates of oppositional defiant disorder (ODD) and sleep disorders in the post-pandemic cohort. This decline might suggest a variety of interpretations, including potential shifts in diagnostic criteria, variations in the contextual factors that contribute to these disorders, or even changes in the environment in which adolescents operate. For instance, with the transition to online learning and decreased traditional school settings, some youth may have experienced reduced external pressures, which could mitigate the expressions of defiant behavior often observed in school contexts [16]. Furthermore, the lower rates of sleep disorders could hint at changes in daily routines and sleep patterns that emerged during lockdowns—such as reduced screen time associated with structured classroom settings and altered family dynamics during this period. However, it is crucial to note that the delayed detection of these disorders may also occur, necessitating the ongoing monitoring of adolescent mental health as the long-term impacts of the pandemic unfold [61].

Complex Interplay of Stressors and Access to Care. Overall, these contrasting findings highlight the pandemic's multifactorial impact on adolescent mental health. They suggest a possible dual effect: while the pandemic has intensified certain stressors (e.g., grief, anxiety, depressive symptoms), it has also altered the context surrounding others, potentially leading to a reduction in some behavior-related disorders. Changes in access to mental health care during this period significantly influenced these outcomes. While some adolescents may have benefited from telehealth services during lockdowns, others encountered barriers, such as technology access, privacy concerns, and reduced in-person support [62]. Implementing online interventions may serve as an effective strategy to support families navigating these challenges [63]. The observed increases in depression and PTSD, alongside demographic shifts and potentially lowered rates of certain disorders, underscore the importance of ongoing surveillance, research, and tailored interventions.

4.4. Predictive Models

Predictive Modeling of Suicidal Behavior. The present study employed logistic regression models (Models 1 and 2) to evaluate the predictive accuracy for suicidal behavior (SB). These models demonstrated significant predictive accuracy, with Model 1 yielding a χ^2 statistic of 236.661 (df = 312, $p < 0.001$) and a Tjur R^2 value of 0.571, while Model 2 offered a slightly improved Tjur R^2 of 0.599. This level of predictive power suggests that the models effectively identified key variables that contribute to the risk of suicidal behavior in the adolescent population assessed.

Through these models, we identified several significant predictors of SB, including depression, prior suicidal ideation, and, intriguingly, school-related conflicts. Specifically, our findings underscored the substantial risk conferred by depressive symptoms, with Model 1 reporting an odds ratio (OR) of 5.700 ($p < 0.001$) and Model 2 indicating an even greater risk at OR = 6.803 ($p < 0.001$). This aligns with the existing literature that consistently underscores the critical role of depression as a precursor to suicidal behaviors in adolescents [38,39,64].

Moreover, our analyses revealed that a history of suicidal ideation was strongly correlated with current suicidal behaviors, with Model 1 reporting an OR of 47.261 ($p < 0.001$) and Model 2 reflecting an even higher OR of 68.410 ($p < 0.001$). These findings reinforce previous studies that have documented the importance of prior suicidal thoughts as a robust predictor of subsequent suicidal actions, illustrating the urgent need for effective monitoring and intervention strategies for individuals presenting with such histories [8,65]. In this regard, a recently published systematic review indicates that dialectical behavior therapy was the only intervention shown to be effective for adolescents at a high risk for suicide and suicide attempts [66].

Interestingly, our models indicated that school-related conflicts were associated with a decreased risk of SB (Model 1: OR = 0.317, $p = 0.023$). This counterintuitive finding necessitates further investigation, as it diverges from most existing literature that associates academic stress and school-related issues with an increased risk of depression and suicidal behavior [67,68]. Potential explanations for this protective effect could include the role of social support systems within academic settings or variations in coping mechanisms among adolescents facing academic challenges. Further qualitative and quantitative research is warranted to explore the nature of these school-related conflicts, as understanding their impact on suicidal risk could inform targeted interventions within educational frameworks.

Novel Risk Factor: Parent Living Abroad. An additional significant finding from Model 2 was the identification of having a parent living abroad as a novel risk factor for suicidal behavior (OR = 11.438, $p = 0.020$). This factor has not been extensively discussed in the literature regarding adolescent suicidal behavior, suggesting a unique area for further exploration. The emotional distance and potential for familial disconnection associated with having a parent reside in a different country could exacerbate feelings of loneliness, abandonment, or instability among adolescents [69,70]. Prior studies have indicated that parental absence or separation can significantly affect a child's emotional well-being and increase vulnerability to mental health issues [71]. Further research focusing on parenting styles, family dynamics, and the emotional ramifications of having a parent living abroad could elucidate the mechanisms contributing to an increased suicidal risk in this demographic.

Predictive Modeling of Non-Suicidal Self-Injury (NSSI). The logistic regression models employed in this study revealed significant predictive capability for non-suicidal self-injury (NSSI), with Model 1 achieving a χ^2 statistic of 197.244 (df = 312, $p < 0.001$) and a Tjur R^2 of 0.510, while Model 2 showed an improved Tjur R^2 of 0.528. These results indicate that our models adeptly identified critical factors contributing to the propensity for NSSI within the adolescent population studied.

Key Predictors of NSSI. Among the most striking findings from our analysis was the identification of a history of self-harm as a potent predictor of current NSSI behavior—with Model 1 reporting an odds ratio (OR) of 42.054 ($p < 0.001$) and Model 2 revealing an even greater OR of 52.437 ($p < 0.001$). This finding aligns with a robust body of literature emphasizing the cyclical nature of self-harm behaviors, whereby individuals with a history of self-injury are at a significantly increased risk for future episodes [7,8,72,73]. The persistence of NSSI among adolescents underscores the necessity for vigilant monitoring and effective intervention targeting this population, as early identification and treatment can prevent the escalation of self-harming behaviors. Results of a systematic review indicate some evidence for a reduction in NSSI relapse among adolescents after dialectical behavior therapy (DBT-A) interventions [74].

In addition to the history of self-harm, our models highlighted the significance of comorbidity, with a greater number of comorbid diagnoses emerging as a notable risk factor for NSSI. Specifically, Model 1 indicated an OR of 1.741 ($p = 0.001$), while Model 2 reported an OR of 1.709 (p=0.003). This result resonates with previous research indicating that adolescents with multiple mental health disorders are particularly vulnerable to engaging in self-injurious behaviors [75,76]. Understanding the interplay between diverse comorbidities, such as depression, anxiety, ADHD, and post-traumatic stress disorder (PTSD), is critical for developing comprehensive treatment plans that address the multifactorial nature of mental health challenges in this demographic [77].

Conduct Disorder and Its Protective Effect. Interestingly, our findings also revealed that conduct disorder exhibited a protective effect regarding NSSI (Model 1: OR = 0.230, $p = 0.001$; Model 2: OR = 0.184, $p < 0.001$). This unexpected result warrants closer examination, as it diverges from prevailing narratives that associate conduct disorder with higher risks of aggressive or self-injurious behavior among adolescents [78,79]. One possible explanation for this protective association could be that adolescents diagnosed with conduct disorder may express their distress through externalizing behaviors rather than self-harm, thereby reducing the likelihood of engaging in NSSI [80]. However, the relationship may be more nuanced: research suggests that externalizing behaviors and suicidality are indirectly linked, mediated by internalizing factors, and that externalizing behaviors may offer an alternative coping mechanism [80]. Further investigation is necessary to clarify this complex interaction. Alternatively, this finding may reflect underlying differences in coping mechanisms or social support systems within this population, deserving extensive studies to elucidate the complexity of these relationships.

The significant association between comorbidity and NSSI highlights the interconnectedness of various mental health challenges within this population. A comprehensive understanding of these relationships can better inform clinical practice and intervention strategies. For instance, mental health practitioners should conduct thorough assessments of adolescents presenting with self-injurious behavior, including a detailed evaluation of comorbid conditions, to ensure that treatment plans holistically address the patient's mental health profile [81,82].

Random Forest Modeling. While exhibiting lower R^2 values than logistic regression, the random forest models offer distinct advantages in assessing relative variable importance for both suicidal behavior (SB) and non-suicidal self-injury (NSSI).

For SB, prior suicidal ideation and depression emerged as the most prominent predictors, consistent with the findings from the logistic regression models. However, the random forest approach revealed the influence of additional factors, such as a history of suicide attempts, school-related conflicts, family conflict, and various demographic variables, which may have been obscured by multicollinearity in the logistic regression analyses [83,84]. This ability to uncover hidden relationships within the data underscores the utility of random forest modeling.

Similarly, for NSSI, prior self-harm remained the strongest predictor, affirming the findings of the logistic regression. Notably, the random forest model highlighted the significance of borderline personality disorder traits (BPDs), a factor that was not statistically significant in the logistic regression analysis. This is particularly relevant, as the literature has established the correlation between BPDs and self-injurious behaviors, further emphasizing the need for vigilant screening and assessments in clinical practice [85,86].

The consistent identification of key predictors across both modeling approaches enhances confidence in their clinical relevance and potential implications for intervention strategies.

The observed lower R^2 values in the random forest models for both outcomes, compared to the logistic regression models, can be attributed to the inherent higher dimensionality of the random forest modeling technique. While logistic regression typically focuses on a selected number of predictor variables, random forest models consider the entire dataset, encompassing a larger number of potential predictors and interactions among them. This complexity, while beneficial for capturing nuanced relationships, can lead to lower R^2 values as a consequence of how R^2 is calculated in high-dimensional contexts [87]. It is crucial to note that lower R^2 values do not imply inferior model performance, particularly regarding the ability of the model to evaluate and rank predictor importance. The implementation of permutation importance in random forest modeling provides a robust method for assessing the contribution of each predictor variable. This approach allows for a comprehensive evaluation of variable importance that can reveal the impact of multiple variables that might otherwise be masked by high collinearity when relying solely on regression coefficients derived from logistic regression [88].

Moreover, the permutation importance method addresses the limitation of traditional significance testing within regression frameworks, where multicollinearity can inflate standard errors and lead to erroneous conclusions about the importance of specific predictors [89]. By revealing hidden relationships and emphasizing the importance of additional factors, like borderline personality disorder traits, the findings from random forest analyses underscore the necessity of utilizing diverse modeling techniques to inform clinical practice and improve outcomes in adolescent mental health.

4.5. Limitations

This retrospective cohort study, while offering valuable insights into adolescent self-harm, has several limitations. First, the reliance on existing clinical records introduces recall bias, particularly regarding the self-harm history, trauma, and family history, and poses challenges related to data quality and completeness. Self-reports and parent-reports are prone to memory errors and social desirability bias, where individuals might under- or overreport particular behaviors or experiences. This can lead to inaccurate data, potentially jeopardizing the reliability of our findings. Furthermore, the data may be incomplete due to missing information or varying levels of detail in the original records, which can affect the thoroughness of our analysis. Diagnostic information, based on ICD-10 codes, may not fully capture the complexity of adolescent presentations, leading to the potential underrepresentation of nuanced conditions.

The sample, drawn from a single emergency department, may not be representative of all adolescents who engage in self-harm, as the predominantly female and urban composition limits generalizability. The focus on emergency admissions introduces selection bias, excluding adolescents with less severe presentations who may not seek emergency care. This problem is likely to be particularly reflected when it comes to the composition of our control group, which also includes only patients who presented under emergency conditions. Thus, although it serves our objective of identifying those factors that cause only a proportion of severe psychiatric cases to resort to SB or NSSI, the inclusion of only these cases limits the comparability with non-emergency populations. Furthermore, the broad age range (6-18 years) used in the sample may obscure age-related differences in self-harm behaviors. Measurement error is also a concern, particularly in key variables, like family conflict, trauma, and the socioeconomic status, which were derived from clinical records and may not have been fully documented or consistently reported. Furthermore, another limitation of our study is that specialized questionnaires were not used to quantify the predictor variables, but only a series of predefined questions was used.

The use of both logistic regression and random forest models introduces inherent assumptions, such as the normality of residuals in regression, which may not have been fully met. While multicollinearity was not significant according to Variance Inflation Factors (VIFs), its potential influence on the logistic regression results cannot be ruled out. The subjective nature of hyperparameter selection in random forest models is another limitation, as this may impact model performance and stability.

Moreover, the pre- and post-pandemic comparison does not fully account for other socio-political or economic factors that could have influenced adolescent mental health. Attributing the observed changes solely to the pandemic risks oversimplification, especially when other external variables may have played a role. The specific impact of COVID-19 lockdown measures on access to mental health services, which could have contributed to changes in self-harm behaviors, was not addressed in the study.

The retrospective design prevents the drawing of definitive causal inferences, and observed associations may be influenced by unmeasured confounders. These limitations should be carefully considered when interpreting the findings. Future research utilizing prospective designs and standardized measures is needed to confirm and extend these results.

5. Conclusions

This retrospective cohort study examined the risk factors and clinical predictors of suicidal behavior (SB) and non-suicidal self-injury (NSSI) in adolescents presenting to a Romanian pediatric psychiatry emergency department, both before and after the COVID-19 pandemic. The study confirmed a high prevalence of both SB and NSSI among the adolescent sample, consistent with the existing literature. The most common methods of self-harm were cutting and scratching, with a significant increase in prevalence observed post-pandemic. Medication ingestion was the most frequent method for suicide attempts, also showing a notable post-pandemic rise.

Our analysis identified several critical individual, family, and environmental risk factors for both SB and NSSI, including depression, a history of self-harm behaviors, conduct disorder, sleep disorders, anxiety disorders, PTSD, borderline personality traits, family conflict, and exposure to potentially psycho-traumatic negative life events. Both logistic regression and random forest models proved effective in predicting SB and NSSI, with logistic regression offering higher R^2 values, while random forest provided valuable insights into the relative importance of various predictors. Notably, random forest highlighted the significance of variables, such as a history of suicide attempts and borderline personality traits—factors obscured by multicollinearity in logistic regression models.

The study also revealed significant shifts in adolescent self-harm behaviors following the COVID-19 pandemic, with increases in depression, suicidal ideation, and exposure to possible psycho-traumatic negative life events. These findings align with growing concerns about the pandemic's detrimental impact on adolescent mental health. Interestingly, we also observed lower rates of family and academic conflict, suggesting a complex interplay of pandemic-related factors that warrant further investigation.

These findings emphasize the need for comprehensive, multidisciplinary approaches to prevent, identify, and treat self-harm behaviors in adolescents. Such interventions should address not only individual-level factors, like depression, anxiety, and other mental health issues, but also the critical role of family and social environments. Early intervention, particularly for adolescents with a history of self-harm, is essential. Further research is needed to better understand the complex and evolving relationships among factors influencing adolescent mental health.

Future studies should focus on prospective longitudinal research to establish definitive causal relationships, expand the sample size to include more diverse populations to improve generalizability, and develop and evaluate culturally sensitive and effective preventive interventions. Additionally, further exploration into how specific pandemic-related factors impacted adolescent mental health and access to care is crucial.

Supplementary Materials: The following supporting information can be downloaded at: https://www.mdpi.com/article/10.3390/children12010081/s1, Table S1: Predictor variables used in the two regression models.; Table S2: Demographic characteristics of the whole sample of participants.; Table S3: Performance of Model 1 in predicting suicidal behaviors.; Table S4: Performance of Model 2 in predicting suicidal behaviors.; Table S5: Performance of Model 1 in predicting non-suicidal self-injurious behaviors.; Table S6: Performance of Model 2 in predicting non-suicidal self-injurious behaviors.; Table S7: Ranking of all variables used by the random forest model predicting suicidal behavior.; Table S8: Ranking of all variables used by the random forest model predicting NSSI.

Author Contributions: Conceptualization, R.Ș. and E.P.; methodology, R.Ș., T.V., and E.P.; software, T.V.; validation, R.Ș. and E.P.; formal analysis, T.V.; investigation, R.Ș., T.V., and E.P.; resources, R.Ș. and E.P.; data curation, R.Ș. and T.V.; writing—original draft preparation, R.Ș. and T.V.; writing—review and editing, R.Ș., T.V., and E.P.; visualization, T.V.; supervision, R.Ș. and E.P.; project administration, R.Ș. and E.P. All authors have read and agreed to the published version of the manuscript.

Funding: This research received no external funding.

Institutional Review Board Statement: The study adhered to the principles of the Declaration of Helsinki and received approval from the Emergency Clinical Hospital for Children Cluj-Napoca Clinical Trials Quality Assurance Commission (Approval No. 80/14.12.2020).

Informed Consent Statement: All participants provided informed consent for the use of their medical data for research purposes. Consent was obtained from patients and from their parents or legal guardians. Patients who exclusively utilized outpatient services, declined consent, or had incomplete medical records were excluded.

Data Availability Statement: Data are available on request due to privacy restrictions.

Conflicts of Interest: The authors declare no conflicts of interest.

References

1. American Psychiatric Association. *Diagnostic and Statistical Manual of Mental Disorders: DSM-5*, 5th ed.; American Psychiatric Association: Arlington, VA, USA, 2013; 947p.
2. Lloyd-Richardson, E.E.; Perrine, N.; Dierker, L.; Kelley, M.L. Characteristics and functions of non-suicidal self-injury in a community sample of adolescents. *Psychol. Med.* **2007**, *37*, 1183–1192. [CrossRef] [PubMed]
3. Plener, P.L.; Schumacher, T.S.; Munz, L.M.; Groschwitz, R.C. The longitudinal course of non-suicidal self-injury and deliberate self-harm: A systematic review of the literature. *Borderline Pers. Disord. Emot. Dysregulation* **2015**, *2*, 2. [CrossRef] [PubMed]
4. Lim, K.S.; Wong, C.H.; McIntyre, R.S.; Wang, J.; Zhang, Z.; Tran, B.X.; Tan, W.; Ho, C.S.; Ho, R.C. Global Lifetime and 12-Month Prevalence of Suicidal Behavior, Deliberate Self-Harm and Non-Suicidal Self-Injury in Children and Adolescents between 1989 and 2018: A Meta-Analysis. *Int. J. Environ. Res. Public Health* **2019**, *16*, 4581. [CrossRef]
5. Kaess, M.; Parzer, P.; Mattern, M.; Plener, P.L.; Bifulco, A.; Resch, F.; Brunner, R. Adverse childhood experiences and their impact on frequency, severity, and the individual function of nonsuicidal self-injury in youth. *Psychiatry Res.* **2013**, *206*, 265–272. [CrossRef] [PubMed]
6. Predescu, E.; Sipos, R. Self-Harm Behaviors, Suicide Attempts, and Suicidal Ideation in a Clinical Sample of Children and Adolescents with Psychiatric Disorders. *Children* **2023**, *10*, 725. [CrossRef] [PubMed]
7. Castellví, P.; Lucas-Romero, E.; Miranda-Mendizábal, A.; Parés-Badell, O.; Almenara, J.; Alonso, I.; Blasco, M.J.; Cebrià, A.; Gabilondo, A.; Gili, M.; et al. Longitudinal association between self-injurious thoughts and behaviors and suicidal behavior in adolescents and young adults: A systematic review with meta-analysis. *J. Affect. Disord.* **2017**, *215*, 37–48. [CrossRef] [PubMed]

8. Ribeiro, J.D.; Franklin, J.C.; Fox, K.R.; Bentley, K.H.; Kleiman, E.M.; Chang, B.P.; Nock, M.N. Self-injurious thoughts and behaviors as risk factors for future suicide ideation, attempts, and death: A meta-analysis of longitudinal studies. *Psychol. Med.* **2016**, *46*, 225–236. [CrossRef]
9. Borschmann, R.; Becker, D.; Coffey, C.; Spry, E.; Moreno-Betancur, M.; Moran, P.; Patton, G.C. 20-year outcomes in adolescents who self-harm: A population-based cohort study. *Lancet Child. Adolesc. Health.* **2017**, *1*, 195–202. [CrossRef] [PubMed]
10. Eadeh, H.M.; Breaux, R.; Nikolas, M.A. A Meta-Analytic Review of Emotion Regulation Focused Psychosocial Interventions for Adolescents. *Clin. Child. Fam. Psychol. Rev.* **2021**, *24*, 684–706. [CrossRef] [PubMed]
11. World Health Organization. *Suicide Worldwide in 2019: Global Health Estimates*; World Health Organization: Geneva, Switzerland, 2021. Available online: https://iris.who.int/bitstream/handle/10665/341728/9789240026643-eng.pdf?sequence=1 (accessed on 12 December 2024).
12. O'Connor, R.C.; Nock, M.K. The psychology of suicidal behaviour. *Lancet Psychiatry* **2014**, *1*, 73–85. [CrossRef]
13. Glenn, C.R.; Klonsky, E.D. Nonsuicidal Self-Injury Disorder: An Empirical Investigation in Adolescent Psychiatric Patients. *J. Clin. Child. Adolesc. Psychol.* **2013**, *42*, 496–507. [CrossRef] [PubMed]
14. Wichstrøm, L. Predictors of Non-Suicidal Self-Injury Versus Attempted Suicide: Similar or Different? *Arch. Suicide Res.* **2009**, *13*, 105–122. [CrossRef] [PubMed]
15. Fegert, J.M.; Vitiello, B.; Plener, P.L.; Clemens, V. Challenges and burden of the Coronavirus 2019 (COVID-19) pandemic for child and adolescent mental health: A narrative review to highlight clinical and research needs in the acute phase and the long return to normality. *Child. Adolesc. Psychiatry Ment. Health* **2020**, *14*, 20. [CrossRef]
16. Oosterhoff, B.; Palmer, C.A.; Wilson, J.; Shook, N. Adolescents' Motivations to Engage in Social Distancing During the COVID-19 Pandemic: Associations With Mental and Social Health. *J. Adolesc. Health* **2020**, *67*, 179–185. [CrossRef]
17. Guessoum, S.B.; Lachal, J.; Radjack, R.; Carretier, E.; Minassian, S.; Benoit, L.; Moro, M.R. Adolescent psychiatric disorders during the COVID-19 pandemic and lockdown. *Psychiatry Res.* **2020**, *291*, 113264. [CrossRef] [PubMed]
18. Hawes, M.T.; Szenczy, A.K.; Klein, D.N.; Hajcak, G.; Nelson, B.D. Increases in depression and anxiety symptoms in adolescents and young adults during the COVID-19 pandemic. *Psychol. Med.* **2022**, *52*, 3222–3230. [CrossRef] [PubMed]
19. Predescu, E.; Calugar, I.; Bibu-Monus, C.; Sipos, R. Trends and Prevalence of Hospital Admissions Related to Deliberate Self-Poisoning and Used Substances in Romanian Adolescents between 2016 and 2022. *Children* **2023**, *10*, 790. [CrossRef] [PubMed]
20. Racine, N.; McArthur, B.A.; Cooke, J.E.; Eirich, R.; Zhu, J.; Madigan, S. Global Prevalence of Depressive and Anxiety Symptoms in Children and Adolescents During COVID-19: A Meta-analysis. *JAMA Pediatr.* **2021**, *175*, 1142–1150. [CrossRef]
21. Warne, N.; Heron, J.; Mars, B.; Solmi, F.; Biddle, L.; Gunnell, D.; Hammerton, G.; Moran, P.; Munafò, M.; Penton-Voak, I.; et al. Emotional dysregulation in childhood and disordered eating and self-harm in adolescence: Prospective associations and mediating pathways. *J. Child. Psychol. Psychiatry* **2023**, *64*, 797–806. [CrossRef]
22. World Health Organization. *Mental Health Atlas 2020*; World Health Organization: Geneva, Switzerland, 2021.
23. Probst, P.; Wright, M.N.; Boulesteix, A. Hyperparameters and tuning strategies for random forest. *WIREs Data Min. Knowl. Discov.* **2019**, *9*, e1301. [CrossRef]
24. Șipoș, R.; Văidean, T.; Răpciuc, A.M.; Poetar, C.R.; Predescu, E. Analysing Digital Engagement Patterns: A Machine Learning Investigation into Social Anxiety Among Adolescents with ADHD. *J. Clin. Med.* **2024**, *13*, 7461. [CrossRef] [PubMed]
25. Hammen, C. Adolescent Depression: Stressful Interpersonal Contexts and Risk for Recurrence. *Curr. Dir. Psychol. Sci.* **2009**, *18*, 200–204. [CrossRef] [PubMed]
26. Kessler, R.C.; Berglund, P.; Demler, O.; Jin, R.; Merikangas, K.R.; Walters, E.E. Lifetime Prevalence and Age-of-Onset Distributions of DSM-IV Disorders in the National Comorbidity Survey Replication. *Arch. Gen. Psychiatry.* **2005**, *62*, 593–602. [CrossRef] [PubMed]
27. Fortune, S.; Cottrell, D.; Fife, S. Family factors associated with adolescent self-harm: A narrative review. *J. Fam. Ther.* **2016**, *38*, 226–256. [CrossRef]
28. Beesdo, K.; Knappe, S.; Pine, D.S. Anxiety and Anxiety Disorders in Children and Adolescents: Developmental Issues and Implications for DSM-V. *Psychiatr. Clin. N. Am.* **2009**, *32*, 483–524. [CrossRef]
29. Tanner, A.K.; Hasking, P.; Martin, G. Suicidality among adolescents engaging in nonsuicidal self-injury (NSSI) and firesetting: The role of psychosocial characteristics and reasons for living. *Child Adolesc. Psychiatry Ment. Health* **2015**, *9*, 33. [CrossRef] [PubMed]
30. Bilsen, J. Suicide and Youth: Risk Factors. *Front. Psychiatry.* **2018**, *9*, 540. [CrossRef] [PubMed]
31. Farooq, S.; Tunmore, J.; Wajid Ali, M.; Ayub, M. Suicide, self-harm and suicidal ideation during COVID-19: A systematic review. *Psychiatry Res.* **2021**, *306*, 114228. [CrossRef]
32. Gilsbach, S.; Herpertz-Dahlmann, B.; Konrad, K. Psychological Impact of the COVID-19 Pandemic on Children and Adolescents With and Without Mental Disorders. *Front. Public Health* **2021**, *9*, 679041. [CrossRef] [PubMed]

33. Cairns, R.; Karanges, E.A.; Wong, A.; Brown, J.A.; Robinson, J.; Pearson, S.A.; Dawson, A.H.; Buckley, N.A. Trends in self-poisoning and psychotropic drug use in people aged 5–19 years: A population-based retrospective cohort study in Australia. *BMJ Open* **2019**, *9*, e026001. [CrossRef] [PubMed]
34. McCabe, D.J.; Egan, H.M.; Theiler, C.A. The incidence of self-harm ingestions in adolescents and young adults at a tertiary care center. *Am. J. Emerg. Med.* **2023**, *63*, 50–54. [CrossRef]
35. Koppen, A.; Thoonen, I.M.J.; Hunault, C.C.; van Velzen, A.G.; de Lange, D.W.; Rietjens, S.J. Significant Increase in Deliberate Self-Poisonings Among Adolescents During the Second Year of the COVID-19 Pandemic. *J. Adolesc. Health* **2023**, *73*, 319–324. [CrossRef] [PubMed]
36. Mann, J.J.; Apter, A.; Bertolote, J.; Beautrais, A.; Currier, D.; Haas, A.; Hegerl, U.; Lonnqvist, J.; Malone, K.; Marusic, A.; et al. Suicide Prevention Strategies: A Systematic Review. *JAMA* **2005**, *294*, 2064–2074. [CrossRef]
37. Zalsman, G.; Hawton, K.; Wasserman, D.; van Heeringen, K.; Arensman, E.; Sarchiapone, M.; Carli, V.; Höschl, C.; Barzilay, R.; Balazs, J.; et al. Suicide prevention strategies revisited: 10-year systematic review. *Lancet Psychiatry* **2016**, *3*, 646–659. [CrossRef]
38. Barrocas, A.L.; Hankin, B.L.; Young, J.F.; Abela, J.R.Z. Rates of nonsuicidal self-injury in youth: Age, sex, and behavioral methods in a community sample. *Pediatrics* **2012**, *130*, 39–45. [CrossRef]
39. Deutz, M.H.F.; Geeraerts, S.B.; van Baar, A.L.; Deković, M.; Prinzie, P. The Dysregulation Profile in middle childhood and adolescence across reporters: Factor structure, measurement invariance, and links with self-harm and suicidal ideation. *Eur. Child Adolesc. Psychiatry* **2016**, *25*, 431–442. [CrossRef]
40. Fang, L.; Tong, Y.; Li, M.; Wang, C.; Li, Y.; Yuan, M.; Zhang, X.; Wang, G.; Wang, J.; Su, P. Anxiety in adolescents and subsequent risk of suicidal behavior: A systematic review and meta-analysis. *J. Affect. Disord.* **2024**, *358*, 97–104. [CrossRef] [PubMed]
41. McRae, E.; Stoppelbein, L.; O'Kelley, S.; Smith, S.; Fite, P. Pathways to Suicidal Behavior in Children and Adolescents: Examination of Child Maltreatment and Post-Traumatic Symptoms. *J. Child. Adolesc. Trauma* **2022**, *15*, 715–725. [CrossRef]
42. Eskander, N.; Vadukapuram, R.; Zahid, S.; Ashraf, S.; Patel, R.S. Post-traumatic Stress Disorder and Suicidal Behaviors in American Adolescents: Analysis of 159,500 Psychiatric Hospitalizations. *Cureus* **2020**, *12*, e8017. [CrossRef] [PubMed]
43. Miranda-Mendizabal, A.; Castellví, P.; Parés-Badell, O.; Alayo, I.; Almenara, J.; Alonso, I.; Blasco, M.J.; Cebrià, A.; Gabilondo, A.; Gili, M.; et al. Gender differences in suicidal behavior in adolescents and young adults: Systematic review and meta-analysis of longitudinal studies. *Int. J. Public Health* **2019**, *64*, 265–283. [CrossRef] [PubMed]
44. Nolen-Hoeksema, S. Emotion regulation and psychopathology: The role of gender. *Annu. Rev. Clin. Psychol.* **2012**, *8*, 161–187. [CrossRef] [PubMed]
45. Lee, J. Mental health effects of school closures during COVID-19. *Lancet Child Adolesc. Health* **2020**, *4*, 421. [CrossRef]
46. Zhang, C.; Ye, M.; Fu, Y.; Yang, M.; Luo, F.; Yuan, J.; Tao, Q. The Psychological Impact of the COVID-19 Pandemic on Teenagers in China. *J. Adolesc. Health.* **2020**, *67*, 747–755. [CrossRef] [PubMed]
47. Halicka-Masłowska, J.; Szewczuk-Bogusławska, M.; Rymaszewska, J.; Adamska, A.; Misiak, B. From Emotional Intelligence to Self-Injuries: A Path Analysis in Adolescents with Conduct Disorder. *Front. Psychiatry* **2021**, *11*, 556278. [CrossRef] [PubMed]
48. Tatnell, R.; Kelada, L.; Hasking, P.; Martin, G. Longitudinal Analysis of Adolescent NSSI: The Role of Intrapersonal and Interpersonal Factors. *J. Abnorm. Child Psychol.* **2014**, *42*, 885–896. [CrossRef] [PubMed]
49. Saccaro, L.F.; Giff, A.; De Rossi, M.M.; Piguet, C. Interventions targeting emotion regulation: A systematic umbrella review. *J. Psychiatr. Res.* **2024**, *174*, 263–274. [CrossRef]
50. Miao, R.; Liu, C.; Zhang, J.; Jin, H. Impact of the COVID-19 pandemic on the mental health of children and adolescents: A systematic review and meta-analysis of longitudinal studies. *J. Affect. Disord.* **2023**, *340*, 914–922. [CrossRef] [PubMed]
51. Golberstein, E.; Wen, H.; Miller, B.F. Coronavirus Disease 2019 (COVID-19) and Mental Health for Children and Adolescents. *JAMA Pediatr.* **2020**, *174*, 819–820. [CrossRef]
52. Xiong, J.; Lipsitz, O.; Nasri, F.; Lui, L.M.W.; Gill, H.; Phan, L.; Chen-Li, D.; Iacobucci, M.; Ho, R.; Majeed, A.; et al. Impact of COVID-19 pandemic on mental health in the general population: A systematic review. *J. Affect. Disord.* **2020**, *277*, 55–64. [CrossRef] [PubMed]
53. Mosheva, M.; Barzilai, Y.; Hertz-Palmor, N.; Mekori-Domachevsky, E.; Avinir, A.; Erez, G.; Vardi, N.; Schoen, G.; Lahav, T.; Sadeh, H.; et al. Child and Adolescent Mental Health during the COVID-19 Pandemic: Challenges of Psychiatric Outpatient Clinics. *Healthcare* **2023**, *11*, 765. [CrossRef]
54. Batchelor, R.; Catanzano, M.; Kerry, E.; Bennett, S.D.; Coughtrey, A.E.; Liang, H.; Curry, V.; Heyman, I.; Shafran, R. Debate: Lessons learned in lockdown—A one-day remotely delivered training on low-intensity psychological interventions for common mental health conditions. *Child Adolesc. Ment. Health* **2020**, *25*, 175–177. [CrossRef]
55. Barbieri, V.; Piccoliori, G.; Mahlknecht, A.; Plagg, B.; Ausserhofer, D.; Engl, A.; Wiedermann, C.J. Adolescent Mental Health during the COVID-19 Pandemic: The Interplay of Age, Gender, and Mental Health Outcomes in Two Consecutive Cross-Sectional Surveys in Northern Italy. *Behav. Sci.* **2023**, *13*, 643. [CrossRef]
56. Wang, S.; Chen, L.; Ran, H.; Che, Y.; Fang, D.; Sun, H.; Peng, J.; Liang, X.; Xiao, Y. Depression and anxiety among children and adolescents pre and post COVID-19: A comparative meta-analysis. *Front. Psychiatry* **2022**, *13*, 917552. [CrossRef]

57. Temple, J.R.; Baumler, E.; Wood, L.; Guillot-Wright, S.; Torres, E.; Thiel, M. The Impact of the COVID-19 Pandemic on Adolescent Mental Health and Substance Use. *J. Adolesc. Health* **2022**, *71*, 277–284. [CrossRef] [PubMed]
58. Pfefferbaum, B.; North, C.S. Mental Health and the Covid-19 Pandemic. *N. Engl. J. Med.* **2020**, *383*, 510–512. [CrossRef] [PubMed]
59. Kataoka, S.; Langley, A.; Wong, M.; Baweja, S.; Stein, B. Responding to Students with PTSD in Schools. *Child. Adolesc. Psychiatr. Clin. N. Am.* **2012**, *21*, 119–x. [CrossRef] [PubMed]
60. Păsărelu, C.R.; Dobrean, A.; Florean, I.S.; Predescu, E. Parental stress and child mental health: A network analysis of Romanian parents. *Curr. Psychol.* **2023**, *42*, 24275–24287. [CrossRef]
61. Zawilska, J.B.; Kuczyńska, K. Psychiatric and neurological complications of long COVID. *J. Psychiatr. Res.* **2022**, *156*, 349–360. [CrossRef]
62. Bakshi, S.; Tandon, U. Understanding barriers of telemedicine adoption: A study in North India. *Syst. Res. Behav. Sci.* **2022**, *39*, 128–142. [CrossRef]
63. Păsărelu, C.R.; David, D.; Dobrean, A.; Noje, A.; Roxana, Ș.; Predescu, E. ADHDCoach—A virtual clinic for parents of children with ADHD: Development and usability study. *Digit. Health* **2023**, *9*, 20552076231161963. [CrossRef] [PubMed]
64. Gili, M.; Castellví, P.; Vives, M.; de la Torre-Luque, A.; Almenara, J.; Blasco, M.J.; Cebrià, A.I.; Gabilondo, A.; Pérez-Ara, M.A.; A, M.-M.; et al. Mental disorders as risk factors for suicidal behavior in young people: A meta-analysis and systematic review of longitudinal studies. *J. Affect. Disord.* **2019**, *245*, 152–162. [CrossRef] [PubMed]
65. Klonsky, E.D.; Muehlenkamp, J.J. Self-injury: A research review for the practitioner. *J. Clin. Psychol.* **2007**, *63*, 1045–1056. [CrossRef] [PubMed]
66. García-Fernández, A.; Bobes-Bascarán, T.; Martínez-Cao, C.; González-Blanco, L.; Fernández-Fernández, J.; Zurrón-Madera, P.; Zazo, E.S.; Jiménez-Treviño, L.; García-Portilla, M.P.; Bobes, J.; et al. Psychological interventions for suicidal behavior in adolescents: A comprehensive systematic review. *Transl. Psychiatry* **2024**, *14*, 438. [CrossRef]
67. Chen, Y.; Xie, R.; Tan, D.; Wang, X.; Fan, R.; Li, W.; Ding, W. Bidirectional longitudinal relationships between victimization, resilience and suicidal ideation of adolescents. *Child Youth Serv. Rev.* **2023**, *154*, 107130. [CrossRef]
68. Kim, M.H.; Min, S.; Ahn, J.S.; An, C.; Lee, J. Association between high adolescent smartphone use and academic impairment, conflicts with family members or friends, and suicide attempts. *PLoS ONE* **2019**, *14*, e0219831. [CrossRef] [PubMed]
69. Graham, E.; Jordan, L.P. Migrant Parents and the Psychological Well-Being of Left-Behind Children in Southeast Asia. *J. Marriage Fam.* **2011**, *73*, 763–787. [CrossRef] [PubMed]
70. Račaitė, J.; Antia, K.; Winkler, V.; Lesinskienė, S.; Sketerskienė, R.; Maceinaitė, R.; Tracevskytė, I.; Dambrauskaitė, E.; Šurkienė, G. Emotional and behavioural problems of left behind children in Lithuania: A comparative analysis of youth self-reports and parent/caregiver reports using ASEBA. *Child. Adolesc. Psychiatry Ment. Health* **2024**, *18*, 33. [CrossRef] [PubMed]
71. Flouri, E.; Buchanan, A. Early father's and mother's involvement and child's later educational outcomes. *Br. J. Educ. Psychol.* **2004**, *74 Pt 2*, 141–153. [CrossRef] [PubMed]
72. Whitlock, J. Self-Injurious Behavior in Adolescents. *PLoS Med.* **2010**, *7*, e1000240. [CrossRef] [PubMed]
73. Bennardi, M.; McMahon, E.; Corcoran, P.; Griffin, E.; Arensman, E. Risk of repeated self-harm and associated factors in children, adolescents and young adults. *BMC Psychiatry* **2016**, *16*, 421. [CrossRef]
74. Witt, K.G.; Hetrick, S.E.; Rajaram, G.; Hazell, P.; Taylor Salisbury, T.L.; Townsend, E.; Hawton, K. Interventions for self-harm in children and adolescents. *Cochrane Database Syst. Rev.* **2021**, *2021*, CD013667.
75. Nock, M.K.; Joiner, T.E.; Gordon, K.H.; Lloyd-Richardson, E.; Prinstein, M.J. Non-suicidal self-injury among adolescents: Diagnostic correlates and relation to suicide attempts. *Psychiatry Res.* **2006**, *144*, 65–72. [CrossRef] [PubMed]
76. McEvoy, D.; Brannigan, R.; Cooke, L.; Butler, E.; Walsh, C.; Arensman, E.; Clarke, M. Risk and protective factors for self-harm in adolescents and young adults: An umbrella review of systematic reviews. *J. Psychiatr. Res.* **2023**, *168*, 353–380. [CrossRef]
77. Berny, L.M.; Mojekwu, F.; Nichols, L.M.; Tanner-Smith, E.E. Investigating the Interplay Between Mental Health Conditions and Social Connectedness on Suicide Risk: Findings from a Clinical Sample of Adolescents. *Child Psychiatry Hum. Dev.* **2024**. [CrossRef]
78. Beautrais, A.L. Risk factors for suicide and attempted suicide among young people. *Aust. N. Z. J. Psychiatry* **2000**, *34*, 420–436. [CrossRef]
79. Ruchkin, V.; Koposov, R.A.; Koyanagi, A.; Stickley, A. Suicidal Behavior in Juvenile Delinquents: The Role of ADHD and Other Comorbid Psychiatric Disorders. *Child Psychiatry Hum. Dev.* **2017**, *48*, 691–698. [CrossRef] [PubMed]
80. Kim, G.; Shin, J.; Kim, J.W. The mediating role of internalizing and externalizing symptoms in the relationship between childhood trauma and suicidality among adolescents: A structural equation model. *Child Adolesc. Psychiatry Ment. Health* **2021**, *15*, 79. [CrossRef] [PubMed]
81. Nock, M.K.; Hwang, I.; Sampson, N.A.; Kessler, R.C. Mental disorders, comorbidity and suicidal behavior: Results from the National Comorbidity Survey Replication. *Mol. Psychiatry* **2010**, *15*, 868–876. [CrossRef] [PubMed]
82. Hamza, C.A.; Stewart, S.L.; Willoughby, T. Examining the link between nonsuicidal self-injury and suicidal behavior: A review of the literature and an integrated model. *Clin. Psychol. Rev.* **2012**, *32*, 482–495. [CrossRef] [PubMed]

83. Hastie, T.; Tibshirani, R.; Friedman, J. Random Forests. In *The Elements of Statistical Learning: Data Mining, Inference, and Prediction*; Hastie, T., Tibshirani, R., Friedman, J., Eds.; Springer: New York, NY, USA, 2009; pp. 587–604. [CrossRef]
84. Bayman, E.O.; Dexter, F. Multicollinearity in Logistic Regression Models. *Anesth. Analg.* **2021**, *133*, 362. [CrossRef] [PubMed]
85. Blaha, Y.; Cavelti, M.; Lerch, S.; Steinhoff, A.; Koenig, J.; Kaess, M. Risk-taking and self-harm behaviors as markers of adolescent borderline personality disorder. *Eur. Child. Adolesc. Psychiatry* **2024**, *33*, 2743–2753. [CrossRef]
86. Gratz, K.L. Measurement of Deliberate Self-Harm: Preliminary Data on the Deliberate Self-Harm Inventory. *J. Psychopathol. Behav. Assess.* **2001**, *23*, 253–263. [CrossRef]
87. Liaw, A.; Wiener, M. Classification and Regression by random Forest. *R News* **2002**, *2*, 18–22. Available online: https://cran.r-project.org/doc/Rnews/Rnews_2002-3.pdf (accessed on 28 December 2024).
88. Breiman, L. Random Forests. *Mach. Learn.* **2001**, *45*, 5–32. [CrossRef]
89. James, G.; Witten, D.; Hastie, T.; Tibshirani, R. *An Introduction to Statistical Learning*; Springer Texts in Statistics; Springer: New York, NY, USA, 2013; Volume 103. Available online: http://link.springer.com/10.1007/978-1-4614-7138-7 (accessed on 28 December 2024).

children

MDPI

Article

Neurodevelopmental Disorders and Connective Tissue-Related Symptoms: An Exploratory Case-Control Study in Children

Leonardo Zoccante [1], Gianfranco Di Gennaro [2], Erika Rigotti [3], Marco Luigi Ciceri [4], Andrea Sbarbati [5] and Marco Zaffanello [3,*]

1 Azienda Ulss 9 Scaligera, 37122 Verona, Italy; leonardo.zoccante@aulss9.veneto.it
2 Science of Health Department, School of Medicine, Magna Graecia University of Catanzaro, 88100 Catanzaro, Italy; gianfranco.digennaro@unicz.it
3 Department of Surgery, Dentistry, Paediatrics and Gynaecology, University of Verona, 37126 Verona, Italy; erika.rigotti@aovr.veneto.it
4 Childhood, Adolescence, Families and Family Health Centers, Via Salvo d'Acquisto 7, 37122 Verona, Italy; marco.ciceri@aulss9.veneto.it
5 Department of Neurosciences, School of Medicine, Biomedicine and Movement Sciences, Anatomy and Histology Section, University of Verona, 37124 Verona, Italy; andrea.sbarbati@univr.it
* Correspondence: marco.zaffanello@univr.it

Abstract: Background/Objectives: Autism spectrum disorder (ASD), attention deficit hyperactivity disorder (ADHD), and Tourette syndrome (TS) are neurodevelopmental disorders (NDDs) with overlapping symptoms, suggesting a partially shared genetic origin. This study investigates the prevalence of connective tissue-related conditions in individuals with ASD, ADHD, or TS. **Methods**: A questionnaire was administered to families of 120 individuals with ASD, ADHD, or TS, collecting sociodemographic data and examining 10 types of disorders affecting various organs and systems. Statistical analyses were performed using STATA 16.0, with the significance level set at 5%. **Results**: Among the 120 patients, 48 had ASD, 36 had ADHD, and 36 had TS. Flat feet were significantly more common in individuals with ASD (52.1%; OR 7.20; $p < 0.001$), ADHD (52.8%; OR 6.73; $p = 0.001$), and TS (38.9%; OR 3.70; $p = 0.034$) compared to controls (13.6%). Hypersensitivity was more frequent in individuals with ASD (56.3%; OR 5.90; $p = 0.001$), ADHD (50.0%; OR 4.11; $p = 0.011$), and TS (58.3%; OR 5.35; $p = 0.003$) compared to controls (18.2%). Myopia and ptosis were more common in ADHD (30.6%). There was a possible trend towards orthodontic device use in TS (OR 3.20; $p = 0.076$). Flat feet and hypersensitivity were also common in fathers (31.0% and 36.4%, respectively), mothers (31.0% and 15.2%), and patients (43.8% and 55%). **Conclusions**: The findings of this study highlight the significant associations between ASD, ADHD, and TS and specific physical symptoms, such as flat feet, sensory hypersensitivity, and other connective tissue-related manifestations. The familial prevalence of these symptoms suggests a potential genetic underpinning, further supporting the hypothesis of shared aetiological pathways. These insights underscore the need for interdisciplinary research to explore the mechanisms linking neurodevelopmental and connective tissue disorders, aiming to improve diagnosis and management strategies.

Keywords: autism spectrum disorder; attention deficit hyperactivity disorder; connective tissue; neurodevelopmental disorders; Tourette syndrome

1. Introduction

Autistic spectrum disorder (ASD), attention deficit hyperactivity disorder (ADHD), and Tourette syndrome (TS) are neurodevelopmental disorders (NDDs) that typically emerge during childhood and persist throughout life. ASD is a complex developmental condition that affects how individuals interact, communicate, and behave. ADHD is an NDD characterised by persistent patterns of inattention, hyperactivity, and impulsivity. TS is a tic disorder involving involuntary, repetitive movements (motor tics) and sounds (vocal tics).

These conditions manifest in diverse ways, leading to impairments in personal, social, academic, and occupational functioning [1,2]. The aetiopathogenesis of these disorders is thought to involve a complex interplay of genetic, epigenetic, and environmental factors. Extensive research into the heritability of NDDs suggests that a substantial proportion of phenotypic variance can be attributed to genetic influences [3,4]. Notably, certain genes associated with ASD have also been implicated in ADHD and TS [4].

Although ASD, ADHD, and TS are traditionally viewed as distinct conditions, differences in the timing of abnormal neurodevelopment and, more importantly, the neural circuits involved distinguish these disorders [5]. However, emerging evidence indicates they may share partially overlapping genetic factors [4,6]. Specific genes and genetic regions have been identified that appear to contribute to a shared genetic predisposition for ASD, ADHD, and TS [4]. This genetic overlap is further supported by the significant symptomatological similarities among these disorders, which include attentional difficulties, impulsivity, repetitive or ritualistic behaviours, deficits in communication and social interaction, obsessive traits, anxiety disorders, and abnormalities in sensory processing [1,4,7].

Moreover, ASD, ADHD, and TS seem to exhibit overlapping neuropathological mechanisms. These disorders share features such as long-range underconnectivity and short-range overconnectivity in brain networks, reflecting similar patterns of neural dysfunction [8]. Long-range underconnectivity refers to weak connections between distant brain regions [9]. Conversely, short-range overconnectivity describes enhanced connections within local brain regions [10]. This pattern reflects distinct neural dysfunctions that can manifest across different conditions. Consequently, it has been hypothesised that ASD, ADHD, and TS may represent a spectrum of related neurodevelopmental disorders, collectively termed "abnormal connectivity spectrum disorders" [11].

Connective tissue diseases are a group of disorders impacting structures such as tendons, ligaments, cartilage, and the extracellular matrix. Several symptoms have a potential association with connective tissue disorders. Chronic fatigue and muscle pain are prevalent in autoimmune diseases and connective tissue disorders [12]. The excessive sweating of hands and feet can be associated with connective tissue disorders [13,14]. Gastrointestinal symptoms (constipation and diarrhoea) are often seen in connective tissue disorders [15,16]. Hypersensitivity to sensory stimuli, including tactile, visual, and auditory inputs, is linked to various connective tissue disorders, such as Ehlers–Danlos syndrome. Sensory processing differences are observed in approximately 90% of individuals with ASD, particularly in response to tactile stimuli. Recent research using ASD mouse models has shed light on the neurobiological mechanisms underlying these sensory alterations [17].

In addition, connective tissue plays a crucial role in supporting the structure and function of the nervous system [18]. The interaction between brain network connectivity disorders and connective tissue abnormalities suggests the existence of a complex relationship in which structural issues may influence functional outcomes [19]. A recent study utilising in vivo confocal microscopy revealed significant changes in the corneal connective tissue structure of adults with ASD compared to typically developing controls [20]. A broader perspective on the central and peripheral connectivity alterations characterising NDDs is proposed through the "Connectivome Theory" [21]. This theory underscores the role of connective tissue in various organs, highlighting its multifunctional properties, including structural support, connection, nourishment, regulation, and modulation among different cellular elements. Therefore, abnormalities in glial function or extracellular matrix composition and alterations in connective tissue can hinder proper neuronal wiring [22].

The primary objective of this study is to examine the prevalence of pathologies associated with connective tissue alterations in individuals diagnosed with ASD, ADHD, or TS and to compare these findings with those from a healthy control group. A secondary aim is to evaluate whether these symptoms are observed at a significant rate among the parents of affected individuals.

2. Materials and Methods

The questionnaire (see Appendix A), designed to investigate symptoms associated with connective tissue disorders, was administered to the families of 120 individuals diagnosed with NDDs, specifically ASD, ADHD, and TS, as well as to a control group attending the Child and Adolescent Neuropsychiatry Outpatient Clinics at the University Hospital of Verona, Italy.

The data collection period spanned from December 2019 to January 2022. Parents or caregivers actively participated in the study by responding to structured questionnaires, contributing to data acquisition.

This study was approved by the Ethical Committee of the University Hospital of Verona under the following codes: CESC 2243 (Paediatric Clinic, University Hospital of Verona) and CESC 2242 (Child and Adolescent Neuropsychiatry Outpatient Clinics, University Hospital of Verona). Written informed consent was obtained from each participant's parents.

The questionnaire gathered sociodemographic data and assessed the presence of 18 symptom categories in both the patients and their parents. These categories were as follows:

- Varicose veins, vasculitis, and haemorrhoids;
- Striae rubrae, skin irregularities, or redness;
- Excessive sweating of the hands and feet;
- Joint inflammation and rheumatism;
- Joint dislocations and subluxations/dislocations;
- Joint pain involving 1 to 3 large joints lasting for more than 3 months;
- Back pain, transient muscle pain in the limbs, or chronic fatigue;
- Hip dysplasia, scoliosis, or kyphosis;
- Inguinal, umbilical, abdominal, or disc hernias;
- Flat feet;
- Constipation, diarrhoea, or alternating bowel patterns;
- Heartburn, gastroesophageal reflux, or hiatal hernia;
- Use of orthodontic appliances;
- Tactile, visual, auditory, olfactory, or gustatory hypersensitivity;
- Myopia or drooping eyelids, including unilateral or bilateral ptosis;
- Immune and/or autoimmune diseases.

The same questionnaire was also administered to a control group comprising 44 families with typically developing, healthy children attending the clinic.

Statistical Analysis

Continuous Gaussian variables were summarised as mean values with standard deviations (S.D.). Categorical variables were described using counts and percentages.

The presence of symptoms was compared across controls, TS, ASD, and ADHD groups using logistic regression models. In these models, the dependent variable was the presence of the symptom, while case–control status served as the independent variable. Age and sex were included as covariates to adjust the estimates.

To address issues of separation and potential convergence difficulties caused by the low prevalence of certain symptoms, Firth's penalised maximum likelihood method was employed in the logistic regression analyses [23,24].

Statistical analyses were conducted using the STATA 16.0 software package (www.stata.com). A significance threshold of 5% was applied for all statistical tests.

3. Results

A total of 164 participants were included in the study. Of these, 44 (26.8%) were healthy controls, while the remaining 120 (73.2%) were cases: there were 48 (29.3%) with ASD, 36 (22.0%) with ADHD, and 36 (22.0%) with TS. The mean age of the cases was 10.1 years (S.D.: 3.6), compared to the 9.5 years (S.D.: 2.5) observed for the controls.

The control group was evenly distributed by sex, with 22 males (50.0%) and 22 females (50.0%). In contrast, most cases were male, comprising 110 participants (91.7%).

The analysis presented in Table 1 demonstrates that flat feet are significantly more prevalent among individuals with ASD (52.1%), ADHD (52.8%), and TS (38.9%) compared to the control group (13.6%), indicating a strong association with the NDDs under investigation. Heartburn, gastro-oesophageal reflux, and hiatus hernia are notably more frequent in individuals with TS (27.8%) relative to the other groups. Similarly, the use of orthodontic appliances is more common in subjects with TS (41.7%) compared to the other cohorts. Hypersensitivity is markedly more prevalent in individuals with ASD (56.3%), ADHD (50.0%), and TS (58.3%) compared to controls (18.2%), further supporting the existence of a strong correlation with the NDDs included in the study. Additionally, myopia and ptosis are observed more frequently in individuals with ADHD (30.6%) compared to the other groups (Table 1, Figure 1).

Table 1. The table shows the prevalence of symptoms in four groups: ASD (autism spectrum disorder), ADHD (attention deficit hyperactivity disorder), TS (Tourette syndrome), and controls (individuals without specific diagnoses). The data are expressed as the percentage of affected individuals in each group and the percentage variation (Δ%) compared to the controls.

Symptoms	ASD (%)	Δ%	ADHD (%)	Δ%	TS (%)	Δ%	Controls (%)
Hypertension	0.0	0	0.0	0	2.8	2.8	0.0
Varicose veins/vasculitis/haemorrhoids	2.1	2.1	0.0	0	0.0	0	0.0
Striae rubrae/skin irregularities/reddened skin	4.2	−7.2	13.9	2.5	11.1	−0.3	11.4
Excessive sweating of hands and feet	14.6	5.5	22.2	13.1	22.2	13.1	9.1
Joint inflammation/rheumatism	2.1	2.1	2.8	2.8	5.6	5.6	0.0
Joint dislocations/subluxations/dislocations	2.1	2.1	2.8	2.8	5.6	5.6	0.0
Joint pain involving 1 to 3 large joints lasting for more than 3 months	2.1	−0.2	5.6	3.3	2.8	0.5	2.3
Back pain/transient muscle pain in the limbs/chronic fatigue	4.2	−14	22.2	4	16.7	−1.5	18.2
Hip dysplasia/scoliosis/curved back	6.3	−2.8	8.3	−0.8	11.1	2	9.1
Inguinal/umbilical, abdominal, or disc hernias	2.1	−2.4	0.0	−4.5	8.3	3.8	4.5

Table 1. *Cont.*

Symptoms	ASD (%)	Δ%	ADHD (%)	Δ%	TS (%)	Δ%	Controls (%)
Flat feet	52.1	38.5	52.8	39.2	38.9	25.3	13.6
Constipation/diarrhoea/alternating bowel	16.7	5.3	11.1	−0.3	13.9	2.5	11.4
Heartburn/gastroesophageal reflux/hiatal hernia	14.6	7.8	5.6	−1.2	27.8	21	6.8
Rectal or uterine prolapse/urinary and/or faecal incontinence	4.2	4.2	2.8	2.8	0.0	0	0.0
Use of orthodontic appliances	20.8	2.6	30.6	12.4	41.7	23.5	18.2
Tactile/visual/auditory/olfactory or gustatory hypersensibility	56.3	38.1	50.0	31.8	58.3	34.8	18.2
Myopia or drooping eyelids/unilateral or bilateral eyelid ptosis	8.3	6	30.6	28.3	13.9	11.6	2.3
Immune and/or autoimmune diseases	0.0	−4.5	0.0	0	0.0	0	4.5

Legend: Δ%, percentage variation in each symptom compared to the controls.

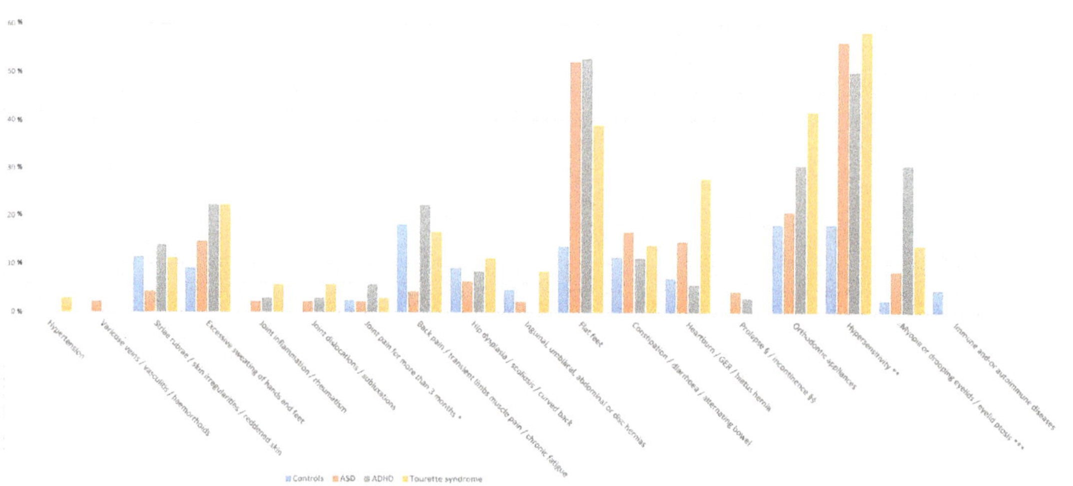

Figure 1. The bar graph illustrates the percentage prevalence of symptoms among children in the control group and those with neurodevelopmental disorders, including autism spectrum disorder, attention deficit hyperactivity disorder, and Tourette syndrome. The categories are colour-coded as follows: ASD (orange), ADHD (green), Tourette syndrome (yellow), and controls (blue). Abbreviations: * Joint pain involving 1 to 3 large joints lasting for more than 3 months; **, Tactile/visual/auditory/olfactory or gustatory hypersensibility; ***, Myopia or drooping eyelids/unilateral or bilateral eyelid ptosis.

The analysis in Table 2 indicates that individuals with ASD exhibit a lower tendency to experience back pain, transient muscle pain in the limbs, and chronic fatigue (OR 0.25; 95% CI: 0.053–1.16; p = 0.076). The data also reveal a strong association between flat feet and various NDDs, including ADHD (OR 6.73; 95% CI: 2.097–21.63; p = 0.001), ASD (OR 7.20; 95% CI: 2.438–21.23; $p < 0.001$), and TS (OR 3.70; 95% CI: 1.107–12.34; p = 0.034). Additionally, there is a potential trend towards the increased use of orthodontic appliances in TS (OR 3.20; 95% CI: 0.887–11.51; p = 0.076).

Table 2. The table presents the results of the regression analysis used to assess the association between symptoms and autism spectrum disorder, attention deficit hyperactivity disorder, and Tourette syndrome.

Symptoms	ASD (OR, 95% CI)	p Value (ASD)	ADHD (OR, 95% CI)	p Value (ADHD)	TS (OR, 95% CI)	p Value (TS)
Hypertension	2.19 (0.021–228.08)	0.740	1.86 (0.011–306.46)	0.812	4.90 (0.033–734.81)	0.534
Varicose veins/vasculitis/haemorrhoids	3.58 (0.069–185.13)	0.526	1.26 (0.011–143.97)	0.924	1.09 (0.009–135.69)	0.973
Striae rubrae/skin irregularities/reddened skin	0.34 (0.062–1.91)	0.222	0.81 (0.188–3.45)	0.771	0.52 (0.107–2.54)	0.419
Excessive sweating of hands and feet	1.78 (0.451–7.01)	0.411	2.12 (0.523–8.56)	0.293	1.79 (0.422–7.62)	0.429
Joint inflammation/rheumatism	2.61 (0.065–105.07)	0.610	2.43 (0.059–99.60)	0.639	3.40 (0.082–141.57)	0.520
Joint dislocations/subluxations	2.79 (0.075–104.34)	0.578	3.10 (0.071–134.14)	0.557	4.82 (0.116–201.07)	0.409
Joint pain involving 1 to 3 large joints for more than 3 months	1.14 (0.083–15.65)	0.922	1.79 (0.151–21.20)	0.645	0.90 (0.053–15.23)	0.942
Back pain/transient muscle pain in the limbs/chronic fatigue	0.25 (0.053–1.16)	0.076	1.21 (0.353–4.12)	0.765	0.82 (0.211–3.15)	0.769
Hip dysplasia/scoliosis/ curved back	0.91 (0.170–4.92)	0.915	0.84 (0.151–4.69)	0.846	0.99 (0.176–5.55)	0.988
Inguinal, umbilical, abdominal or disc hernias	0.55 (0.060–5.03)	0.596	0.18 (0.007–4.70)	0.306	1.21 (0.150–9.71)	0.860
Flat feet	7.20 (2.438–21.23)	<0.001	6.73 (2.097–21.63)	0.001	3.70 (1.107–12.34)	0.034
Constipation/diarrhoea/ alternating bowel	2.07 (0.579–7.44)	0.263	1.45 (0.325–6.49)	0.625	1.85 (0.414–8.28)	0.421
Heartburn/gastroesophageal reflux/hiatus hernia	1.92 (0.460–7.98)	0.372	0.63 (0.105–3.75)	0.609	3.05 (0.697–13.37)	0.138
Rectal or uterine prolapse/urinary and/or faecal incontinence	4.34 (0.144–131.51)	0.399	2.58 (0.068–97.84)	0.609	0.71 (0.009–56.36)	0.880
Use of orthodontic appliances	2.02 (0.602–6.77)	0.255	2.36 (0.650–8.57)	0.192	3.20 (0.887–11.51)	0.076
Tactile, visual, auditory, olfactory or gustatory hypersensitivity	5.90 (2.160–16.12)	0.001	4.11 (1.385–12.19)	0.011	5.35 (1.738–16.47)	0.003
Myopia or drooping eyelids/unilateral or bilateral eyelid ptosis	3.18 (0.433–23.37)	0.255	13.12 (1.859–92.56)	0.010	5.01 (0.615–40.81)	0.132
Immune and/or autoimmune diseases	0.38 (0.018–8.18)	0.537	0.30 (0.010–9.11)	0.488	0.38 (0.011–13.29)	0.594

Legend: CI, confidence interval; OR, odds ratio; TS, Tourette syndrome. Yellow colour: statistically significant.

A significant association between hypersensitivity and NDDs was also identified. Individuals with hypersensitivity demonstrate a higher propensity for ADHD (OR 4.11; 95% CI: 1.385–12.19; $p = 0.011$), ASD (OR 5.90; 95% CI: 2.160–16.12; $p = 0.001$), and TS (OR 5.35; 95% CI: 1.738–16.47; $p = 0.003$), confirming that there is a robust association between hypersensitivity and these disorders. Finally, the analysis revealed that there was a significant association between myopia or eyelid ptosis and ADHD (OR 13.12; 95% CI: 1.859–92.56; $p = 0.01$).

Given that both flat feet and hypersensitivity were more prevalent in each NDD under investigation, we performed a familial analysis across the entire cohort of parents (Table 3; Figure 2). Flat feet were common (OR 8.3) among fathers (31.0%), mothers (31.0%), and patients (43.8%; $p < 0.001$). The symptoms of tactile, visual, auditory, olfactory, or gustatory hypersensitivity were more frequent (OR 3.31) among fathers (36.4%) compared to mothers (15.2%) and were associated with a high prevalence of the symptoms in patients (55%; $p = 0.006$).

Table 3. The table presents a comparative analysis of the percentage distribution of symptoms among all patients, their fathers, and their mothers, alongside the statistical significance of the observed associations.

Symptoms		Controls	Overall Patients (ASD + ADHD + TS)	Father's Patients	Mother's Patients	Statistical Analysis		
		n (%)	*n* (%)	*n* (%)	*n* (%)	OR	*p*-Value	*p*-Overall
Totals		44	120					
Striae rubrae/skin irregularities/reddened skin	absent	39 (88.6)	109 (90.8)	15 (13.8)	7 (6.4)	2.44	0.206	0.330
	present	55 (11.4)	11 (9.2)	5 (45.5)	0 (0)			
Excessive sweating of hands and feet	absent	40 (90.9)	97 (80.8)	11 (11.3)	10 (10.3)	1.49	0.480	0.299
	present	4 (9.1)	23 (19.2)	4 (17.4)	2 (8.7)			
Back pain/transient muscle pain in the limbs/ chronic fatigue	absent	36 (81.8)	110 (91.7)	21 (19.1)	19 (17.3)	2.08	0.283	0.862
	present	8 (18.2)	10 (8.3)	3 (30.0)	3 (30.0)			
Flat feet	absent	38 (86.4)	62 (51.7)	5 (8.1)	4 (4.5)	8.3	<0.001	<0.001
	present	6 (13.6)	58 (48.3)	18 (31.0)	18 (31.0)			
Constipation/diarrhoea/ abdominal discomfort	absent	39 (88.6)	103 (85.8)	23 (22.3)	8 (7.8)	3.01	0.041	0.302
	present	55 (11.4)	17 (14.2)	8 (47.1)	4 (23.5)			
Heartburn/gastroesophageal reflux/hiatus hernia	absent	41 (93.2)	101 (84.2)	33 (32.7)	25 (24.8)	1.68	0.344	0.389
	present	3 (6.8)	19 (15.8)	9 (47.4)	6 (31.6)			
Use of orthodontic appliances	absent	36 (81.8)	84 (70.0)	23 (27.4)	10 (11.9)	1.48	0.372	0.109
	present	8 (18.2)	36 (30.0)	12 (33.3)	10 (27.8)			
Tactile, visual, auditory, olfactory or gustatory hypersensitivity	absent	36 (81.8)	54 (45.0)	8 (14.8)	3 (5.6)	3.31	0.006	<0.001
	present	8 (18.2)	66 (55.0)	24 (36.4)	10 (15.2)			
Myopia or drooping eyelids/unilateral or bilateral eyelid ptosis	absent	43 (97.7)	100 (83.3)	28 (28.0)	26 (26.0)	1.27	0.635	0.059
	present	1 (2.3)	20 (16.7)	9 (45.0)	6 (30.0)			

Legend: ASD, autism spectrum disorder; ADHD, attention deficit hyperactivity disorder; NDDs, neurodevelopmental disorders; OR, odds ratio; TS, Tourette's syndrome. Yellow colour: statistically significant; green colour: borderline significance ($0.05 < p < 0.100$).

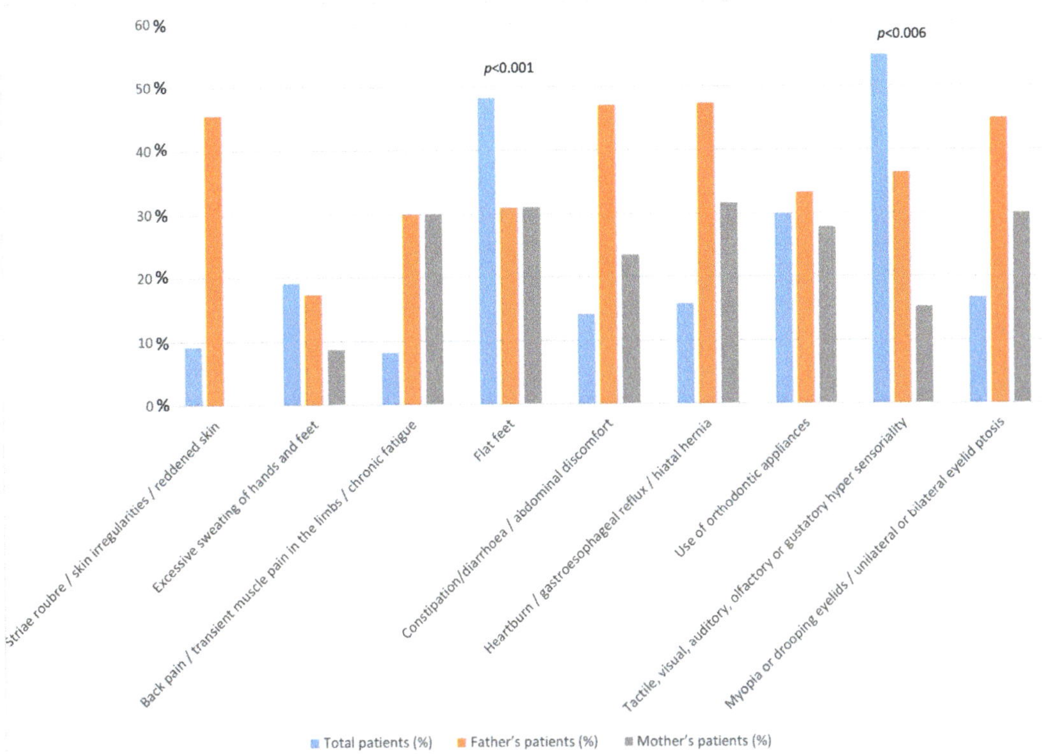

Figure 2. The figure presents the percentage distribution of symptoms among all patients, their fathers, and their mothers. The statistically positive significance of the observed associations is shown.

4. Discussion

In our study, we identified a strong association between flat feet, hypersensitivity, and the neuropsychiatric conditions of ASD, ADHD, and TS. The use of orthodontic appliances was more frequent in individuals with TS, and myopia and ptosis were notably prevalent in those with ADHD. Additionally, flat feet and hypersensitivity were more common among the parents affected by the NDDs under investigation.

Recent studies have indicated that there is a potential link between NDDs and connective tissue-related symptoms. The underlying mechanisms linking NDDs and connective tissue-related symptoms may involve immune dysregulation, chronic inflammation, and vascular issues that impact brain function [25,26]. For example, a condition characterised by cognitive and behavioural challenges and notable physical features linked to connective tissue disorders is Fragile X Syndrome. Individuals with Fragile X Syndrome often exhibit distinct physical traits associated with connective tissue dysregulation, such as joint hypermobility, hyperextensible skin, and increased tissue fragility [27,28].

Our findings revealed a significantly higher prevalence of flat feet in individuals with ASD (52.1%), ADHD (52.8%), and TS (38.9%) compared to the control group (13.6%). In a study analysing children aged 3 to 10 years, the overall prevalence of flat feet was reported to be 15.7% [29]. A systematic review indicated that the detection rate of flat feet in children over the past two decades was approximately 25% [30]. Previous research indicated that 52–53% of children with ADHD had exhibit mild to severe flat feet, in contrast to only 8–13% of their typically developing peers [31].

The causes of flat feet can be categorised as either congenital or acquired, but identifying the specific aetiology in paediatric cases is challenging. Flat feet may present as an isolated condition or as part of a broader syndrome [32]. For instance, certain congenital disorders, including Ehlers–Danlos syndrome, are characterised by both flat feet and NDDs due to underlying connective tissue abnormalities [33]. Notably, genetic syndromes impacting connective tissue, such as Marfan syndrome and Ehlers–Danlos syndrome, are linked to neurodevelopmental challenges and mitral cardiovascular issues, including valve prolapse and aortic aneurysms [34–36]. The shared pathophysiological mechanism underlines the clinical overlap between connective tissue anomalies and associated cardiovascular complications.

In connective tissues, elastic fibres play a crucial role in the extracellular matrix, contributing to the elasticity and resilience of tissues. These fibres give connective tissues elasticity and resilience [37]. Although no direct evidence links flat feet to alterations in the extracellular matrix, the structural integrity of the foot is mainly dependent on connective tissues, primarily composed of extracellular matrix components.

In our study, we observed that hypersensitivity was significantly more prevalent in individuals with TS (58.3%; OR 5.35, 95% CI 1.738–16.47), ASD (56.3%; OR 5.9, 95% CI 2.160–16.12), and ADHD (50.0%; OR 4.11, 95% CI 1.385–12.19) compared to controls (18.2%). In a representative sample of elementary school-aged children (ages 7–11), 16% of parents reported that their children had at least four tactile or auditory sensations [38]. Among children with ASD, the prevalence of sensory abnormalities was significantly higher at 53.6% compared to 8.0% in non-ASD children [39].

In the context of ASD, hypersensitivity refers to an increased sensitivity to stimuli such as sound, light, touch, taste, and smell. Research has suggested that this heightened sensitivity is associated with abnormalities in glial cells, which may disrupt the development of the myelin sheath, leading to delays in response times [40,41]. There is a substantial body of literature supporting the association between sensory alterations and ASD [21,42–44]. Tactile hypersensitivity and auditory hypersensitivity have been identified as predictors of an ASD diagnosis [39]. Moreover, connective tissue plays a crucial role in the structure and function of the outer, middle, and inner ear and the central auditory pathways.

In our study, myopia and ptosis were more prevalent in subjects with ADHD (30.6%; OR 13.12, 95% CI 1.859–92.56) compared to those with TS (13.9%) and ASD (8.3%) and compared to controls (2.3%). A systematic review covering data from 2000 to 2022 reported the overall pooled prevalence of childhood myopia was 5.2% [45].

Previous studies have not identified a significant association between myopia and ptosis [46]. However, individuals with ASD often exhibit defects in oculomotor activity and the pupillary sphincter response to the light reflex [47] and frequently display refractive deficits [48]. The most common ocular issues in ASD include difficulties with eye alignment (convergence insufficiency) and refractive errors [44]. The connective tissue in the eyes plays a crucial role in supporting the blood vessels and nerves that comprise the retina [49]. Additionally, the corneal–scleral framework primarily comprises connective tissue [49,50].

The use of orthodontic appliances was more common in individuals with TS (41.7%) compared to other groups and controls (OR 3.20, 95% CI 0.887–11.51). A study conducted in Germany revealed that approximately 33.5% of children aged 11–14 years were undergoing orthodontic treatment [51]. In Denmark, a retrospective study indicated that 27% of children were undergoing orthodontic appliance therapy [52]. Factors influencing treatment frequency included age, gender, and socio-economic status.

Orthodontic appliances (oral orthotics, occlusal splints) have been investigated as potential treatments for reducing tics in individuals with TS. Some studies have explored the use of customised oral splints and dental orthodontic devices to manage tics [53,54]. In recent years, reports have suggested that dental orthodontic devices, typically used for treating temporomandibular joint (TMJ) disorders, may also effectively reduce tics when worn by individuals with TS [54].

Family history is strongly associated with the risk of ASD. The individual risk of ASD increases with closer genetic relationships [3]. A reanalysis of a previous study on the familial risk of ASD estimated that 83% of the risk could be attributed to genetic factors, suggesting that genetics play a pivotal role in the development of ASD [55]. In the familial analysis of our study, which included patients diagnosed with ASD, ADHD, and TS, flat feet were observed frequently in fathers (31%), mothers (31%), and patients (48.3%). Sensory hypersensitivity, which was commonly observed in patients (55%), was more prevalent in fathers (24%) compared to mothers (10%). Myopia and ptosis, which were present in 16.7% of the patients, were more frequently found in fathers (45%) than in mothers (30%). To date, the search results have not provided specific data regarding the prevalence of hypersensitivity and flat feet in the parents of children with NDDs.

The recent literature suggests that ptosis, myopia, and flat feet can manifest as features of connective tissue disorders. Flat feet have been found to be significantly more prevalent in individuals with ASD, while myopia and ptosis are more common among children with ADHD. Additionally, the use of orthodontic appliances has been observed to be more frequently in individuals with TS, which may be linked to underlying connective tissue abnormalities. Notably, orthodontic appliance use has been associated with connective tissue disorders, particularly in conditions like Ehlers–Danlos syndrome [56]. These findings indicate that ptosis, flat feet, and the use of orthodontic appliances, as potential manifestations of connective tissue disorders, may have significant genetic and phenotypic overlaps with specific NDDs.

In the context of ASD, ADHD, and TS, abnormalities in connective tissue may represent a shared underlying factor. This hypothesis is supported by emerging research that underscores the interconnectedness of these NDDs through physical manifestations [57,58].

Official symmetry refers to the balanced arrangement of features, which is significant in understanding neurodevelopmental disorders (NDDs) such as ASD, ADHD, and TS [59]. Research highlights the role of brain symmetry in diagnosing and treating these disorders [59], linking structural abnormalities to symptom severity [60]. Associations between NDDs and physical traits, like flat feet and hypersensitivity, underscore the need to explore genetic and developmental pathways to achieve better outcomes [61,62]. This holistic perspective integrates behavioural and physical characteristics as interconnected aspects of NDDs.

Several limitations may affect the validity and generalisability of the present study. The small sample size of each NDD subgroup and the gender imbalance may introduce bias into the results. Clinic-based recruitment could lead to selection bias, and the control group may not represent the general population. Additionally, reliance on self-reported questionnaires without evaluating their reliability and validity may result in recall bias. The subjective nature of some symptoms also lacks clinical verification. The use of multiple testing increases the risk of false positives. This study does not account for all potential confounders, and its cross-sectional design prevents the establishment of causal inferences. Furthermore, while the familial analysis suggests a genetic component, it is limited by the absence of genetic testing.

Finally, our study did not directly compare the prevalence of physical findings, such as flat feet, between individuals with NDDs and the general population. This limits the generalizability of our findings. Future research should focus on direct comparative analyses to clarify these associations.

5. Conclusions

In conclusion, the study identified significant associations between certain NDDs (ASD, ADHD, and TS) and physical symptoms, such as flat feet and sensory hypersensitivity. These symptoms were also frequently observed in parents, suggesting the existence of a strong familial component. This finding implies that overlapping aetiological factors may manifest in various ways, with connective tissue abnormalities potentially serving as a common underlying factor. Further research is required to confirm and expand upon these findings.

Author Contributions: Conceptualisation, L.Z. and M.L.C.; methodology, G.D.G.; software, G.D.G.; validation, L.Z. and M.Z.; formal analysis, G.D.G.; investigation, L.Z. and M.L.C.; resources, L.Z.; data curation, M.Z. and E.R.; writing—original draft preparation, M.Z.; writing—review and editing, A.S., M.L.C. and E.R.; visualisation, A.S. and E.R.; supervision, L.Z. All authors have read and agreed to the published version of the manuscript.

Funding: This research received no external funding.

Institutional Review Board Statement: The study was approved by the Ethical Committee of the University Hospital of Verona: CESC 2243 (Pediatric Clinic, University Hospital of Verona) and CESC 2242 (Child and Adolescent Neuropsychiatry Outpatient Clinics, University Hospital of Verona) on 10 December 2019.

Informed Consent Statement: Written informed consent was obtained from each participant's parents.

Data Availability Statement: Data are unavailable due to privacy and ethical restrictions.

Acknowledgments: We thank Antonio Maria Persico for the helpful discussion.

Conflicts of Interest: The authors declare no conflicts of interest.

Appendix A

Questionnaire used for the study, in English language and Italian language.

Paediatric Laxity Questionnaire

Subject's gender:
Male
Female
Subject's diagnosis:
Autism
ADHD
Tourette's syndrome
Control
How many brothers does the subject have?
How many sisters does the subject have?
Has the child or their parents had high blood pressure on two or three occasions?
Has the child or their parents had varicose veins, vasculitis, or haemorrhoids?
Has the child or their parents had stretch marks, skin discolouration, or unexplained reddened skin?
Has the child or their parents had excessive sweating of the palms and/or soles of the feet?
Has the child or their parents had joint inflammation or rheumatism (bursitis, tenosynovitis, etc.)?
Has the child or their parents had dislocations, subluxations, or luxation of one or more joints on more than one occasion?
Has the child or their parents had joint pain involving 1 to 3 large joints for more than 3 months?

Has the child or their parents had back pain, transient muscle aches in the limbs (e.g., growing pains), or symptoms of chronic fatigue?
Has the child or their parents had hip dysplasia, scoliosis, or a curved spine?
Has the child or their parents had inguinal, umbilical, or abdominal hernias, or herniated discs?
Has the child or their parents had flat feet?
Has the child or their parents had constipation, diarrhoea, or alternating bowel habits?
Has the child or their parents had heartburn, gastro-oesophageal reflux, or a hiatus hernia?
Has the child or their parents had rectal or uterine prolapse, or urinary or faecal incontinence?
Has the child or their parents worn or wear orthodontic appliances?
Has the child or their parents had hypersensitivity to touch (feeling tags on trousers, discomfort with a belt, feeling of tight trousers), sight (perception of bright lights, glare), hearing (perception of reverberations, amplified noises), smell (heightened perception of odours, dysosmia), or taste?
Has the child or their parents had a diagnosis of myopia or drooping eyelids (ptosis), either unilateral or bilateral? Has the child or their parents had any immune or autoimmune diseases? (e.g., type 1 diabetes, coeliac disease, thyroiditis, rheumatoid arthritis, Crohn's disease, polyneuropathy, multiple sclerosis, etc.)
Has the child or have the parents had, or do they currently have, any immune or autoimmune diseases? (e.g., type 1 diabetes, coeliac disease, thyroiditis, rheumatoid arthritis, Crohn's disease, polyneuropathies, multiple sclerosis, etc.)

Questionario lassità pediatrica (Italian version)

Genere del soggetto:
Maschio
Femmina
Patologia del soggetto:
Autismo
ADHD
Sindrome di Tourette
Controllo
Quanti fratelli ha il soggetto?
Quante sorelle ha il soggetto?
Il bambino o i genitori hanno presentato o presentano ipertensione arteriosa in due o tre rilevazioni?
Il bambino o i genitori hanno presentato o presentano vene varicose, vasculiti o emorroidi?
Il bambino o i genitori hanno presentato o presentano striae rubre, smagliature e segni cutanei, cute arrossata senza apparente causa?
Il bambino o i genitori hanno presentato o presentano un eccesso di sudorazione ai palmi delle mani e/o alle piante dei piedi?
Il bambino o i genitori hanno presentato o presentano infiammazioni o reumatismi articolari (borsiti, tenosinoviti, ecc.)?
Il bambino o i genitori hanno presentato o presentano dislocazioni, sublussazioni o lussazioni di una o più articolazioni in più di una occasione?
Il bambino o i genitori hanno presentato o presentano dolore articolare coinvolgente da 1 a 3 grosse articolazioni lamentato per più di 3 mesi?
Il bambino o i genitori hanno presentato o presentano dolore alla schiena, dolori muscolari transitori agli arti (ad es. dolori della crescita) o sintomi da affaticamento cronico?
Il bambino o i genitori hanno presentato o presentano displasia dell'anca, scoliosi o dorso curvo?

Il bambino o i genitori hanno presentato o presentano ernie inguinali, ombelicali, addominali oppure ernie discali?
Il bambino o i genitori hanno presentato o presentano piedi piatti?
Il bambino o i genitori hanno presentato o presentano stipsi, diarrea o alvo alterno?
Il bambino o i genitori hanno presentato o presentano pirosi retrosternale, reflusso gastroesofageo o ernia iatale?
Il bambino o i genitori hanno presentato o presentano prolassi rettali/uterini oppure incontinenza urinaria e/o fecale?
Il bambino o i genitori hanno utilizzato o utilizzano apparecchi ortodontici?
Il bambino o i genitori hanno presentato o presentano ipersensorialità a livello tattile (percepiscono etichette dei pantaloni, fastidio per cintura, senso di pantaloni stretti), a livello visivo (percezione di luci intense, abbagliamenti), a livello uditivo (percezione di rimbombi, rumori accentuati), a livello olfattivo (percezioni accentuate di odori, disosmie) a livello gustative?
Il bambino o i genitori hanno presentato o presentano un quadro oculistico di miopia oppure un rilievo di palpebre cadenti o ptosi palpebrale mono o bi laterale?
Il bambino o i genitori hanno presentato o presentano malattie immunitarie e/o autoimmunitarie? (es. diabete di tipo 1, celiachia, tiroiditi, artrite reumatoide, morbo di Crohn, polineuropatie, sclerosi multipla, etc.)

References

1. Huisman-van Dijk, H.M.; Schoot, R.; Rijkeboer, M.M.; Mathews, C.A.; Cath, D.C. The relationship between tics, OC, ADHD and autism symptoms: A cross- disorder symptom analysis in Gilles de la Tourette syndrome patients and family-members. *Psychiatry Res.* **2016**, *237*, 138–146. [CrossRef] [PubMed]
2. Morris-Rosendahl, D.J.; Crocq, M.A. Neurodevelopmental disorders—The history and future of a diagnostic concept. *Dialogues Clin. Neurosci.* **2020**, *22*, 65–72. [CrossRef] [PubMed]
3. Xie, S.; Karlsson, H.; Dalman, C.; Widman, L.; Rai, D.; Gardner, R.M.; Magnusson, C.; Sandin, S.; Tabb, L.P.; Newschaffer, C.J.; et al. The Familial Risk of Autism Spectrum Disorder with and without Intellectual Disability. *Autism Res.* **2020**, *13*, 2242–2250. [CrossRef]
4. Yang, Z.; Wu, H.; Lee, P.H.; Tsetsos, F.; Davis, L.K.; Yu, D.; Lee, S.H.; Dalsgaard, S.; Haavik, J.; Barta, C.; et al. Investigating Shared Genetic Basis Across Tourette Syndrome and Comorbid Neurodevelopmental Disorders Along the Impulsivity-Compulsivity Spectrum. *Biol. Psychiatry* **2021**, *90*, 317–327. [CrossRef] [PubMed]
5. Hollander, E. Obsessive-compulsive disorder and spectrum across the life span. *Int. J. Psychiatry Clin. Pract.* **2005**, *9*, 79–86. [CrossRef] [PubMed]
6. Darrow, S.M.; Grados, M.; Sandor, P.; Hirschtritt, M.E.; Illmann, C.; Osiecki, L.; Dion, Y.; King, R.; Pauls, D.; Budman, C.L.; et al. Autism Spectrum Symptoms in a Tourette's Disorder Sample. *J. Am. Acad. Child Adolesc. Psychiatry* **2017**, *56*, 610–617.e1. [CrossRef] [PubMed]
7. Petti, T.; Gupta, M.; Fradkin, Y.; Gupta, N. Management of sleep disorders in autism spectrum disorder with co-occurring attention-deficit hyperactivity disorder: Update for clinicians. *BJPsych Open* **2023**, *10*, e11. [CrossRef]
8. Lau-Zhu, A.; Fritz, A.; McLoughlin, G. Overlaps and distinctions between attention deficit/hyperactivity disorder and autism spectrum disorder in young adulthood: Systematic review and guiding framework for EEG-imaging research. *Neurosci. Biobehav. Rev.* **2019**, *96*, 93–115. [CrossRef]
9. Vasa, R.A.; Mostofsky, S.H.; Ewen, J.B. The Disrupted Connectivity Hypothesis of Autism Spectrum Disorders: Time for the Next Phase in Research. *Biol. Psychiatry Cogn. Neurosci. Neuroimaging* **2016**, *1*, 245–252. [CrossRef]
10. Tomasi, D.; Volkow, N.D. Reduced Local and Increased Long-Range Functional Connectivity of the Thalamus in Autism Spectrum Disorder. *Cereb. Cortex* **2019**, *29*, 573–585. [CrossRef] [PubMed]
11. Kern, J.K.; Geier, D.A.; King, P.G.; Sykes, L.K.; Mehta, J.A.; Geier, M.R. Shared Brain Connectivity Issues, Symptoms, and Comorbidities in Autism Spectrum Disorder, Attention Deficit/Hyperactivity Disorder, and Tourette Syndrome. *Brain Connect.* **2015**, *5*, 321–335. [CrossRef] [PubMed]
12. Staines, D.R. Is chronic fatigue syndrome an autoimmune disorder of endogenous neuropeptides, exogenous infection and molecular mimicry? *Med. Hypotheses* **2004**, *62*, 646–652. [CrossRef] [PubMed]
13. Coon, E.A.; Cheshire, W.P., Jr. Sweating Disorders. *Continuum* **2020**, *26*, 116–137. [CrossRef]

14. Parvaneh, V.J.; Shahvaladi, H.; Rahmani, K.; Yekta, S.J.; Gorji, F.A.; Shiari, R.; Abdollahimajd, F. Correlation between benign joint hypermobility syndrome and primary focal hyperhidrosis in children: A novel concept. *BMC Musculoskelet. Disord.* **2020**, *21*, 268. [CrossRef] [PubMed]
15. Fikree, A.; Chelimsky, G.; Collins, H.; Kovacic, K.; Aziz, Q. Gastrointestinal involvement in the Ehlers-Danlos syndromes. *Am. J. Med. Genet. C Semin. Med. Genet.* **2017**, *175*, 181–187. [CrossRef] [PubMed]
16. Marshall, J.B.; Kretschmar, J.M.; Gerhardt, D.C.; Winship, D.H.; Winn, D.; Treadwell, E.L.; Sharp, G.C. Gastrointestinal manifestations of mixed connective tissue disease. *Gastroenterology* **1990**, *98 Pt 1*, 1232–1238. [CrossRef] [PubMed]
17. Balasco, L.; Provenzano, G.; Bozzi, Y. Sensory Abnormalities in Autism Spectrum Disorders: A Focus on the Tactile Domain, From Genetic Mouse Models to the Clinic. *Front. Psychiatry* **2019**, *10*, 1016. [CrossRef] [PubMed]
18. Cikes, N. Central nervous system involvement in systemic connective tissue diseases. *Clin. Neurol. Neurosurg.* **2006**, *108*, 311–317. [CrossRef]
19. Kurosinski, P.; Götz, J. Glial cells under physiologic and pathologic conditions. *Arch. Neurol.* **2002**, *59*, 1524–1528. [CrossRef]
20. Chien, Y.L.; Wu, P.Y.; Wu, J.H.; Huang, W.L.; Hsiao, C.C.; Hsieh, Y.T.; Cheng, T.; Gau, S.S.; Chen, W.L. Corneal structural alterations in autism spectrum disorder: An in vivo confocal microscopy study. *Autism Res.* **2023**, *16*, 2316–2325. [CrossRef]
21. Zoccante, L.; Ciceri, M.L.; Gozzi, L.A.; Gennaro, G.D.; Zerman, N. The "Connectivome Theory": A New Model to Understand Autism Spectrum Disorders. *Front. Psychiatry* **2021**, *12*, 794516. [CrossRef] [PubMed]
22. Rahman, M.M.; Islam, M.R.; Yamin, M.; Islam, M.M.; Sarker, M.T.; Meem, A.F.K.; Akter, A.; Emran, T.B.; Cavalu, S.; Sharma, R. Emerging Role of Neuron-Glia in Neurological Disorders: At a Glance. *Oxid. Med. Cell. Longev.* **2022**, *2022*, 3201644. [CrossRef] [PubMed]
23. Heinze, G.; Puhr, R. Bias-reduced and separation-proof conditional logistic regression with small or sparse data sets. *Stat. Med.* **2010**, *29*, 770–777. [CrossRef] [PubMed]
24. Heinze, G.; Schemper, M. A solution to the problem of separation in logistic regression. *Stat. Med.* **2002**, *21*, 2409–2419. [CrossRef]
25. Guinchat, V.; Baeza-Velasco, C.; Bulbena, A.; Castori, M. Editorial: Neurodevelopmental, neuropsychiatric and psychosocial correlates of joint hypermobility and related disorders. *Front. Psychiatry* **2022**, *13*, 1109515. [CrossRef]
26. Poshattiwar, R.S.; Acharya, S.; Shukla, S.; Kumar, S. Neurological Manifestations of Connective Tissue Disorders. *Cureus* **2023**, *15*, e47108. [CrossRef] [PubMed]
27. Butler, M.G.; Hossain, W.A.; Steinle, J.; Gao, H.; Cox, E.; Niu, Y.; Quach, M.; Veatch, O.J. Connective Tissue Disorders and Fragile X Molecular Status in Females: A Case Series and Review. *Int. J. Mol. Sci.* **2022**, *23*, 9090. [CrossRef] [PubMed]
28. Ramírez-Cheyne, J.A.; Duque, G.A.; Ayala-Zapata, S.; Saldarriaga-Gil, W.; Hagerman, P.; Hagerman, R.; Payán-Gómez, C. Fragile X syndrome and connective tissue dysregulation. *Clin. Genet.* **2019**, *95*, 262–267. [CrossRef] [PubMed]
29. Pfeiffer, M.; Kotz, R.; Ledl, T.; Hauser, G.; Sluga, M. Prevalence of flat foot in preschool-aged children. *Pediatrics* **2006**, *118*, 634–639. [CrossRef]
30. Xu, L.; Gu, H.; Zhang, Y.; Sun, T.; Yu, J. Risk Factors of Flatfoot in Children: A Systematic Review and Meta-Analysis. *Int. J. Environ. Res. Public Health* **2022**, *19*, 8247. [CrossRef]
31. Kaya Mutlu, E.; Birinci, T.; Kaya Aytutuldu, G.; Mutlu, C.; Razak Ozdincler, A. The investigation of foot structure within children who have attention-deficit hyperactivity disorder: A case-controlled study. *J. Pediatr. Orthop. B* **2022**, *31*, e24–e30. [CrossRef] [PubMed]
32. Lee, J.S.; Kim, K.B.; Jeong, J.O.; Kwon, N.Y.; Jeong, S.M. Correlation of foot posture index with plantar pressure and radiographic measurements in pediatric flatfoot. *Ann. Rehabil. Med.* **2015**, *39*, 10–17. [CrossRef]
33. Pezaro, S.; Brock, I.; Buckley, M.; Callaway, S.; Demirdas, S.; Hakim, A.; Harris, C.; High Gross, C.; Karanfil, M.; Le Ray, I.; et al. Management of childbearing with hypermobile Ehlers-Danlos syndrome and hypermobility spectrum disorders: A scoping review and expert co-creation of evidence-based clinical guidelines. *PLoS ONE* **2024**, *19*, e0302401. [CrossRef] [PubMed]
34. Loblein, H.J.; Vukmirovich, P.W.; Donofrio, M.T.; Sanz, J.H. Prevalence of neurodevelopmental disorders in a clinically referred sample of children with CHD. *Cardiol. Young* **2023**, *33*, 619–626. [CrossRef]
35. Morton, P.D.; Ishibashi, N.; Jonas, R.A. Neurodevelopmental Abnormalities and Congenital Heart Disease: Insights Into Altered Brain Maturation. *Circ. Res.* **2017**, *120*, 960–977. [CrossRef]
36. Nattel, S.N.; Adrianzen, L.; Kessler, E.C.; Andelfinger, G.; Dehaes, M.; Côté-Corriveau, G.; Trelles, M.P. Congenital Heart Disease and Neurodevelopment: Clinical Manifestations, Genetics, Mechanisms, and Implications. *Can. J. Cardiol.* **2017**, *33*, 1543–1555. [CrossRef] [PubMed]
37. Kielty, C.M.; Sherratt, M.J.; Shuttleworth, C.A. Elastic fibres. *J. Cell Sci.* **2002**, *115*, 2817–2828. [CrossRef] [PubMed]
38. Ben-Sasson, A.; Carter, A.S.; Briggs-Gowan, M.J. Sensory over-responsivity in elementary school: Prevalence and social-emotional correlates. *J. Abnorm. Child Psychol.* **2009**, *37*, 705–716. [CrossRef] [PubMed]
39. Jussila, K.; Junttila, M.; Kielinen, M.; Ebeling, H.; Joskitt, L.; Moilanen, I.; Mattila, M.L. Sensory Abnormality and Quantitative Autism Traits in Children With and Without Autism Spectrum Disorder in an Epidemiological Population. *J. Autism Dev. Disord.* **2020**, *50*, 180–188. [CrossRef] [PubMed]

40. Gage, N.M.; Siegel, B.; Callen, M.; Roberts, T.P. Cortical sound processing in children with autism disorder: An MEG investigation. *Neuroreport* **2003**, *14*, 2047–2051. [CrossRef] [PubMed]
41. Hitoglou, M.; Ververi, A.; Antoniadis, A.; Zafeiriou, D.I. Childhood autism and auditory system abnormalities. *Pediatr. Neurol.* **2010**, *42*, 309–314. [CrossRef]
42. Guimarães-Souza, E.M.; Joselevitch, C.; Britto, L.R.G.; Chiavegatto, S. Retinal alterations in a pre-clinical model of an autism spectrum disorder. *Mol. Autism* **2019**, *10*, 19. [CrossRef]
43. Lindly, O.J.; Chan, J.; Fenning, R.M.; Farmer, J.G.; Neumeyer, A.M.; Wang, P.; Swanson, M.; Parker, R.A.; Kuhlthau, K.A. Vision care among school-aged children with autism spectrum disorder in North America: Findings from the Autism Treatment Network Registry Call-Back Study. *Autism* **2021**, *25*, 840–853. [CrossRef]
44. Longo, R.; Allegrini, F.; Gusson, E.; Morbio, R.; Di Gennaro, G.; Gozzi, L.A.; Marchini, G.; Zoccante, L. Visual-motor involvement in autism spectrum disorder: Could the stereopsis deficit affect motor coordination? *Front. Psychiatry* **2023**, *14*, 1130185. [CrossRef]
45. Alrasheed, S.H.; Alghamdi, W. Systematic review and meta-analysis of the prevalence of myopia among school-age children in the Eastern Mediterranean Region. *East. Mediterr. Health J.* **2024**, *30*, 312–322. [CrossRef] [PubMed]
46. Chou, W.P.; Chen, Y.L.; Hsiao, R.C.; Lai, Y.H.; Yen, C.F. Bidirectional associations between hyperopia, myopia, astigmatism, and strabismus, and attention-deficit/hyperactivity disorder in children: A national population-based cohort study. *Braz. J. Psychiatry* **2023**, *45*, 397–404. [CrossRef] [PubMed]
47. Johnson, C.R.; DeMand, A.; Lecavalier, L.; Smith, T.; Aman, M.; Foldes, E.; Scahill, L. Psychometric properties of the children's sleep habits questionnaire in children with autism spectrum disorder. *Sleep Med.* **2016**, *20*, 5–11. [CrossRef] [PubMed]
48. Ikeda, J.; Davitt, B.V.; Ultmann, M.; Maxim, R.; Cruz, O.A. Brief report: Incidence of ophthalmologic disorders in children with autism. *J. Autism Dev. Disord.* **2013**, *43*, 1447–1451. [CrossRef] [PubMed]
49. Asif, M.I.; Kalra, N.; Sharma, N.; Jain, N.; Sharma, M.; Sinha, R. Connective tissue disorders and eye: A review and recent updates. *Indian J. Ophthalmol.* **2023**, *71*, 2385–2398. [CrossRef]
50. Sridhar, M.S. Anatomy of cornea and ocular surface. *Indian J. Ophthalmol.* **2018**, *66*, 190–194. [CrossRef] [PubMed]
51. Krey, K.F.; Hirsch, C. Frequency of orthodontic treatment in German children and adolescents: Influence of age, gender, and socio-economic status. *Eur. J. Orthod.* **2012**, *34*, 152–157. [CrossRef] [PubMed]
52. Rölling, S. Orthodontic treatment-service studied retrospectively in a group of Danish children aged 15–16 years. *Community Dent. Oral Epidemiol.* **1984**, *12*, 355–357. [CrossRef] [PubMed]
53. Bennett, S.M.; Hindin, J.S.; Mohatt, J.; Bauer, C.; Schild, J.; Falk, A.; Specht, M.; Woods, D.; Walkup, J. Proof of Concept Study of an Oral Orthotic in Reducing Tic Severity in Tourette Syndrome. *Child Psychiatry Hum. Dev.* **2022**, *53*, 953–963. [CrossRef] [PubMed]
54. Murakami, J.; Tachibana, Y.; Akiyama, S.; Kato, T.; Taniguchi, A.; Nakajima, Y.; Shimoda, M.; Wake, H.; Kano, Y.; Takada, M.; et al. Oral splint ameliorates tic symptoms in patients with tourette syndrome. *Mov. Disord.* **2019**, *34*, 1577–1578. [CrossRef] [PubMed]
55. Sandin, S.; Lichtenstein, P.; Kuja-Halkola, R.; Hultman, C.; Larsson, H.; Reichenberg, A. The Heritability of Autism Spectrum Disorder. *JAMA* **2017**, *318*, 1182–1184. [CrossRef]
56. Arun, T.; Nalbantgil, D.; Sayinsu, K. Orthodontic treatment protocol of Ehlers-Danlos syndrome type VI. *Angle Orthod.* **2006**, *76*, 177–183.
57. Csecs, J.L.L.; Iodice, V.; Rae, C.L.; Brooke, A.; Simmons, R.; Quadt, L.; Savage, G.K.; Dowell, N.G.; Prowse, F.; Themelis, K.; et al. Joint Hypermobility Links Neurodivergence to Dysautonomia and Pain. *Front. Psychiatry* **2021**, *12*, 786916. [CrossRef] [PubMed]
58. Zoccante, L.; Zaffanello, M.; Di Gennaro, G. Editorial: The "Connectivome Theory": Psyche, soma and the systemic involvement of connective tissue in neurodivergence. *Front. Psychiatry* **2024**, *15*, 1436796. [CrossRef] [PubMed]
59. Damianidou, E.; Mouratidou, L.; Kyrousi, C. Research models of neurodevelopmental disorders: The right model in the right place. *Front. Neurosci.* **2022**, *16*, 1031075. [CrossRef] [PubMed]
60. Hadders-Algra, M. Early Diagnostics and Early Intervention in Neurodevelopmental Disorders—Age-Dependent Challenges and Opportunities. *J. Clin. Med.* **2021**, *10*, 861. [CrossRef] [PubMed]
61. Kushki, A.; Anagnostou, E.; Hammill, C.; Duez, P.; Brian, J.; Iaboni, A.; Schachar, R.; Crosbie, J.; Arnold, P.; Lerch, J.P. Examining overlap and homogeneity in ASD, ADHD, and OCD: A data-driven, diagnosis-agnostic approach. *Transl. Psychiatry* **2019**, *9*, 318. [CrossRef] [PubMed]
62. Ma, S.L.; Chen, L.H.; Lee, C.C.; Lai, K.Y.C.; Hung, S.F.; Tang, C.P.; Ho, T.P.; Shea, C.; Mo, F.; Mak, T.S.H.; et al. Genetic Overlap Between Attention Deficit/Hyperactivity Disorder and Autism Spectrum Disorder in SHANK2 Gene. *Front. Neurosci.* **2021**, *15*, 649588. [CrossRef]

children

MDPI

Article

Development and Psychometric Properties of the Pain and Sensitivity Reactivity Scale in a Diverse Sample of Autistic People

Agustín E. Martínez-González [1,*], Matti Cervin [2], José A. Piqueras [3], Lidia Infante-Cañete [4] and Susana Pérez-Sánchez [5]

1 Department of Developmental Psychology and Didactics, University of Alicante, Carretera San Vicente del Raspeig, s/n, 03690 San Vicente del Raspeig, Spain
2 Department of Clinical Sciences Lund, Lund University, 221 00 Lund, Sweden; matti.cervin@med.lu.se
3 Department of Health Psychology, Miguel Hernández University of Elche, Edificio Altamira, Avda. de la Universidad, s/n, 03202 Elche, Spain; jpiqueras@umh.es
4 Department of Developmental and Educational Psychology, Faculty of Psychology, University of Malaga, 29010 Malaga, Spain; lidiainfante@uma.es
5 Hospital Pediatric Service University General "Los Arcos", 30739 San Javier, Spain; susanaperezsanchez@gmail.com
* Correspondence: agustin.emartinez@ua.es

Abstract: Background: Recent studies indicate the need to examine how the gut microbiota–brain axis is implicated in pain, sensory reactivity and gastro-intestinal symptoms in autism spectrum disorder (ASD), but no scale exists that assesses all these constructs simultaneously. Methods: We created a pool of 100 items based on the real-world experience of autistic people, and a multidisciplinary team and stakeholders reduced this pool to 50 items assessing pain, sensory hypersensitivity, and sensory hyposensitivity. In the present study, we present this new assessment tool, the Pain and Sensitivity Reactivity Scale (PSRS), and examine its psychometric properties in a sample of 270 individuals with autism spectrum disorder (ASD; mean age = 9.44, SD = 4.97), of which almost half (45%) had intellectual disability (ID). Results: A factorial model of three factors (pain, hyporeactivity, and hyperreactivity) and five specific factors for sensory hypo- and hyperreactivity, respectively, fitted the data well. Good to excellent internal consistency and adequate test–retest reliability was found for most PSRS scales. Sound psychometric properties were found in individuals with and without ID. Correlations with other measures of sensory sensitivity and pain indicated sound convergent validity. Conclusions: PSRS shows promise as a reliable measure to analyze pain and sensory reactivity in autistic people regardless of whether they have ID or not. The measure overcomes several limitations of previous assessment tools and includes variables that are important for the understanding of the gut microbiota–brain axis in ASD.

Keywords: autism; pain; sensitivity reactivity; sensory hyporeactivity; sensory hyperreactivity; sensory-over responsivity; sensory-under reactivity

1. Introduction

Autism spectrum disorder (ASD) is a neurodevelopmental disorder that is diagnosed based on two main criteria: (1) deficits in social communication and interaction skills, and (2) the presence of restricted and repetitive patterns of behavior [1]. Restricted and repetitive behaviors (RRBs) can be caused by hyper- or hyporesponsiveness to sensory stimuli or unusual interest in sensory aspects of the environment in ASD [1,2].

Altered sensory responsiveness refers to impairments in modulating outputs in relation to sensory stimuli, including in visual, auditive, tactile, smell, taste and proprioceptive modalities [3]. Individuals with sensory difficulties have difficulties regulating and organizing behavioral responses to sensory inputs to match environmental demands. Sensory responsiveness can be classified into three patterns: sensory over-responsivity (SOR: e.g., covering one's ears in response to sounds), sensory under-responsivity (SUR: e.g., a lack of sensation of loud sounds, slow reaction to pain), and sensation-seeking/sensory interests, repetitions and seeking behaviors (SIRS) [4]. Nonverbal children with ASD are more likely to demonstrate SUR and SIRS compared to peers [5], but few measures of sensory functioning in ASD include SUR and SIRS [3,6]. Research also suggests that SOR, SUR and SIRS commonly co-occur in autistic people, creating significant phenotypic heterogeneity, and both SOR and SUR are included in the diagnostic criteria of ASD [1,3,7,8].

A recent review identified several limitations of current assessment tools of sensory functioning in ASD, with major limitations being (1) that items had not been developed in collaboration with stakeholders, and (2) lack of structural validity analyses (e.g., confirmatory factor analysis) [9]. On the other hand, age, the presence of intellectual disability (ID) and who reports the data (e.g., caregiver versus self-report) are significant moderators in the assessment of SOR [3].

The review also highlighted the difficulty of conducting external validity analyses since the validator measures themselves had unclear psychometric properties. Further, no measure was identified that met the criteria of sufficient psychometric quality according to the COSMIN guidelines [10]. Further, there was a lack of consensus around the terminology (e.g., sensory hyper-reactivity, hyperresponsiveness, SOR) and which components are most relevant to sensory functioning [9]. Last, most current assessment tools do not include specific sensory factors, such as auditory hypersensitivity and auditory hyposensitivity. Thus, there is a need for assessment tools of sensory functioning in ASD that are developed in accordance with leading theories of sensory functioning, in collaboration with stakeholders (e.g., psychologists, pediatricians, educators, families) and where the structural validity of the measure is comprehensively examined.

Uljarević et al. [11] point out that a three-pronged approach should be used when developing measures of sensory reactivity: (1) consider sensory features as dimensional constructs (e.g., tactile hyposensitivity vs. tactile hyperreactivity), (2) examine differences across relevant groups of people (e.g., in people with ASD with and without ID), and (3) move towards comprehensive, multidimensional, and multimodal approaches to the measurement of sensory features, for example, by including pain dimensions.

For the latter, pain is of relevance to sensory functioning in ASD. First, autistic people are at greater risk of experiencing unrecognized pain, especially children with impaired cognitive ability and limited language skills [12]. Second, the frequency and severity of repetitive behavior has a high association with pain [13]. Third, there appears to be a relation between hyposensitivity and pain in ASD, as individuals with ASD show hyposensitivity to subjective pain intensity and affective aspects of pain sensitivity compared to controls [14]. That is, an apparent indifference to pain may be expressed by some autistic people, but this phenomenon has rarely been examined [12], and the relation between sensory reactivity and pain should be analyzed with specific measures [15].

In conclusion, anxiety, SOR, and gastro-intestinal symptoms (abdominal pain and constipation) are possibly interrelated in ASD, and may share underlying mechanisms [16,17]. Further, these variables are all related to the "gut–microbiota–brain axis" [18–21]. The microbiota–gut–brain axis is a novel field of study where sensory reactions, pain (gastrointestinal symptoms), and gut microbiota can be studied in ASD [18,19].

The present study evaluates the Pain and Sensitivity Reactivity Scale (PSRS), which was developed, in collaboration with stakeholders, to assess sensory hypersensitivity, sensory hyposensitivity, and pain and in autistic individuals with and without ID.

2. Materials and Methods

2.1. Participants

Caregivers of 270 individuals with ASD (mean age = 9.44, SD = 4.97) participated in this research. The participants were from Spain and came from both urban and rural areas of the following regions: Valencian Community, Murcia region, Madrid, Castilla la Mancha, Castilla y León, Galicia, and Andalusia. Participants with ASD and ID were included when ASD was the primary diagnosis. Table 1 shows the sociodemographic and diagnostic characteristics of the sample.

Table 1. Sociodemographic characteristics of the ASD sample.

Variables	*n* (%)
Age	
4–41 years old	270
Gender	
Female	92 (34.1%)
Male	177 (65.6%)
Other	1 (0.4%)
Country/region of birth	
Spain	254 (94.1%)
Ecuador	4 (1.5%)
Colombia	1 (0.4%)
Argentina	2 (0.7%)
Chile	1 (0.4%)
Dominican Republic	1 (0.4%)
Other	4 (1.5%)
Reported diagnosis	
ASD w/o ID	149 (55.2%)
ASD w Mild ID	37 (13.7%)
ASD w Moderate ID	51 (18.9%)
ASD w Severe ID	32 (11.9%)
Context	
Regular class in a regular school	132 (48.9%)
Special class in a regular school	46 (17%)
Special School	52 (19.3%)
Residence	0 (0%)
Residence and Special School	0 (0%)
Day center	0 (0%)
Regular class and Special School	2 (0.7%)
Open classroom	21 (7.8%)
Other	11 (4.1%)

Note. w = with; w/o = without; ASD = Autism Spectrum Disorder; ID = Intellectual Disability.

2.2. Measures

2.2.1. Sociodemographic Questionnaire

Lam and Aman's [22] sociodemographic questionnaire was adapted for the online data collection used in the present study. The questionnaire includes a series of sociodemographic items (e.g., age, sex, country of birth) as well as information on the specific ASD diagnosis and co-occurring diagnoses (e.g., ID).

2.2.2. Social Communication Questionnaire (SCQ)

The SCQ [23,24] is an instrument oriented towards parents or caregivers, with 40 items determining the possible presence of ASD. This instrument has been used for the assessment of ASD in children and adults [25]. It provides a total overall score and three additional scores (Social Interaction Problems, Communication Difficulties, and restricted, Repetitive, and Stereotyped Behaviors). Only the overall score was used in the present study. The present study used Form B of the scale, which assesses behaviors during the past three months. The SCQ has good psychometric properties [24], and showed adequate internal consistency in the present sample (∝ = 0.80).

2.2.3. Repetitive Behaviors Scale-Revised (RBS-R)

The RBS-R is a 43-item instrument oriented to caregivers and mental health professionals which assesses six different dimensions of repetitive behaviors in individuals with ASD and ID: (a) stereotypic, (b) self-injurious, (c) compulsive, (d) ritualistic, (e) sameness, and (f) restrictive [26]. Responses are recorded on a 4-point rating scale ranging from 0 to 3. This scale has been used in both children and adults with ASD [26]. RBS-R has demonstrated adequate psychometric properties for use with individuals with ASD from different countries [27,28]. The internal consistency of this scale in this sample was high (a = 0.95; ω = 0.95).

2.2.4. Short Sensory Profile (SSP)

The SSP [29] is a 38-item caregiver-reported instrument comprised of the items that demonstrated the highest discriminative power of atypical sensory processing based on the Sensory Profile (SP) [30]. Items are scored on a six-point Likert scale. The seven domains of the SSP were based on factor analysis of reported responding in daily life with a normative sample of typically developing children and include tactile sensitivity, taste/smell sensitivity, movement sensitivity, underresponsive/seeks sensation, auditory filtering, low energy/weak, and visual/auditory sensitivity. Studies have shown adequate psychometric properties of the SSP, with internal consistency estimates ranging from 0.70 to 0.90 [31–33]. The SSP has been used in children and adults with ASD [33]. In the present study, we used the full scale as well as the tactile sensitivity, taste/smell sensitivity, visual/auditory sensitivity scales, and underresponsive/seeks sensation subscales. The internal consistency of the full scale in the present sample was excellent (∝ = 0.92; ω = 0.91) and all subscales showed adequate internal consistency (∝/ω > 0.70).

2.2.5. Non-Communicating Children's Pain Checklist—Revised (NCCPC)

McGrath et al. [34] originally developed the NCCPC to measure pain in nonverbal, cognitively impaired children (age range, 3 to 17 years). The NCCPC has been used in children, adults, and patients with varying degrees of cognitive impairment (mean age = 42) [35]. The scale contains 30 items, each rated on a 4-point Likert. Observers are asked to rate the frequency of each item [34]. Studies have found adequate internal consistency in individuals with ASD (Cronbach's a = 0.72) [36] and ID [37]. The NCCPC-R has shown high internal consistency (Cronbach's a = 0.93), significant correlations with pain intensity ratings provided by carers, consistency over time, and good sensitivity and specificity in relation to pain [36]. In the present sample, the internal consistency of the NCCPC-R was excellent (∝ = 0.92; ω = 0.92).

2.2.6. Pain and Sensitivity Reactivity Scale (PSRS)

The PSRS is an assessment tool that evaluates reactivity to pain and sensory stimuli using 50 items. The scale is composed of three broad dimensions: pain, sensory hyporeactivity, and sensory hyperreactivity. All items are rated on a 4-point Likert scale ranging from 0 (the behavior does not occur) to 3 (the behavior occurs and is a severe problem). The broader dimensions of hyposensitivity and hypersensitivity include tactile, olfactory, visual, gustatory, and auditory subscales. In addition, the PSRS includes a pain reactivity domain that is assessed using seven items. The PSRS draws in part from the theory of Miller et al. [4] and from neuroscience research showing that pain and sensory reactivity are closely linked [14]. The development of PSRS is described below and its psychometric properties evaluated in the present study.

2.3. Procedures

Development of PSRS: The purpose of the development of the PSRS was to create a measure that allows for measuring sensory reactivity and pain in non-autistic and autistic people as well as in individuals with ASD and ID. We adhered to the theoretical model of Miller et al. [4] of SOR and SUR when developing PSRS. Each item is rated on a similar scale to what has been used successfully in other instruments developed for autistic populations (e.g., RBS-R). Items ask for how often a sensation is experienced and to what extent the sensation is a problem. Sensations are indicated as a problem when they are very annoying, very frequent and negatively affect life activities and generate negative consequences for the person or for others.

The PSRS was developed by a multidisciplinary team (3 pediatric specialists, a psychiatrist, two doctoral neuropsychologists, a doctoral psychologist, a neurodevelopmental psychologist, a doctor in chemistry specialized in gut microbiota, a nurse, and two special education teachers). In an initial phase, a pool of 100 SOR, SUR, and pain situations reported by autistic people and their families was generated. Four experts carried out the evaluation (a neuropsychologist with clinical experience in instrument validation; a psychiatrist; a nurse; and a pediatrician). Regarding the pain factor, initially, descriptions of different types of physical pain were included according to the records of the pediatric and psychiatric services. Initially, 32 items related to different physical and medical situations that caused pain were obtained which were then reduced to a shorter item list that included: (1) abdominal pain (e.g., constipation, bloating; 5 items); (2) infectious conditions-related pain (e.g., fever, otalgia; 4 items); (3) skin-related pain (e.g., ulcers, wounds, chafing, eczema, bruises; 5 items); (4) functional pain (e.g., occult fractures, deformities, hangnails, hip/shoulder dislocations, subluxations, spasticity; 3 items); (5) sight and taste-related pain (Eyes: irritation, conjunctivitis, ulcers, wounds; Teeth/Mouth/Throat: caries, canker sores, gingivostomatitis, tonsillitis, abscesses; 4 items). Subsequently, three doctors (two pediatricians and one psychiatrist) screened the items and found that many items were redundant in each of the painful situations, rendering a final set of 7 pain items.

In a second phase, the evaluation of the items was carried out until a total of 50 items were retained. Thus, the examples that were included in each of the 50 items were reviewed and refined. This process was carried out by two special education teachers who are experts in ASD, a pediatrician, a neuropsychologist, and a psychologist.

In a third phase, the clarity of the items was analyzed by three experts. Two were autism experts with experience in instrument development and one expert with more than twenty years of experience in medical assessment. All of them were doctors. The Dunn et al. [38] protocol was applied to all experts to evaluate the items. Judges rated the relevance of each item on a 5-point scale (1: low item clarity; 5: high item clarity), and sought consensus among the experts. Mean item clarity scores were calculated, considering as adequate those items with a score equal to or higher than 3 out of 5 [39]. Items were considered to have an adequate degree of relevance if the V-index was above this cut-off point and the 95% confidence interval did not include the value 0.70 [40]. The mean item clarity scores were above 3.54 in all cases, indicating that the experts considered the items to be clearly worded. In addition, the clinical opinion of the experts was taken into account to indicate the items that were most frequent in individuals with ASD.

Finally, the items were reviewed by caregivers of individuals with ASD. These caregivers had a child with ASD and were aware of situations of sensory reactivity and pain in their children. Their life experience helped improve some examples and clarifications included in the PSRS items. Finally, minor adjustments were made to increase clarity of items.

Recruitment: Causal or incidental sampling was used. Families who had children with ASD in 15 Spanish centers participated. Two centers were specific special education schools; one was residence for people with ASD and ID; eleven were early intervention centers; and one was a regular school with open classrooms. The sample belonged to different sized urban areas, with representation from both rural and urban areas.

A letter with information about the study was sent to a host of stakeholder organizations including education centers, special education centers and associations for families with children with ASD. The center's director informed the families that they could participate in the study with an online version survey or a paper-and-pencil version. Researchers had an online meeting or a phone call with centers to explain the purpose of the research. Subsequently, the institutions contacted the families to organize a meeting and explain the purpose of the study. Similarly, some institutions facilitated family contacts so that the researchers could directly explain the purpose of the study, and social networks were used to show an explanatory video of the study.

All participating families and caregivers had a child diagnosed with ASD according to DSM-5 criteria [1]. Individuals with ASD with or without ID were diagnosed according to DSM-5 criteria using standardized scales (e.g., Wechsler Nonverbal Scale of Ability, Leiter-3 scale, etc.). The subjects were previously diagnosed by the mental health services and institutions in charge of establishing each country's degree of disability and dependency. The diagnosis of ASD was made at the early care centers and the pediatric services of the mental health centers of each region. Families with children with another type of neurodevelopmental disorder (e.g., ADHD) were excluded from the study.

The researchers organized a training session for all participating schools in which the purpose of the research study, the instruments used and the administration instructions were described. The tests were administered by experienced psychologists who gave instructions and provided individual assistance to families who needed it. Appropriate instructions were provided for each scale. Participating families completed the protocol at home, and in some cases in a room set up at the center. The researchers could help families resolve doubts about the diagnosis in the first part of the survey, and an explanatory video highlighted the need for the families to consult the psychological and psychiatric reports in case of doubt about the diagnosis. However, the diagnostic part of the protocol was reviewed by the center's psychologist to detect possible omissions or errors in the severity level of the ASD.

The total time to complete all instruments included in the study was approximately 25 min. After one month, a random sample of 83 caregivers who had a child with ASD completed the study instruments again; this was done to examine test–retest reliability. Participating families did not receive financial compensation for their participation in the study. The study was conducted between June 2020 and May 2022 and was approved by the Ethics Committee of the University of Alicante in Spain (reference: UA-2020-03-27). Caregivers provided informed consent.

2.4. Data Analysis

COSMIN Taxonomy of Measurement Properties has been used in the development of the PSRS instrument. First, we evaluated the structural validity of the PSRS (explained above). In short, the PSRS includes a pain scale with 7 indicators/items, a broad sensory hyporeactivity scale with 5 subscales (4–6 items each), and a broad sensory hyperreactivity scale, also with 5 subscales (4–5 items each). In the factor model, we defined the 5 first-order sensory hypo- and hyperreactivity factors to be indicators of the higher, second-order hypo- and hypersensitivity scales, which were then modeled as indicators of a broad third-order sensory reactivity scale (see Figure 1).

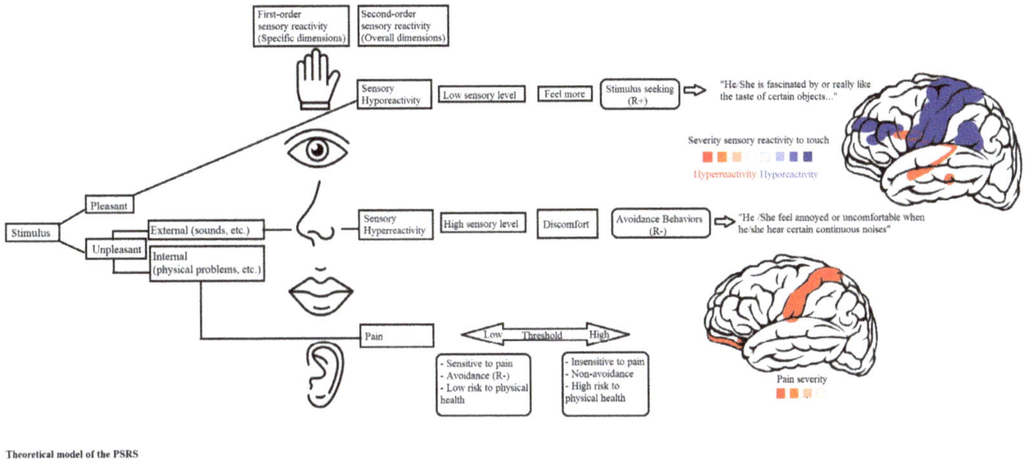

Figure 1. Theoretical model and structure of the PSRS. Copyright © 2023 Martinez-González A.E. [41].

To test how well the proposed factor structure explained covariance among responses from the participants, we used the R library lavaan and confirmatory factor analysis (CFA). Because the items of PSRS are ordinal, the diagonally weighted least squares estimator was used. A global evaluation of four fit indices were used to evaluate overall model/data fit: Comparative Fit Index (CFI), Root Mean Square Error of Approximation (RMSEA) and Standardized Mean Square Residual (SRMR). An RMSEA below 0.06, an SRMR below 0.08 and CFI and TLI estimates greater than 0.90 are indicative of acceptable model-data fit; CFI and TLI estimates above 0.95 are indicative of good model-data fit [42]. Scaled fit indices were estimated because of the ordinal nature of the items. Modification indices were evaluated to highlight sources of misfit. The internal consistency of the items of the latent factors were examined by estimating the Cronbach's alpha (α) and McDonald's omega (ω) coefficients, and we considered coefficients above 0.70 to indicate adequate internal consistency. The average variance extracted (AVE) was also computed, which estimates the degree of item variance that can be explained by a latent factor. CFA was selected above exploratory factor analysis as the scale had a clear theoretical structure and all items were developed to be used as indicators of pre-defined latent factors.

Construct validity was examined by correlating the empirically derived scores of the measure with the total score of the SSP (convergent validity in relation to the PSRS sensory reactivity scale), the subscale scores of the SSP (convergent and divergent validity in relation to the sensory subscales of PSRS), NCCPC (convergent validity in relation to the PSRS pain scale), RBSR (divergent validity), and SCQ (divergent validity). We expected the corresponding scales (e.g., scales assessing sensory processing) to be more strongly correlated than non-corresponding scale (e.g., scales assessing sensory processing and RRBs). To statistically compare correlations, we used the method presented in Hittner et al. [42], which is implemented in the R library cocor. Test–retest reliability was examined by computing the intraclass correlation coefficient (ICC [2,k]) [43] for the repeated assessments, with values between 0.50 and 0.75 representing moderate reliability, values between 0.75 and 0.90 good reliability, and values greater than 0.90 excellent reliability [10].

3. Results

3.1. Structural Validity of PSRS

The proposed model explained sample patterns in the data adequately (RMSEA = 0.05, CFI = 0.91, TLI = 0.91, SRMR = 0.10). All item and factor loadings are presented in Table 2. All indicators loaded significantly ($p < 0.001$) onto their proposed first-order latent factor (all standardized loadings > 0.50), and each of the specific hypo- and hypersensitivity factors loaded significantly onto the second-order factors (all standardized loadings > 0.50), which loaded significantly onto the third-order Broad Sensory Reactivity factor. The pain and the broad sensory reactivity factor had a statistically significant positive association/correlation (r = 0.42, $p < 0.001$).

Modification indices suggested that correlated residuals for items 12 and 13 ("Likes touching things and people" and "Hugs people hard"), for the hypo- and hypersensitivity olfactory factors, and for items 9 and 31 ("Scratches wounds until they bleed" and "Feels discomfort by imperfections in the skin") would improve model/data fit. When adding these parameters, model/data fit was improved (RMSEA = 0.04, CFI = 0.93, TLI = 0.92, SRMR = 0.09) and all additions were statistically significant and showed meaningful parameter estimations (i.e., standardized parameters > 0.30).

Table 2. Standardized loading of model indicators. All items load statistically significantly ($p < 0.001$) onto the proposed factor.

First-Order	Pain	Hypo Tactile	Hypo Olfactory	Hypo Visual	Hypo Taste	Hypo Audio	Hyper Tactile	Hyper Olfactory	Hyper Visual	Hyper Taste	Hyper Audio
Item 1 [He/she hurts or feels discomfort when he/she has stomach problems]	0.65										
Item 2 [He/she hurts or feels discomfort when he/she has inflammation problems]	0.79										
Item 3 [He/she hurts or feels discomfort when he/she has eye irritation, conjunctivitis, etc.]	0.74										
Item 4 [He/she hurts or feels discomfort when he/she has a fever]	0.63										
Item 5 [He hurts or feels discomfort when he/she has had a fracture or have gone to rehabilitation]	0.52										
Item 6 [He/she hurts or feels discomfort when they prick you for an analysis]	0.70										
Item 7 [He/she hurts or feels discomfort when he/she has fallen or been hit.]	0.54										
Item 8 [He/She prefers very hot or cold water]		0.60									
Item 9 [He/She scratches his wounds until they bleed again.]		0.57									
Item 10 [He/She likes to dress in tight clothes, socks, and shoes.]		0.50									
Item 11 [Squeezes the pen or pencil down a lot when writing.]		0.68									
Item 12 [He/She likes to touch things and people.]		0.64									
Item 13 [Hugs people tight.]		0.59									

Table 2. *Cont.*

First-Order	Pain	Hypo Tactile	Hypo Olfactory	Hypo Visual	Hypo Taste	Hypo Audio	Hyper Tactile	Hyper Olfactory	Hyper Visual	Hyper Taste	Hyper Audio
Item 14 [He/She is fascinated by certain smells.]			0.94								
Item 15 [He/She smells myself, people and objects.]			0.89								
Item 16 [He/She prefers or likes intense or strong odors.]			0.77								
Item 17 [He/She has a hard time perceiving unpleasant odors or bad odors.]			0.60								
Item 18 [He/She is fascinated by moving or spinning objects.]				0.77							
Item 19 [He/She prefers or likes intense or bright colors.]				0.80							
Item 20 [He/She is attracted to light and reflections.]				0.61							
Item 21 [He/She has a hard time perceiving the strong light before his eyes]				0.59							
Item 22 [He/She is fascinated or really likes the taste of certain objects or parts of the body]					0.77						
Item 23 [He/She likes food with strong flavors.]					0.52						
Item 24 [He/She likes to suck or lick objects, food, etc.]					0.66						
Item 25 [He/She doesn't feel full/satiated after eating a lot.]					0.66						
Item 26 [He/She is attracted to certain sounds.]						0.64					
Item 27 [He/She listens to TV or music at a very high volume.]						0.60					
Item 28 [He/She likes to make noises or loud sounds.]						0.76					
Item 29 [He/She has a hard time listening to what others are saying, etc.]						0.66					
Item 30 [He/She feels discomfort or discomfort when touched.]							0.64				
Item 31 [He/She feels discomfort or discomfort when he/she notices skin imperfections]							0.69				
Item 32 [He/She feels discomfort or discomfort when touching certain textures.]							0.87				

Table 2. *Cont.*

First-Order	Pain	Hypo Tactile	Hypo Olfactory	Hypo Visual	Hypo Taste	Hypo Audio	Hyper Tactile	Hyper Olfactory	Hyper Visual	Hyper Taste	Hyper Audio
Item 33 [He/She feels discomfort or discomfort when certain elements or objects come into contact that can touch my head or nails]							0.70				
Item 34 [He/She feels upset or uncomfortable when his/her favorite or usual clothes are not ready.]							0.72				
Item 35 [He/She gets upset or uncomfortable when he/she smells certain odors that other people don't mind.]								0.91			
Item 36 [He/She feels discomfort or discomfort when he/she smells certain places]								0.95			
Item 37 [He/She feels discomfort or discomfort when he/she smells certain foods.]								0.93			
Item 38 [He/She feels annoyed or uncomfortable when he/she smells certain people.]								0.89			
Item 39 [He/She feels upset or uncomfortable when he/she sees certain colors of food on a plate]									0.87		
Item 40 [He/She feels upset or uncomfortable when he/she sees the physical appearance of some people.]									0.72		
Item 41 [He/she feels upset or uncomfortable when he/she sees a change in something or someone]									0.78		
Item 42 [He/she feels annoyed or uncomfortable when seeing high-intensity light stimuli or bright light.]									0.69		
Item 43 [He/she feels sick or uncomfortable about the taste of certain foods, so he/she only accepts some flavors.]										0.89	
Item 44 [He/she is bothered or uncomfortable by foods with specific textures]										0.79	
Item 45 [He/she feels discomfort or discomfort from foods that are new]										0.86	
Item 46 [He/she feels discomfort or discomfort when changes, even small or subtle, occur in his/her favorite foods]										0.88	

Table 2. *Cont.*

First-Order	Pain	Hypo Tactile	Hypo Olfactory	Hypo Visual	Hypo Taste	Hypo Audio	Hyper Tactile	Hyper Olfactory	Hyper Visual	Hyper Taste	Hyper Audio
Item 47 [He/she feels annoyed or uncomfortable when he/her hears certain continuous noises]											0.89
Item 48 [He/she feels annoyed or uncomfortable when he/she hears certain sudden, unexpected and intense noises.]											0.89
Item 49 [He/she feels annoyed or uncomfortable when he/she hears loud noises]											0.87
Item 50 [He/she feels annoyed or uncomfortable when he/she listens to music that is not what he/she usually listens to.]											0.78
Second-Order	Sensory hyporeactivity	Sensory hyperreactivity									
Hypo Tactile	0.68										
Hypo Olfactory	0.59										
Hypo Visual	0.83										
Hypo Taste	0.69										
Hypo Audio	0.84										
Hyper Tactile		0.93									
Hyper Olfactory		0.65									
Hyper Visual		0.83									
Hyper Taste		0.73									
Hyper Audio		0.78									
Third-Order	Broad Sensory Reactivity										
Sensory hyporeactivity	0.83										
Sensory hyperreactivity	0.85										

3.2. Internal Consistency

Internal consistency coefficients for all first- and second-order factors (estimated without the first-order level) are presented in Table 3. All factors showed adequate to good internal consistency except for the hyposensitivity tactile and the hyposensitivity gustatory factors. The internal consistency of the broader factors was good to excellent, but the AVE for the hyposensitivity factor was low.

3.3. Convergent and Divergent Validity

The correlations between the two broad PSRS scales (pain and sensory reactivity) and convergent and divergent validator measures are presented at the top panel of Table 4. The correlations between the sensory subscales of the PSRS and the subscales of the SSP are at the bottom panel of Table 4. The PSRS pain scale was significantly and moderately correlated with NCCPC, but this correlation was not significantly stronger than the correlation between the PSRS pain scale and SSP and RBSR. The PSRS pain scale was not significantly correlated with SCQ, and the PSRS pain scale was significantly more strongly correlated with NCCPC than with SCQ.

Table 3. Internal consistency of model factors.

	α	ω	AVE
Pain	0.83	0.79	44%
Broad Sensory hyporeactivity	0.90	0.89	30%
Hypo Tactile	0.68	0.55	26%
Hypo Olfactory	0.84	0.82	65%
Hypo Visual	0.76	0.73	49%
Hypo Taste	0.69	0.67	43%
Hypo Auditory	0.74	0.70	44%
Broad Sensory hyperreactivity	0.93	0.93	56%
Hyper Tactile	0.85	0.80	53%
Hyper Olfactory	0.95	0.92	84%
Hyper Visual	0.84	0.78	59%
Hyper Taste	0.91	0.88	73%
Hyper Auditory	0.89	0.88	74%

Notes. AVE = Average variance explained.

Table 4. Correlations between the broad PSRS scales and validator measures.

	SSP	NCCPC	RBS-R	SCQ
PSRS Pain	0.33 **	0.29 **	0.37 **	−0.12
PSRS Broad Sensory Reactivity	0.71 **	0.48 **	0.73 **	−0.16 *
	SSP Tactile	**SSP Taste/Smell**	**SSP Under Responsivity**	**SSP Visual/Auditory**
PSRS Hypo Tactile	0.52 **	0.43 **	0.58 **	0.45 **
PSRS Hypo Olfactory	0.34 **	0.25 **	0.29 **	0.30 **
PSRS Hypo Visual	0.48 **	0.40 **	0.49 **	0.44 **
PSRS Hypo Taste	0.39 **	0.34 **	0.48 **	0.37 **
PSRS Hypo Auditory	0.48 **	0.37 **	0.53 **	0.44 **
PSRS Hyper Tactile	0.59 **	0.56 **	0.42 **	0.48 **
PSRS Hyper Olfactory	0.38 **	0.41 **	0.23 **	0.31 **
PSRS Hyper Visual	0.51 **	0.53 **	0.34 **	0.47 **
PSRS Hyper Taste	0.43 **	0.77 **	0.29 **	0.36 **
PSRS Hyper Auditory	0.48 **	0.41 **	0.33 **	0.60 **

Note. * $p < 0.05$. ** $p < 0.01$. SSP = Short Sensory Profile. NCCPC = Non-Communicating Children's Pain Checklist—Revised. RBS-R = Repetitive Behavior Scale—Revised. SCQ = Social Communication Questionnaire. PSRS = Pain and Sensitivity Reactivity Scale.

The PSRS sensory reactivity scale was strongly and significantly correlated with SSP and this correlation was significantly stronger than between the PSRS and all other validator scales except RBS-R. Moreover, moderate to high correlations were found between the sensory hyperreactivity subscales of the PSRS and the hypersensitivity scales of the SSP (between 0.31 and 0.77) and strong correlations between corresponding scales for tactile (r = 0.59), taste (r = 0.77) and auditory (r = 0.60) domains, while moderate correlations emerged for the olfactory (r = 0.41) and visual (r = 0.47) domains. Similarly, moderate to strong correlations were observed in the sensory hyporesponsiveness subscales of the PSRS and the under-responsive/seeks sensation subscale of the SSP (rs between 0.29 and 0.58). The strongest correlations emerged for the tactile (r = 0.58) and auditory (r = 0.53) domains.

3.4. PSRS in Participants with and Without Intellectual Disability

We were underpowered to examine measurement invariance (i.e., whether the proposed factor structure was similar) in participants with and without ID. Instead, we examined the internal consistency for the factors in each sample separately. The pain scale showed slightly better coefficients in participants with (α = 0.84, ω = 0.83) versus without (α = 0.72, ω = 0.69) ID. For sensory hyporeactivity, the two groups showed very similar coefficients: with ID ($\alpha = 0.85$, $\omega = 0.83$); without ID ($\alpha = 0.85$, $\omega = 0.85$). Similar results emerged for sensory hyperreactivity: with ID ($\alpha = 0.90$, $\omega = 0.89$); without ID ($\alpha = 0.93$, $\omega = 0.93$). We also examined whether the two groups differed in their scores using linear regression models accounting for age and sex differences. No significant differences in PSRS factor/scale scores were present.

3.5. Test–Retest Reliability

The test–retest coefficients (ICCs) for the pain, sensory hyporeactivity, sensory hyperreactivity, and full sensory reactivity PSRS scales are in Table 5. ICCs were estimated for the full sample and for participants with and without ID, respectively. ICCs for most scales were good to excellent. Of note, the ICCs for the broad sensory reactivity scale as well as the hypo- and hypersensitivity scale were lower for participants with ID.

Table 5. Intraclass correlation coefficients and their 95% confidence intervals for the PSRS scales in the full test–retest sample and in participants with and without intellectual disability, respectively.

	ASD Full Sample $n = 83$	**ASD with ID** $n = 23$	**ASD Without ID** $n = 60$
Pain	0.78 (0.73, 0.82)	0.80 (0.72, 0.85)	0.75 (0.68, 0.81)
Broad Sensory Reactivity	0.90 (0.88, 0.92)	0.61 (0.47, 0.71)	0.96 (0.95, 0.97)
Sensory hyporeactivity	0.90 (0.87, 0.91)	0.77 (0.69, 0.83)	0.93 (0.91, 0.95)
Sensory hyperreactivity	0.87 (0.84, 0.89)	0.56 (0.40, 0.67)	0.94 (0.92, 0.95)

Note. ASD = Autism Spectrum Disorder; ID = Intellectual Disability.

4. Discussion

Sensory reactivity and pain are linked in ASD, and SOR predicts abdominal pain in autistic people [17]. Similarly, children with ASD who have gastro-intestinal symptoms exhibit more irritable and agitated behaviors [44] and significantly higher rates of both anxiety and sensory hyperreactivity [16]. For these reasons, pain and sensory reactivity are important to include in assessment tools of the gut–microbiota–brain relationship in ASD [45].

In the present study, we present a new transdisciplinary and multidimensional instrument that addresses an important gap in the current instrument pool, the PSRS. First, the PSRS includes both sensory sensitivity and pain scales. Second, each scale is derived from leading theories of sensory functioning and developed in collaboration with stakeholders. Overall, our findings support the proposed factor structure of PSRS, with two broad factors (pain and sensory sensitivity), with the sensory factors including a more complex hierarchical structure with separate scales for hypo- and hypersensitivity, which in turn includes subfactors measuring difficulties within each sensory modality (Tactile, Olfactory, Visual, Taste and Audio). Although fit indices were not excellent, small adjustments, accounting for correlations between items with similar content, substantially improved fit, suggesting that the major sources of misfit are not on the structural level. The multilevel structure of PSRS makes it useful in research since it is possible to analyze data on the level that is most beneficial in relation to the research question. The multilevel structure also makes PSRS useful in general practice as it provides specific information about multidimensional sensory and pain difficulties, which is known to be unidentified in many autistic people.

Findings also supported sound internal consistency of most PSRS scales and the internal consistency of the broader factors (sensory hyporeactivity, sensory hyperreactivity and pain) was good to excellent. Lower internal consistency was found for the tactile hyporeactivity factor. These findings are consistent with previous studies that have found lower internal consistency for tactile sensory reactivity scales [46] as well as weak correlations between measure of ASD and tactile sensitivity [47]. However, there is a paucity of studies that analyze the psychometric properties of scales measuring specific sensory dimensions in ASD [32,48]. An explanation of the lower internal consistency of the sensory hyporeactivity scales may be that such difficulties are more difficult for the caregiver to observe and report. In fact, sensory hyporeactivity is less common at younger ages and may be associated with stimulus-seeking behaviors [49,50].

The sensory hypo- and hyperreactivity factors were moderately to strongly correlated, which is in line with our theoeretical framework (see Figure 1) and suggests that alterations in broader underlying mechanisms are involved in the regulation and modulation of sensory processing. The notion of shared underlying mechanisms was further supported by a moderate correlation between the broad sensory sensitivity factor and pain [17].

Convergent validity was supported since the broad PSRS sensory reactivity scale correlated strongly with SSP. However, the moderate correlations in the olfactory and visual dimensions may be due to the fact that the taste-smell and visual-auditory domains are collapsed in the SSP. The broad PSRS sensory reactivity scale also correlated strongly with the RBS-R scale, which assesses RRBs. Although we expected a stronger correlation with SSP than with RBS-R, these results are in line with results showing a clear association between sensory reactivity and RRBs [2]. In fact, sensory reactivity often precedes the onset of repetitive behaviors [1].

We found only a moderate correlation between the pain subscale of the PSRS and the NCCPC, which suggests that the PSRS pain scale assesses aspects that are quite dissimilar to what is measured via NCCPC. Indeed, while the NCCPC only measures the frequency of pain through facial, vocal, and body expressions [34], the PSRS addresses pain through a multidomain measurement framework where frequency, discomfort, and interference are included. Further, the PSRS pain scale is designed for specific pain situations that occur in ASD, and items were developed in collaboration with experienced pediatricians.

A strength of the present study is the inclusion of many individuals with ID and we wanted to examine whether the PSRS was suitable regardless of whether an individual had ID. While we were underpowered to conduct formal invariance tests (e.g., multigroup confirmatory factor analysis), we estimated internal consistency of the broad factors separately in those with and without ID, with internal consistency generally being high in both samples. This is promising and suggests that the items of the broad factors hang together well regardless of ID status. Future studies should include larger samples and conduct formal invariance test. However, it is a challenge to include participants with ID in research since individuals with ID themselves may be unable to report on measures and since families are often burdened. The PSRS includes both self- and observer-reported version, which may help overcome some of these obstacles.

Last, the test–retest reliability, measured approximately one month apart, supported sound psychometric properties of the PSRS. Again, similar results were found in those with and without ID. Test–retest reliability was slightly lower for the sensory hyperreactivity factor in individuals with ID. This may suggest that sensory experiences may vary more over time in this group or that it is harder for observers to adequately report hyperreactivity phenomena in individuals meeting criteria for ID.

The PSRS has a clinical scope in the field of nursing, medicine and psychology because it has an integrative perspective on sensory responses by including sensitivity to pain. Therefore, the pain sensitivity dimension is the greatest contribution of the PSRS. On the other hand, the possibility to obtain different sub-dimensions of SUR with the PSRS (olfactory, gustatory hypo-reactivity, etc.) is another contribution that will help to understand possible subtypes or profiles of sensory reactivity in ASD, and specifically for SUR in the ASD.

The recent literature points to the major limitations of instrument validation studies on sensory reactivity, indicating a lack of research on structural and convergent validity [9]. The present study overcomes some of the limitations of previous studies, including both structural, convergent and discriminate validity. Nevertheless, some limitations merit mention. First, as mentioned above, we were underpowered to conduct formal invariance tests (e.g., invariance by sex, age and ID status). Second, no inter-rater validation of the scale was conducted as all informants were the main caregiver. Third, including a measure of gastro-intestinal symptoms would have further helped validate the PSRS. Fourthly, although attempts have been made to justify that there is a relationship between sensation-seeking and SUR, and that other scales do not include the sensation-seeking variable, it may be that this is an added limitation to the PSRS.

5. Conclusions

In conclusion, the PSRS shows promise as a robust measure that can be used to assess sensory reactivity across several domains and pain in individuals with ASD regardless of whether they have ID or not. Future research should expand samples to examine whether the measure works similarly across sexes and age groups. Further, the psychometric properties of the instrument should be analyzed in non-autistic samples. Although the PSRS has fewer items than other similar instruments, a shorter version could be explored, not the least since several items were strongly correlated.

Author Contributions: Conceptualization, A.E.M.-G.; methodology, M.C.; formal analysis, M.C.; investigation, A.E.M.-G.; data curation, J.A.P. and S.P.-S.; writing—original draft preparation, A.E.M.-G. and M.C.; writing—review and editing, A.E.M.-G., J.A.P. and L.I.-C. All authors have read and agreed to the published version of the manuscript.

Funding: This research received no external funding.

Institutional Review Board Statement: The study was conducted between June 2020 and May 2022 and was approved by the Ethics Committee of the University of Alicante in Spain (reference: UA-2020-03-27) on 27 March 2020.

Informed Consent Statement: Informed consent was obtained from all subjects involved in the study.

Data Availability Statement: The original contributions presented in this study are included in the article. Further inquiries can be directed to the corresponding author.

Conflicts of Interest: The authors declare no conflicts of interest.

References

1. American Psychiatric Association. *Diagnostic and Statistical Manual of Mental Disorders*, 5th ed.; Text Revision; American Psychiatric Association (APA): Washington, DC, USA, 2022.
2. Glod, M.; Riby, D.M.; Rodgers, J. Short report: Relationships between sensory processing, repetitive behaviors, anxiety, and intolerance of uncertainty in autism spectrum disorder and Williams syndrome. *Autism Res.* **2019**, *12*, 759–765. [CrossRef]
3. Ben-Sasson, A.; Gal, E.; Fluss, R.; Katz-Zetler, N.; Cermak, S.A. Update of a Meta-analysis of Sensory Symptoms in ASD: A New Decade of Research. *J. Autism Dev. Disord.* **2019**, *49*, 4974–4996. [CrossRef] [PubMed]
4. Miller, L.J.; Coll, J.R.; Schoen, S.A. A Randomized Controlled Pilot Study of the Effectiveness of Occupational Therapy for Children With Sensory Modulation Disorder. *Am. J. Occup. Ther.* **2007**, *61*, 228–238. [CrossRef]
5. Patten, E.; Ausderau, K.K.; Watson, L.R.; Baranek, G.T. Sensory Response Patterns in Nonverbal Children with ASD. *Autism Res. Treat.* **2013**, *2013*, 1–9. [CrossRef]
6. Baranek, G.T.; Watson, L.R.; Boyd, B.A.; Poe, M.D.; David, F.J.; McGuire, L. Hyporesponsiveness to social and nonsocial sensory stimuli in children with autism, children with developmental delays, and typically developing children. *Dev. Psychopathol.* **2013**, *25*, 307–320. [CrossRef]
7. Cárcel López, M.D.; Ferrando-Prieto, M. La estimulación multisensorial para mejorar el procesamiento sensorial en las personas con TEA. *Rev. Discapac. Clínica Neurocienc.* **2024**, *11*, 41–54. [CrossRef]
8. Martínez-González, A.E.; Rodríguez-Jiménez, T.; Piqueras, J.A.; Cañete, L.I.; Berutich, S.H.; Andreo-Martínez, P.; Ordóñez-Rubio, T.; Lillo, V.M.B.; Cubi, M.D.M.; Navarro-Soria, I. Cross-disorder comparison of sensory reactivity, pain, gastro-intestinal symptoms and obsessive-compulsive symptoms in adolescents and young adults with autism and other neurodevelopmental disorders. *Int. J. Dev. Disabil.* **2024**, 1–12. [CrossRef]
9. Gunderson, J.; Worthley, E.; Byiers, B.; Symons, F.; Wolff, J. Self and caregiver report measurement of sensory features in autism spectrum disorder: A systematic review of psychometric properties. *J. Neurodev. Disord.* **2023**, *15*, 5. [CrossRef]
10. Prinsen, C.A.C.; Mokkink, L.B.; Bouter, L.M.; Alonso, J.; Patrick, D.L.; De Vet, H.C.W.; Terwee, C.B. COSMIN guideline for systematic reviews of patient-reported outcome measures. *Qual. Life Res.* **2018**, *27*, 1147–1157. [CrossRef]
11. Uljarević, M.; Baranek, G.; Vivanti, G.; Hedley, D.; Hudry, K.; Lane, A. Heterogeneity of sensory features in autism spectrum disorder: Challenges and perspectives for future research. *Autism Res.* **2017**, *10*, 703–710. [CrossRef]
12. Duerden, E.G.; Taylor, M.J.; Lee, M.; McGrath, P.A.; Davis, K.D.; Roberts, S.W. Decreased Sensitivity to Thermal Stimuli in Adolescents With Autism Spectrum Disorder: Relation to Symptomatology and Cognitive Ability. *J. Pain* **2015**, *16*, 463–471. [CrossRef] [PubMed]

13. Courtemanche, A.B.; Black, W.R.; Reese, R.M. The Relationship Between Pain, Self-Injury, and Other Problem Behaviors in Young Children With Autism and Other Developmental Disabilities. *Am. J. Intellect. Dev. Disabil.* **2016**, *121*, 194–203. [CrossRef] [PubMed]
14. Simon, D.M.; Damiano, C.R.; Woynaroski, T.G.; Ibañez, L.V.; Murias, M.; Stone, W.L.; Wallace, M.T.; Cascio, C.J. Neural Correlates of Sensory Hyporesponsiveness in Toddlers at High Risk for Autism Spectrum Disorder. *J. Autism Dev. Disord.* **2017**, *47*, 2710–2722. [CrossRef] [PubMed]
15. Yasuda, Y.; Hashimoto, R.; Nakae, A.; Kang, H.; Ohi, K.; Yamamori, H.; Fujimoto, M.; Hagihira, S.; Takeda, M. Sensory cognitive abnormalities of pain in autism spectrum disorder: A case-control study. *Ann. Gen. Psychiatry* **2016**, *15*, 8. [CrossRef]
16. Mazurek, M.O.; Vasa, R.A.; Kalb, L.G.; Kanne, S.M.; Rosenberg, D.; Keefer, A.; Murray, D.S.; Freedman, B.; Lowery, L.A. Anxiety, Sensory Over-Responsivity, and Gastrointestinal Problems in Children with Autism Spectrum Disorders. *J. Abnorm. Child. Psychol.* **2013**, *41*, 165–176. [CrossRef]
17. Mazurek, M.O.; Keefer, A.; Shui, A.; Vasa, R.A. One-year course and predictors of abdominal pain in children with autism spectrum disorders: The role of anxiety and sensory over-responsivity. *Res. Autism Spectr. Disord.* **2014**, *8*, 1508–1515. [CrossRef]
18. Martínez-González, A.E.; Andreo-Martínez, P. The Role of Gut Microbiota in Gastrointestinal Symptoms of Children with ASD. *Medicina* **2019**, *55*, 408. [CrossRef] [PubMed]
19. Andreo-Martínez, P.; García-Martínez, N.; Sánchez-Samper, E.P.; Quesada-Medina, J.; MacFabe, D. Metabolitos de la microbiota intestinal implicados en el trastorno del espectro autista. *Rev. Discapac. Clínica Neurocienc.* **2018**, *5*, 39. [CrossRef]
20. Andreo-Martínez, P.; Rubio-Aparicio, M.; Sánchez-Meca, J.; Veas, A.; Martínez-González, A.E. A Meta-analysis of Gut Microbiota in Children with Autism. *J. Autism Dev. Disord.* **2022**, *52*, 1374–1387. [CrossRef]
21. Mayer, E.A.; Labus, J.; Aziz, Q.; Tracey, I.; Kilpatrick, L.; Elsenbruch, S.; Schweinhardt, P.; Van Oudenhove, L.; Borsook, D. Role of brain imaging in disorders of brain–gut interaction: A Rome Working Team Report. *Gut* **2019**, *68*, 1701–1715. [CrossRef] [PubMed]
22. Lam, K.S.L.; Aman, M.G. The Repetitive Behavior Scale-Revised: Independent Validation in Individuals with Autism Spectrum Disorders. *J. Autism Dev. Disord.* **2007**, *37*, 855–866. [CrossRef] [PubMed]
23. Rutter, M.; Bailey, A.; Lord, C. *The Social Communication Questionnaire: Manual*; Western Psychological Services: Los Ángeles, CA, USA, 2003.
24. Pereña, J.; Santamaría, P. *Cuestionario de Comunicación Social: SCQ: Manual. [Social Communication Questionnaire: Handbook]*; TEA: Madrid, Spain, 2005.
25. Wigham, S.; Rodgers, J.; Berney, T.; Le Couteur, A.; Ingham, B.; Parr, J.R. Psychometric properties of questionnaires and diagnostic measures for autism spectrum disorders in adults: A systematic review. *Autism* **2019**, *23*, 287–305. [CrossRef]
26. Bodfish, J.W.; Symons, F.J.; Parker, D.E.; Lewis, M.H. Varieties of repetitive behavior in autism: Comparisons to mental retardation. *J. Autism Dev. Disord.* **2000**, *30*, 237–243. [CrossRef] [PubMed]
27. Martínez-González, A.E.; Piqueras, J.A. Validation of the Repetitive Behavior Scale-Revised in Spanish-Speakers Participants with Autism Spectrum Disorder. *J. Autism Dev. Disord.* **2018**, *48*, 198–208. [CrossRef]
28. He, H.; Ye, N.; Yi, L.; Yang, C. Validating the Repetitive Behavior Scale-Revised for Children in China Aged 3 to 8 with Autism Spectrum Disorder. *J. Autism Dev. Disord.* **2019**, *49*, 4941–4956. [CrossRef]
29. McIntosh, D.N.; Miller, L.; Shyu, V.; Dunn, W. Overview of the Short Sensory Profile. In *Sensory Profile User's Manual*; Dunn, W., Ed.; Pearsons: San Antonio, TX, USA, 1999; pp. 59–73.
30. Dunn, W. *Short Sensory Profile*; Psychological Corporation: San Antonio, TX, USA, 1999.
31. Tomchek, S.D.; Huebner, R.A.; Dunn, W. Patterns of sensory processing in children with an autism spectrum disorder. *Res. Autism Spectr. Disord.* **2014**, *8*, 1214–1224. [CrossRef]
32. Williams, Z.J.; Failla, M.D.; Gotham, K.O.; Woynaroski, T.G.; Cascio, C. Psychometric Evaluation of the Short Sensory Profile in Youth with Autism Spectrum Disorder. *J. Autism Dev. Disord.* **2018**, *48*, 4231–4249. [CrossRef] [PubMed]
33. Kaneko, A.; Ohshima, R.; Noda, H.; Matsumaru, T.; Iwanaga, R.; Ide, M. Sensory and Social Subtypes of Japanese Individuals with Autism Spectrum Disorders. *J. Autism Dev. Disord.* **2023**, *53*, 3133–3143. [CrossRef] [PubMed]
34. McGrath, P.J.; Rosmus, C.; Canfield, C.; Campbell, M.A.; Hennigar, A. Behaviours caregivers use to determine pain in non-verbal, cognitively impaired individuals. *Dev. Med. Child. Neurol.* **1998**, *40*, 340–343. [PubMed]
35. Liu, J.; Chen, L.L.; Shen, S.; Mao, J.; Lopes, M.; Liu, S.; Kong, X. Challenges in the Diagnosis and Management of Pain in Individuals with Autism Spectrum Disorder. *Rev. J. Autism Dev. Disord.* **2020**, *7*, 352–363. [CrossRef]
36. Breau, L.M.; McGrath, P.J.; Camfield, C.S.; Finley, A.G. Psychometric properties of the non-communicating children's pain checklist-revised. *Pain* **2002**, *99*, 349–357. [CrossRef] [PubMed]
37. Lotan, M.; Ljunggren, E.A.; Johnsen, T.B.; Defrin, R.; Pick, C.G.; Strand, L.I. A Modified Version of the Non-Communicating Children Pain Checklist-Revised, Adapted to Adults With Intellectual and Developmental Disabilities: Sensitivity to Pain and Internal Consistency. *J. Pain* **2009**, *10*, 398–407. [CrossRef] [PubMed]
38. Dunn, J.G.H.; Bouffard, M.; Rogers, W.T. Assessing Item Content-Relevance in Sport Psychology Scale-Construction Research: Issues and Recommendations. *Meas. Phys. Educ. Exerc. Sci.* **1999**, *3*, 15–36. [CrossRef]
39. Alarcón, R.; Blanca, M.J. Development and Psychometric Properties of the Questionnaire for Assessing Educational Podcasts (QAEP). *Front. Psychol.* **2020**, *11*, 579454. [CrossRef] [PubMed]
40. Aiken, L.R. Content Validity and Reliability of Single Items or Questionnaires. *Educ. Psychol. Meas.* **1980**, *40*, 955–959. [CrossRef]

41. Martínez-González, A.E. *Theoretical Model and Structure of the Pain and Sensitivity Reactivity Scale*; Intellectual Property Registration: Murcia, Spain, 2023.
42. Hittner, J.B.; May, K.; Silver, N.C. A Monte Carlo Evaluation of Tests for Comparing Dependent Correlations. *J. Gen. Psychol.* **2003**, *130*, 149–168. [CrossRef]
43. Hu, L.; Bentler, P.M. Cutoff criteria for fit indexes in covariance structure analysis: Conventional criteria versus new alternatives. *Struct. Equ. Model. Multidiscip. J.* **1999**, *6*, 1–55. [CrossRef]
44. Rose, D.R.; Yang, H.; Serena, G.; Sturgeon, C.; Ma, B.; Careaga, M.; Hughes, H.K.; Angkustsiri, K.; Rose, M.; Hertz-Picciotto, I.; et al. Differential immune responses and microbiota profiles in children with autism spectrum disorders and co-morbid gastrointestinal symptoms. *Brain Behav. Immun.* **2018**, *70*, 354–368. [CrossRef] [PubMed]
45. Koo, T.K.; Li, M.Y. A Guideline of Selecting and Reporting Intraclass Correlation Coefficients for Reliability Research. *J. Chiropr. Med.* **2016**, *15*, 155–163. [CrossRef]
46. Kuiper, M.W.; Verhoeven, E.W.; Geurts, H.M. The Dutch Glasgow Sensory Questionnaire: Psychometric properties of an autism-specific sensory sensitivity measure. *Autism* **2019**, *23*, 922–932. [CrossRef]
47. Newton, E.; Schosheim, A.; Patel, S.; Chitkara, D.K.; Van Tilburg, M.A.L. The role of psychological factors in pediatric functional abdominal pain disorders. *Neurogastroenterol. Motil.* **2019**, *31*, e13538. [CrossRef]
48. Simpson, K.; Adams, D.; Alston-Knox, C.; Heussler, H.S.; Keen, D. Exploring the Sensory Profiles of Children on the Autism Spectrum Using the Short Sensory Profile-2 (SSP-2). *J. Autism Dev. Disord.* **2019**, *49*, 2069–2079. [CrossRef] [PubMed]
49. Sapey-Triomphe, L.A.; Moulin, A.; Sonié, S.; Schmitz, C. The Glasgow Sensory Questionnaire: Validation of a French Language Version and Refinement of Sensory Profiles of People with High Autism-Spectrum Quotient. *J. Autism Dev. Disord.* **2018**, *48*, 1549–1565. [CrossRef] [PubMed]
50. Tomchek, S.D.; Little, L.M.; Myers, J.; Dunn, W. Sensory Subtypes in Preschool Aged Children with Autism Spectrum Disorder. *J. Autism Dev. Disord.* **2018**, *48*, 2139–2147. [CrossRef]

children

MDPI

Article

Linking Mechanisms in the Intergenerational Transmission of Mental Health: The Role of Sex in Parent–Adolescent Dynamics

Hye-Jung Yun [1,*], Jungyeong Heo [2] and Cynthia B. Wilson [1]

1 The Florida Center for Prevention Research, Florida State University, Tallahassee, FL 32301, USA; cbwilson2@fsu.edu
2 Counseling & Psychological Services, Purdue University, West Lafayette, IN 47907, USA; heo42@purdue.edu
* Correspondence: hyun@fsu.edu

Abstract: Background/Objectives: This study addresses the significance of mental health concerns by examining the intergenerational transmission of mental health between parents and adolescents. It investigates the serial mediating effects of family resilience, adolescents' adverse childhood experiences (ACEs), and their ability to flourish in the transmission of mental health from parents to adolescents, with a focus on sex differences. Methods: This study used a sample of 54,434 adolescents aged 12–17 from the 2016–2020 National Survey of Children's Health (NSCH). Mothers reported on their mental health status and family resilience, and adolescents' ACEs, flourishing, and mental health problems including depression and anxiety. Serial mediation models were used to assess the hypotheses. Results: The findings revealed that better parental mental health status was associated with fewer mental health problems in adolescents, with significant sex differences observed in these associations. Specifically, in both maternal and paternal models, better parental mental health was linked to higher family resilience, which was associated with fewer ACEs, greater flourishing, and ultimately fewer adolescent mental health problems. Furthermore, maternal mental health had a stronger association with daughters' mental health, while paternal mental health more strongly influenced sons'. Conclusions: These results highlight the importance of targeted prevention and clinical interventions to disrupt the intergenerational transmission of mental health issues.

Keywords: adverse childhood experiences (ACEs); family resilience; ability to flourish; mental health

1. Introduction

The intergenerational transmission of mental health has garnered increasing attention from researchers over the past decade [1]. According to the National Alliance on Mental Illness [2], 20% of adults and 17% of adolescents aged 12–17 in the United States have a mental illness, and globally, 15–23% of children live with a parent who has a mental health diagnosis. The link between the mental health of parents and their children is well established, with poor parental mental health being associated with an increased risk of mental health issues in children's mental health, including anxiety and depression [3–5]. Given these factors, the intergenerational transmission of mental health concerns is particularly important during adolescence, a developmental period marked by significant emotional and cognitive changes.

Adverse childhood experiences (ACEs) encompass a wide range of traumatic and stressful events that can negatively impact children's lives. While much of the research on ACEs has focused on children and adults, there is a growing need to explore adolescence, a developmental stage marked by rapid physical, cognitive, social, and emotional changes [6]. Adolescents exposed to ACEs face heightened mental health challenges, as traumatic experiences can disrupt emotional and cognitive development and are often compounded by a lack of positive family support [7]. Although studies have consistently shown a strong link between ACEs and mental health issues [8], there is limited understanding of the effect of ACEs on the intergenerational transmission of mental health between parents and adolescents. Thus, this study examined the mediating role of adolescents' ACEs in the intergenerational transmission of mental health.

In contrast to research demonstrating the negative effects of ACEs, some studies have identified the protective roles of family and adolescent resilience in mitigating mental health issues [9,10]. Given the potential of resilience as a prevention or intervention tool, it is important to explore its role in the intergenerational transmission of mental health. Thus, this study investigated how family resilience and adolescents' ability to flourish mediate the associations between parental mental health, adolescents' ACEs, and their mental health outcomes.

1.1. Intergenerational Transmission of Mental Health

Although mental health symptoms are generally characterized by their impact on an individual's functioning [11], substantial research highlights the relational nature of mental health issues. Family systems theory [12] offers a useful framework for understanding the intergenerational transmission of mental health, emphasizing that symptoms are often shaped by dynamic interactions within family systems. Research demonstrated that children of parents with poor mental health are more likely to experience mental health problems themselves [3]. A systemic lens emphasizes the interrelatedness of parents' and adolescents' mental health, suggesting that "symptoms represent recursive feedback cycles of escalated behavior and experience that are organized into an interactional system" (p. 124) [13]. For example, Reid [14] found that children living with a parent with poor mental health are more likely to have mood or anxiety disorders compared to those living with a parent without mental health symptoms. Similarly, Lui et al. [15] found that parental mental health directly impacted their children's emotional outcomes. The systemic concept of nonsummativity suggests that "the behavior of an element is different within the system from what it is in isolation" (p. 58) [16]. Building on this, Zhou et al. [17] differentiate between general mental health challenges, which broadly impact a range of psychological and social outcomes, and specific issues, such as internalizing problems (e.g., depression, anxiety) and externalizing problems (e.g., behavioral issues), which are more closely linked to similar outcomes in children, including depression, anxiety, and conduct disorders. Therefore, a comprehensive understanding of the transmission of mental health should also consider additional factors, such as risk and protective factors, within the parent–adolescent subsystem.

1.2. Linking Mechanisms for Transmission of Mental Health Between Parents and Adolescents

While parental mental health plays a significant role in their children's mental health, external risk factors, such as adverse childhood experiences (ACEs), can exacerbate mental health challenges for adolescents. On the other hand, protective factors, like family resilience and adolescents' ability to flourish may help buffer the negative impacts of these experiences. Exploring the interaction between these factors offers a deeper understanding of how mental health is transmitted across generations.

Adolescents' ACEs: ACEs are defined as traumatic experiences during childhood that can impact individuals' health and functioning throughout their lifetime [18,19]. These experiences include parental divorce/separation, the death of a parent or guardian, domestic violence, substance abuse, mental illness, financial hardship, exposure to violence, discrimination, and the incarceration of a family member before the age of 18 [20].

Parental mental illness, a specific type of ACE, can directly impact adolescents' mental health. Further, ACEs can act as a pathway linking parental mental health to adolescents' mental health outcomes. For example, when parents suffer from mental illness, it can lead to an increase in ACEs for their children. In turn, adolescents exposed to ACEs are more likely to exhibit poor mental health outcomes [21,22]. That is, ACEs can lead to a decline in adolescents' mental health, putting them at a higher risk for psychological disorders such as anxiety and depression. Thus, this study examined the mediating effect of adolescents'

ACEs on the relationship between parental mental health status and adolescents' mental health problems.

Family Resilience: Given the negative health outcomes associated with ACEs, it is important to identify protective factors for adolescents who have experienced adversities. In resilience research, the terms "promotive" and "protective" factors have been used to describe variables that contribute to adaptive outcomes under conditions of adversity. Promotive factors are associated with positive outcomes regardless of the level of risk, while protective factors specifically mitigate the adverse effects of high-risk environments [23]. In this study, we adopt the term "protective factors" to emphasize their buffering role in reducing the negative impact of adversity, while acknowledging that these factors may also possess promotive qualities in broader contexts. A growing body of research suggests that high levels of family resilience can serve as a protective factor in the face of adverse experiences [9,24]. Family resilience refers to the ability of the family to adapt to change and overcome significant stressors [25]. Factors associated with family resilience include frequent family communication, effective problem-solving, family strength, and positivity. Recent efforts in clinical practices advocate that family resilience has the potential to mitigate the adverse effects of ACEs on adolescents' mental health. For example, Uddin et al. [9] found that family resilience could reduce the impact of ACEs on children's mental health. However, it remains unclear how family resilience mediates the association among parental mental health status, adolescents' ACEs, and their mental health problems. Therefore, this study examined the mediating role of family resilience in such associations.

Adolescents' Ability to Flourish: Adolescents' ability to flourish is recognized as a foundational component of positive well-being and as a protective factor against mental health problems [26,27]. In 2011/12, the National Survey of Children's Health (NSCH) introduced indicators of flourishing to provide positive measures of health, as recommended by a Technical Expert Panel (TEP). This concept of flourishing in adolescents includes curiosity in learning, resilience, and self-regulation. Bethell et al. [10] found that adolescents exposed to ACEs who displayed demonstrated resilience were significantly less likely to experience emotional, mental, and behavioral problems compared to those with lower resilience. This suggests that the ability to flourish could act as a possible mediator between adolescents' ACEs and mental health outcomes. Therefore, this study examined the mediating effect of adolescents' ability to flourish in the relationship between parental mental health status, adolescents' ACEs, and their mental health problems.

1.3. Sex-Specific Pathways

Previous research indicated that parental mental health may affect sons and daughters differently during adolescence. Connell and Goodman's meta-analysis [28] found that while maternal mental health generally had a stronger association with children's outcomes than paternal mental health, the differences were relatively small, suggesting the importance of both parents' mental health. Specifically, Goodman et al. [29] found that maternal mental health problems have a stronger impact on daughters compared to sons, potentially due to sex-specific modeling and identification processes [30]. These sex-specific pathways highlight the importance of considering child sex within broader family dynamics, such as family resilience, adolescents' ACEs, and their ability to flourish, to fully understand how parental mental health influences adolescent outcomes. Thus, this study examined the sex differences within our research model.

1.4. The Present Study

Given the importance of intergenerational transmission of mental health, this study aims to address existing gaps in the literature by examining how family resilience, adolescents' ACEs, and their ability to flourish mediate the relationship between parental and adolescent mental health. Based on previous theoretical and empirical research, we proposed three hypotheses: First, based on family systems theory [12], parental mental health status would be negatively associated with adolescents' mental health problems (H1). Second, the relationship between parental mental health status and adolescent mental health problems would be serially mediated by family resilience, adolescents' ACEs, and their ability to flourish (H2), as shown in Figure 1. Lastly, based on sex-specific modeling [30], the strength of these relationships would vary by parent and adolescent sex. Specifically, we hypothesized that maternal mental health would have a stronger association with daughters' mental health problems than sons', while paternal mental health would have a stronger association with sons' mental health problems than daughters' (H3).

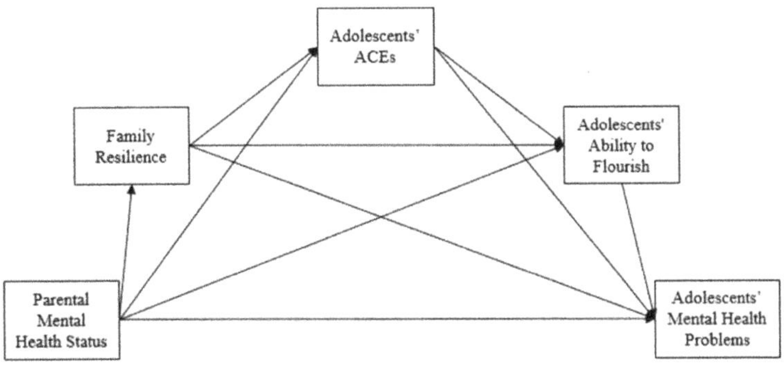

Figure 1. The proposed serial mediation model.

2. Methods

2.1. Samples and Procedures

Data for this study were derived from the 2016–2020 National Survey of Children's Health (NSCH), a nationally representative, cross-sectional survey conducted annually by the U.S. Census Bureau, sponsored by the U.S. Maternal and Child Health Bureau, and maintained by the Child and Adolescent Health Measurement Initiative (CAHMI) [31]. The NSCH assesses various aspects of child and family health-related experiences across the United States. Following the NSCH Guide to Multi-Year Analysis [32], we merged data from five consecutive years (2016–2020) to increase the sample size and enhance the representativeness of the findings. Sampling weights from the NSCH public-use dataset were applied to account for non-response and selection probabilities, ensuring results could be generalized to the U.S. parent and adolescent population. The final sample size was 54,434 parents with adolescents aged 12–17.

2.2. Measures

2.2.1. Parental Mental Health Status

Paternal and maternal mental health were each assessed with a single item, where each parent reported their mental health status. Responses were rated on a three-point Likert scale, recoded as 1 = fair/poor, 2 = good, and 3 = excellent/very, so that higher scores indicated better overall paternal or maternal mental health.

2.2.2. Adolescents' Mental Health Problems

Parents reported on their adolescent children's (ages 12–17) depression and anxiety symptoms. These two items were combined to create an overall indicator of adolescents' mental health problems. Responses were coded as 0 = does not have a condition and 1 = does have a condition. The items of anxiety and depression were summed, with higher scores indicating greater levels of mental health problems in adolescents.

2.2.3. Adolescents' ACEs

Parents reported their adolescent children's ACEs through nine items assessing exposures to (1) financial hardship, (2) parent/guardian separation or divorce, (3) death of parent/guardian, (4) parent/guardian incarceration, (5) domestic violence, (6) victim/witness of neighborhood violence, (7) mental health issues, (8) alcohol/drug abuse, and (9) race/ethnicity discrimination. All items were recoded as 0 = no and 1 = yes, and the items were summed to create the ACE scores, with higher scores indicating a greater number of ACEs. Previous studies have demonstrated good internal consistency reliability (e.g., $\alpha = 0.86$) [33] and validity of ACEs scales, showing a significant association with adolescent depression ($\beta = 0.29$, $p < 0.001$) and anxiety ($\beta = 0.26$, $p < 0.001$) in a variety of samples [34]. McDonald's omega for this measure was 0.66.

2.2.4. Family Resilience

Family resilience was measured using four items that captured qualities of how families respond to difficulties. Participants rated how often their family engages in the following behaviors: (1) talk together about what to do; (2) work together to solve our problems; (3) know we have strengths to draw on; and (4) stay hopeful even in difficult times. Each item was scored on a three-point Likert scale, recoded as 1 = some/none of the time, 2 = most of the time, and 3 = all of the time. Items were summed to create a total family resilience score, with higher scores indicating greater family resilience. Previous studies have demonstrated strong internal reliability (e.g., $\alpha = 0.92$) [35] and construct validity, showing a significant association with adolescent depression ($\beta = -0.71$, $p < 0.001$) [36]. In the current sample, McDonald's omega was 0.89.

2.2.5. Adolescents' Ability to Flourish

Three questions were used to assess adolescents' curiosity about learning, resilience, and self-regulation for adolescents aged 12–17. These questions asked parents if their adolescent children (1) show interest and curiosity in learning new things, (2) work to finish tasks he or she start, and (3) stay calm and in control when faced with a challenge. Each item was recoded as 0 = no and 1 = yes, then summed to create an adolescent's flourishing scores. A higher score reflected a higher level of an adolescent's ability to flourish. Earlier studies have demonstrated good internal reliability (e.g., $\alpha = 0.75$) [37] and validity, showing a significant association with family resilience ($\beta = 0.29$, $p < 0.001$) [38]. McDonald's omega for this measure was 0.73.

2.2.6. Adolescent Sex

Adolescent sex (coded as 1 = female, 0 = male) was added as a moderator to investigate potential sex differences in the research model, given evidence that sex may influence the intergenerational transmission of mental health. Previous research suggests that maternal and paternal mental health may impact sons and daughters differently [28].

2.3. *Analytical Plan*

We conducted path analyses using Mplus 8 [38] to test our hypotheses. The analysis proceeded in three stages.

First, we evaluated the direct effect of parental mental health status on adolescents' mental health problems, expecting a significant path coefficient. This would suggest that better parental mental health is associated with fewer mental health problems in adolescents (H1). Second, we tested the serial mediation model, investigating whether the relationship between parental mental health status (maternal and paternal mental health status, separately) and adolescent mental health problems was mediated through three sequential pathways: family resilience, adolescents' ACEs, and ability to flourish (H2). Each indirect path coefficient was examined to confirm the role of these mediating factors. Lastly, to test sex differences (H3), we conducted multi-group path analyses comparing the path coefficients across sex groups, allowing us to determine whether the strength or direction of associations varied by sex. To achieve this, we conducted a χ^2 difference test between an unrestricted model, in which all path coefficients were freely estimated for each sex, and 10 separate restricted models, each constraining a single path coefficient to be equal across sexes. A significant χ^2 difference between the unrestricted and restricted models indicates that the constrained path coefficient significantly differs by sex.

The significance of indirect effects was evaluated using bootstrap confidence intervals based on 5000 resamples. Cases with missing data on parental mental health status (independent variable) were excluded from analyses while missing data on other variables were handled using Full Information Maximum Likelihood (FIML). Model fits were assessed using chi-square (χ^2), the root mean square error (RMSEA), the comparative index (CFI), and the Tucker–Lewis index (TLI). Models with an RMSEA below 0.05, along with CFI and TLI above 0.95, are considered to have great model fits [39].

3. Results

3.1. Preliminary Results

Descriptive statistics and correlations among the variables are shown in Table 1. From the correlations, both maternal and paternal mental health status was significantly and negatively correlated with adolescents' mental health ($r = -0.21$ for maternal and $r = -0.16$ for paternal, $p < 0.01$), providing preliminary support for H1. Additionally, both maternal and paternal mental health status was significantly and negatively associated with adolescents' ACEs ($r = -0.31$ for maternal and $r = -0.27$ for paternal, $p < 0.01$). Parental mental health was also significantly and positively associated with family resilience ($r = 0.27$ for maternal and $r = 0.26$ for paternal, $p < 0.01$) and adolescents' ability to flourish ($r = 0.15$ for maternal and $r = 0.11$ for paternal; $p < 0.01$). Furthermore, adolescents' ACEs were negatively associated with both family resilience ($r = -0.16$, $p < 0.01$) and adolescent flourishing ($r = -0.16$, $p < 0.01$), while family resilience was positively correlated with adolescents' ability to flourish ($r = 0.21$, $p < 0.01$). These correlations offered preliminary support for H2. Adolescent sex (female =1) is associated with adolescents' mental health problems ($r = 0.08$, $p < 0.01$) and adolescents' ability ($r = 0.05$, $p < 0.01$). Based on these preliminary findings, we proceeded to hypothesis testing.

Table 1. Descriptive statistics and correlations among study variables.

Variables	M or % (SD)	1	2	3	4	5	6
1. Maternal/paternal mental health status	M: 2.71 (0.55) P: 2.76 (0.51)	–	−0.16 **	−0.27 **	0.26 **	0.11 **	0.00
2. Adolescents' mental health problems	0.21 (0.53)	−0.21 **	–	0.23 **	−0.13 **	−0.17 **	0.08 **
3. Adolescents' ACEs	1.34 (1.48)	−0.31 **	0.23 **	–	−0.16 **	−0.16 **	0.01
4. Family resilience	9.22 (2.35)	0.27 **	−0.13 **	−0.16 **	–	0.21 **	0.00
5. Adolescents' ability to flourish	2.43 (0.95)	0.15 **	−0.17 **	−0.16 **	0.21 **	–	0.05 **
6. Adolescent sex (1 = female)	48.5%	0.00	−0.08 **	0.01	0.00	0.05 **	–

Note: Correlations for the maternal sample are shown below the diagonal (N = 48,424); correlations for the paternal sample are shown above the diagonal (N = 42,279). ** $p < 0.01$; two-tailed tested.

3.2. Hypothesis Testing for the Association Between Parental Mental Health Status and Adolescents' Mental Health Problems (H1)

Path analysis results indicated that maternal/paternal mental health statuses were significantly and negatively associated with adolescents' mental health problems ($\beta = -0.20$, $p < 0.01$ for maternal; $\beta = -0.16$, $p < 0.01$ for paternal), after controlling for other influential variables including adolescent sex. In other words, better maternal and paternal mental health were associated with fewer adolescent mental health problems.

3.3. Hypothesis Testing for the Mediating Effects of Family Resilience, Adolescents' ACEs, and Their Ability to Flourish in the Intergenerational Transmission of Mental Health (H2)

The serial mediation model for maternal mental health demonstrated a good fit ($\chi^2(3) = 142.22$, RMSEA $= 0.03$ [95% CI(0.03, 0.04)], CFI $= 0.99$, TLI $= 0.96$). In the model, all regression paths were significant (see Figure 2). Specifically, maternal mental health status positively influenced familial resilience ($\beta = 0.27$, $p < 0.001$) and adolescents' ability to flourish ($\beta = 0.07$, $p < 0.001$), while reducing adolescents' ACEs ($\beta = -0.29$, $p < 0.001$) and mental health problems ($\beta = -0.13$, $p < 0.001$). Family resilience was associated with fewer adolescents' ACEs ($\beta = -0.08$, $p < 0.001$) and mental health problems ($\beta = -0.04$, $p < 0.001$), and it increased adolescents' ability to flourish ($\beta = 0.17$, $p < 0.001$). Additionally, adolescents' ACEs were linked to a decrease in their ability to flourish ($\beta = -0.11$, $p < 0.001$) but an increase in mental health problems ($\beta = 0.16$, $p < 0.001$). Adolescents' ability to flourish was inversely related to their mental health problems ($\beta = -0.12$, $p < 0.001$). As shown in Table 2, the bootstrapping results revealed significant indirect effects from maternal mental health status to adolescents' mental health problems. These findings indicate that family resilience, adolescents' ACEs, and their ability to flourish sequentially mediated the relationship between maternal mental health and adolescents' mental health problems ($\beta = 0.00$, $z = -12.17$, $p < 0.001$).

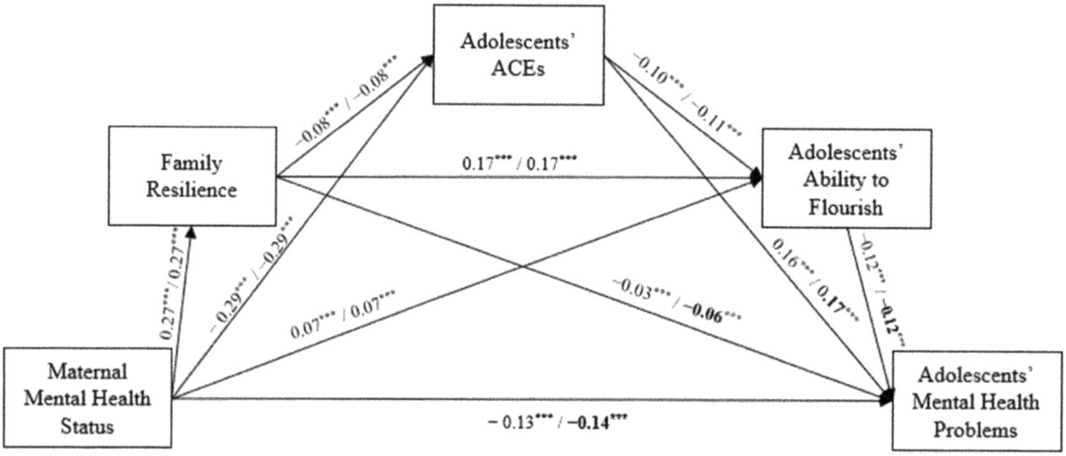

Figure 2. The serial mediation model from maternal mental health status to adolescents' mental health problems. Note: The path coefficients are shown separately for adolescent sex (boys/girls). Bold indicates a significantly higher coefficient compared to the other sex. *** $p < 0.001$.

Table 2. Indirect, direct, and total effects of maternal mental health status on adolescents' mental health problems.

Model Pathway	Estimate [95% CI †]	
	Boys	Girls
Maternal MH → ACEs → adolescent MHP	−0.045 *** (−0.049, −0.041)	−0.047 *** (−0.052, −0.043)
Maternal MH → flourish → adolescent MHP	−0.009 *** (−0.010, −0.007)	−0.008 *** (−0.010, −0.006)
Maternal MH → family resilience → adolescent MHP	−0.008 *** (−0.011, −0.004)	−0.015 *** (−0.019, −0.012)
Maternal MH → family resilience → ACES → adolescent MHP	−0.003 *** (−0.004, −0.003)	−0.004 *** (−0.004, −0.003)
Maternal MH → ACES → flourish → adolescent MHP	−0.003 *** (−0.004, −0.003)	−0.004 *** (−0.005, −0.003)
Maternal MH → family resilience → flourish → adolescent MHP	−0.005 *** (−0.006, −0.005)	−0.006 *** (−0.006, −0.005)
Maternal MH → family resilience → ACES → flourish → adolescent MHP	0.000 *** (0.000, 0.000)	0.000 *** (0.000, 0.000)
Total indirect effect: maternal MH → adolescent MHP	−0.074 *** (−0.079, −0.068)	−0.084 *** (−0.090, −0.079)
Direct effect: maternal MH → adolescent MHP	−0.131 *** (−0.144, −0.118)	−0.135 *** (−0.149, −0.122)
Total effect of maternal MH: total indirect effect + direct effect	−0.205 *** (−0.217, −0.193)	−0.220 *** (−0.232, −0.208)

Note: *** $p < 0.001$; two-tailed tested. † Symmetric confidence interval.

The serial mediation model for paternal mental health demonstrated a good model fit ($\chi^2(3) = 100.05$, RMSEA $= 0.03$ [95% CI(0.023, 0.032)], CFI $= 0.99$, TLI $= 0.96$). The regression coefficients in the serial mediation model of paternal mental health status mirrored those in the maternal model, with all regression paths showing significant effects (see Figure 3). Specifically, paternal mental health status positively influenced family resilience ($\beta = 0.26$, $p < 0.001$) and adolescents' ability to flourish ($\beta = 0.04$, $p < 0.001$) while reducing adolescents' ACEs ($\beta = -0.24$, $p < 0.001$) and mental health problems ($\beta = -0.09$, $p < 0.001$). Family resilience was associated with lower levels of adolescents' ACEs ($\beta = -0.11$, $p < 0.001$) and mental health problems ($\beta = -0.05$, $p < 0.001$) while increasing adolescents' ability to flourish ($\beta = 0.17$, $p < 0.001$). Adolescents' ACEs reduced their ability to flourish ($\beta = -0.12$, $p < 0.001$) and were linked to increased mental health problems ($\beta = 0.14$, $p < 0.001$). Additionally, adolescents' ability to flourish was negatively associated with mental health problems ($\beta = -0.12$, $p < 0.001$). As shown in Table 3, the bootstrapping results revealed significant indirect effects from paternal mental health status to adolescents' mental health problems. These findings show that family resilience, adolescents' ACEs, and their ability to flourish sequentially mediated the association between paternal mental health status and adolescents' mental health problems ($\beta = 0.00$, $z = -13.36$, $p < 0.001$).

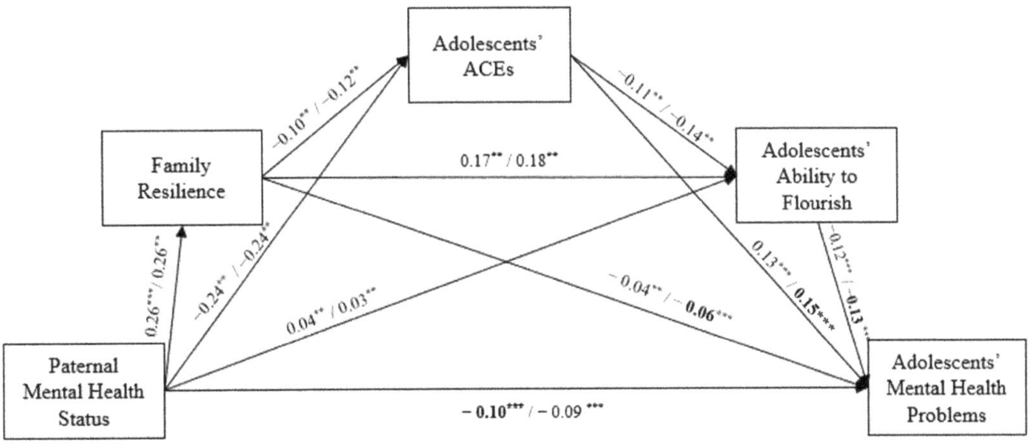

Figure 3. The serial mediation model from paternal mental health status to adolescents' mental health problems. Note: The path coefficients are shown separately for adolescent sex (boys/girls). Bold indicates a significantly higher coefficient compared to the other sex. ** $p < 0.01$, *** $p < 0.001$.

Table 3. Indirect, direct, and total effects of paternal mental health status on adolescents' mental health problems.

Model Pathway	Estimate [95% CI†]	
	Boys	Girls
Paternal MH → ACEs → adolescent MHP	−0.031 *** (−0.034, −0.027)	−0.036 *** (−0.040, −0.033)
Paternal MH → flourish → adolescent MHP	−0.005 *** (−0.007, −0.003)	−0.004 *** (−0.005, −0.002)
Paternal MH → family resilience → adolescent MHP	−0.009 *** (−0.013, −0.006)	−0.016 *** (−0.019, −0.012)
Paternal MH → family resilience → ACES → adolescent MHP	−0.003 *** (−0.004, −0.003)	−0.005 *** (−0.005, −0.004)
Paternal MH → ACES → flourish → adolescent MHP	−0.003 *** (−0.004, −0.003)	−0.004 *** (−0.005, −0.003)
Paternal MH → family resilience → flourish → adolescent MHP	−0.006 *** (−0.006, −0.005)	−0.006 *** (−0.007, −0.005)
Paternal MH → family resilience → ACES → flourish → adolescent MHP	0.000 *** (0.000, 0.000)	−0.001 *** (−0.001, 0.000)
Total indirect effect: paternal MH → adolescent MHP	−0.057 *** (−0.063, −0.052)	−0.071 *** (−0.076, −0.065)
Direct effect: paternal MH → adolescent MHP	−0.096 *** (−0.109, −0.082)	−0.135 *** (−0.034, −0.027)
Total effect of paternal MH: total indirect effect + direct effect	−0.153 *** (−0.166, −0.140)	−0.163 *** (−0.176, −0.149)

Note: *** $p < 0.001$; two-tailed tested. † Symmetric confidence interval.

3.4. Hypothesis Testing for Sex Difference in the Serial Mediation Model (H3)

Some regression coefficients revealed sex differences. In the maternal mental health model, maternal mental health ($\Delta\chi^2$ = 47.88), family resilience ($\Delta\chi^2$ = 47.28), adolescents' ACEs ($\Delta\chi^2$ = 49.77), and their ability to flourish ($\Delta\chi^2$ = 47.51) similarly impact adolescent mental health problems, with stronger effects observed among girls (maternal mental health status: $\beta = -0.14$; family resilience: $\beta = -0.06$; adolescents' ACEs: $\beta = 0.17$; and adolescents' ability to flourish: $\beta = -0.12$) than boys (maternal mental health status: $\beta = -0.13$; family resilience: $\beta = -0.03$; adolescents' ACEs: $\beta = 0.16$; and adolescents' ability to flourish: $\beta = -0.12$).

In the paternal mental health model, family resilience ($\Delta\chi^2$ = 35.73), adolescents' ACEs ($\Delta\chi^2$ = 52.11), and adolescents' ability to flourish ($\Delta\chi^2$ = 37.84) also have similar impacts on adolescents' mental health problems across sex. However, paternal mental health ($\Delta\chi^2$ = 21.39) has a slightly stronger impact on boys' mental health problems ($\beta = -0.10$) than on girls ($\beta = -0.09$)

4. Discussion

Given the public health importance of mental health, this study examined the intergenerational transmission of mental health, focusing on the mediating roles of family resilience, adolescents' ACEs, and their ability to flourish in the association between parental mental health and adolescents' mental health problems. Ground in family systems theory [11], we hypothesized that parental mental health status would directly influence adolescent mental health (H1). Furthermore, we proposed that family resilience, adolescents' ACEs, and their ability to flourish would mediate the intergenerational transmission of mental health between parents and adolescents (H2). Additionally, we explored sex differences in these pathways (H3), hypothesizing that maternal mental health would have a stronger impact on daughters' mental health, while paternal mental health would more strongly affect sons'.

4.1. The Impact of Parental Mental Health on Adolescent Mental Health (H1)

Consistent with our hypothesis and previous research [3–5], we found that both maternal and paternal mental health were significantly and negatively associated with adolescents' mental health problems. This finding underscores the critical influence of parental mental health on adolescent well-being, aligning with family systems theory [12], which emphasizes the interconnectedness of family members' mental health. The relational nature of mental health within families suggests that improving parental mental health may have a beneficial impact on adolescents, potentially reducing the risk of developing mental health issues.

4.2. Mediating Effects of Family Resilience, Adolescents' ACEs, and Adolescents' Ability to Flourish (H2)

Our findings support the second hypothesis, showing that family resilience, adolescents' ACEs, and their ability to flourish serve as serial mediators in the relationship between parental and adolescent mental health. In both maternal and paternal models, better parental mental health was associated with higher family resilience, which in turn was related to fewer ACEs and greater flourishing in adolescents, ultimately resulting in fewer adolescent mental health problems.

As a risk factor, the significant mediating role of ACEs in the relationship between parental mental health and adolescent outcomes aligns with previous research on how adverse experiences impact mental health [21,22]. The negative association between parental mental health and adolescents' ACEs suggests that better parental mental health may serve as a protective factor against adverse experiences, possibly through more effective parenting practices or resilient home environments [9,24].

These findings further support the notion that family resilience can serve as a protective factor [9,24], helping to mitigate the adverse effects of ACEs on adolescent mental health. Defined as a family's capacity to adapt to stress and work together to overcome challenges [25], family resilience is essential for buffering adolescents against the negative impacts of ACEs. This resilience likely creates an environment that promotes positive coping strategies and emotional support, reducing the risk of adolescents developing mental health problems in the face of adversities.

Additionally, the adolescents' ability to flourish, which encompasses curiosity, resilience, and self-regulation, emerged as a significant mediator, supporting previous research on its protective role in mental health outcomes [26,27]. This finding highlights the importance of fostering positive well-being indicators in adolescents as a protective factor against mental health issues. Adolescents who exhibit greater resilience and self-regulation may be better equipped to manage stress, reducing the likelihood of experiencing mental health problems. Together, these mediating factors provide insight into specific protective mechanisms that could help interrupt the transmission of mental health problems across generations.

4.3. Sex-Specific Pathways in the Intergenerational Transmission of Mental Health (H3)

Our findings also support the hypothesis that the pathways linking parental mental health to adolescent mental health outcomes vary by sex. In the maternal health model, the effects of maternal mental health, family resilience, adolescents' ACEs, and their flourishing on adolescent mental health problems were stronger for girls than for boys. This is consistent with research suggesting that maternal mental health often has a more pronounced impact on daughters, potentially due to closer emotional bonds, sex-specific socialization, or identification processes [30]. However, the differences were relatively modest, suggesting that maternal mental health significantly influences both sons and daughters and that improving maternal mental health could have a more substantial protective effect on their adolescent children's well-being.

In the paternal mental health model, family resilience, adolescents' ACEs, and their flourishing had similar impacts on adolescent mental health for both sexes. However, paternal mental health had a slightly stronger effect on boys' mental health problems compared to girls'. This aligns with previous research suggesting that sons may be more influenced by their fathers' mental health, possibly due to sex-specific identification processes [29]. These findings underscore the importance of considering both parental and adolescent sex in understanding the transmission of mental health within families.

4.4. Limitations and Future Directions

Despite its contributions and strengths, this study has limitations primarily due to the use of secondary data. First, the cross-sectional nature of the data limits causal inferences about the observed relationships. Future studies could consider longitudinal designs to better capture the temporal sequences of intergenerational transmission of mental health, e.g., [40,41]. Specifically, previous longitudinal studies provided contrasting insights into cross-lagged effects between parent and child mental health. Griffith et al. [42] found contemporaneous cofluctuation of depressive symptoms but no evidence of bidirectional effects over time. In contrast, Yirmiya et al. [43] identified bidirectional influences between maternal and child anxiety, particularly in trauma-exposed families, with early childhood as a sensitive period. These findings highlight the complexity of intergenerational mental health transmission and the importance of contextual factors like trauma and developmental stages. Future longitudinal studies would benefit from incorporating complex contextual factors when examining intergenerational transmission of mental health. Second, the reliance on parent-reported measures may introduce reporting bias, particularly for adolescent outcomes. Future research could improve accuracy by incorporating multiple informants, objective measures, and adolescent self-reports [44,45]. Third, each maternal and paternal mental health status was accessed using single measures, which may not fully capture the complexity of mental health status. Future studies could benefit from more comprehensive assessments of parental mental health, as well as additional contextual factors that may influence family dynamics. Fourth, while this study focused on examining sex differences within the serial mediation model, we did not include covariates. Future studies could consider sociodemographic factors such as adolescent age, race/ethnicity, educational background, and income, which may further influence the relationships between parental mental health, family resilience, adolescents' ACEs, and their flourishing. Lastly, while this study focuses on adolescents, future research could explore how sex-specific pathways operate across different developmental stages for a more comprehensive understanding.

4.5. Conclusions and Implications

Using a large nationally representative sample from the combined 2016–2020 NSCH data, this study provides significant contributions to understanding the intergenerational transmission of mental health by examining the mediating roles of family resilience, adolescents' ACEs, and their flourishing in the association between parental and adolescent mental health. By identifying key mediating mechanisms and exploring sex-specific pathways, this study enhances our understanding of the complex dynamics through which parental mental health influences adolescent mental health outcomes. The findings emphasize the importance of addressing parental mental health, enhancing family resilience, and fostering adolescents' ability to flourish as protective strategies to mitigate mental health risks across generations. Specifically, the role of family resilience suggests that interventions focusing on family level protective factors could be effective in preventing the transmission of mental health problems. Programs that enhance family communication, problem-solving skills, and collective coping strategies may be particularly impactful, helping families manage stress and reducing adolescent susceptibility to mental health challenges in the context of ACEs.

These findings carry practical implications for policymakers and practitioners seeking to reduce the intergenerational transmission of mental health issues. First, policies and programs that support parental mental health can foster a more resilient family environment, reducing children's exposure to adverse experiences and promoting family dynamics. Access to mental health resources for parents could be prioritized to interrupt the type of mental health challenges across generations. Second, clinicians and practitioners are encouraged to implement family centered prevention strategies that enhance resilience at the family level. Also, programs aimed at fostering positive well-being indicators in adolescents, such as curiosity, resilience, and self-regulation, are vital for mental health prevention. Schools, community organizations, and mental health services can support adolescents in developing these attributes, which may enhance their capacity to handle stress and reduce the risk of mental health issues. Lastly, the observed sex differences suggest that tailored interventions may be necessary to address the distinct needs of sons and daughters. For example, programs that support maternal mental health may focus on enhancing mother–daughter interactions, while those targeting paternal mental health may prioritize father–son dynamics, recognizing the unique influences of each parental role on adolescent mental health.

In conclusion, this study offers important insights into the mechanisms of intergenerational mental health transmission and highlights the protective roles of family resilience and adolescents' flourishing. Targeted policies and interventions that enhance family resilience, support parental mental health, and foster adolescents' well-being may be critical in reducing the transmission of mental health issues across generations. These findings provide a foundation for developing evidence-based strategies aimed at promoting family resilience and mental health stability across generations.

Author Contributions: Conceptualization, H.-J.Y. and J.H.; data curation, H.-J.Y. and J.H.; formal analysis, H.-J.Y. and J.H.; writing—original draft, H.-J.Y. and J.H.; writing—review and editing, C.B.W. All authors have read and agreed to the published version of the manuscript.

Funding: This research received no external funding.

Institutional Review Board Statement: Ethical review and approvals were waived for this study as it involved secondary data analysis with no direct involvement of human subjects.

Informed Consent Statement: Informed consent was obtained from all subjects involved in this study during the initial data collection of the National Survey of Children's Health (NSCH); however, participant consent was waived due to the present study conducting secondary data analysis using publicly available, de-identified data from the NSCH.

Data Availability Statement: Data used in this study are publicly accessible through the National Survey of Children's Health website at https://www.childhealthdata.org/help/dataset (accessed on 20 June 2022).

Acknowledgments: This study utilized data from the National Survey of Children's Health (NSCH), which is funded and directed by the Maternal and Child Health Bureau (MCHB) of the Health Resources and Services Administration (HRSA) and collected and maintained by the U.S. Census Bureau. We are grateful to all the families who participated in the survey, making this research possible.

Conflicts of Interest: The authors declare no conflicts of interest. The funder had no role in the design of this study; in the collection, analysis, or interpretation of the data; in the writing of the manuscript, or in the decision to publish the results.

References

1. Leijdesdorff, S.; van Doesum, K.; Popma, A.; Klaassen, R.; van Amelsvoort, T. Prevalence of psychopathology in children of parents with mental illness and/or addiction: An up to date narrative review. *Curr. Opin. Psychiatry* **2017**, *30*, 312–317. [CrossRef]
2. National Alliance on Mental Illness (NAMI). Mental Health by the Numbers. 2020. Available online: https://www.nami.org/mhstats (accessed on 15 January 2023).
3. Landstedt, E.; Almquist, Y.B. Intergenerational patterns of mental health problems: The role of childhood peer status position. *BMC Psychiatry* **2019**, *19*, 286. [CrossRef]
4. Paananen, R.; Tuulio-Henriksson, A.; Merikukka, M.; Gissler, M. Intergenerational transmission of psychiatric disorders: The 1987 Finnish Birth Cohort study. *Eur. Child Adolesc. Psychiatry* **2021**, *30*, 381–389. [CrossRef]
5. van Santvoort, F.; Hosman, C.M.; Janssens, J.M.; van Doesum, K.T.; Reupert, A.; van Loon, L.M. The Impact of Various Parental Mental Disorders on Children's Diagnoses: A Systematic Review. *Clin. Child Fam. Psychol. Rev.* **2015**, *18*, 281–299. [CrossRef]
6. Soleimanpour, S.; Geierstanger, S.; Brindis, C.D. Adverse childhood experiences and resilience: Addressing the unique needs of adolescents. *Acad. Pediatr.* **2017**, *17*, S108–S114. [CrossRef]
7. Bomysoad, R.N.; Francis, L.A. Adverse childhood experiences and mental health conditions among adolescents. *J. Adolesc. Health* **2020**, *67*, 868–870. [CrossRef]
8. Sciaraffa, M.A.; Zeanah, P.D.; Zeanah, C.H. Understanding and promoting resilience in the context of adverse childhood experiences. *Early Child. Educ. J.* **2018**, *46*, 343–353. [CrossRef]
9. Uddin, J.; Alharbi, N.; Uddin, H.; Hossain, M.B.; Hatipoğlu, S.S.; Long, D.L.; Carson, A.P. Parenting stress and family resilience affect the association of adverse childhood experiences with children's mental health and attention-deficit/hyperactivity disorder. *J. Affect. Disord.* **2020**, *272*, 104–109. [CrossRef]
10. Bethell, C.D.; Gombojav, N.; Whitaker, R.C. Family resilience and connection promote flourishing among US children, even amid adversity. *Health Aff.* **2019**, *38*, 729–737. [CrossRef]
11. Nietzel, M.T.; Wakefield, J.C. American psychiatric association diagnostic and statistical manual of mental disorders. *Contemp. Psychol.* **1996**, *41*, 642–651. [CrossRef]
12. Bowen, M. The use of family theory in clinical practice. *Compr. Psychiatry* **1966**, *7*, 345–374. [CrossRef] [PubMed]
13. Keeney, B. *Aesthetics of Change*; Guildford Press: New York, NY, USA, 1983.
14. Reid, K.M. The relationship between parents' poor emotional health status and childhood mood and anxiety disorder in Florida children, National Survey of Children's health, 2011–2012. *Matern. Child Health J.* **2015**, *19*, 1071–1077. [CrossRef] [PubMed]
15. Lui, M.; Lau, G.K.; Tam, V.C.; Chiu, H.M.; Li, S.S.; Sin, K.F. Parents' Impact on children's school performance: Marital satisfaction, parental involvement, and mental health. *J. Child. Fam. Stud.* **2020**, *29*, 1548–1560. [CrossRef]
16. von Bertalanffy, L. *General System Theory: Foundations, Development, Applications*; George Braziller Inc.: New York, NY, USA, 1968.
17. Zhou, M.; Larsson, H.; D'Onofrio, B.M.; Landén, M.; Lichtenstein, P.; Pettersson, E. Intergenerational Transmission of Psychiatric Conditions and Psychiatric, Behavioral, and Psychosocial Outcomes in Offspring. *JAMA Netw Open* **2023**, *6*, e2348439. [CrossRef] [PubMed]
18. Felitti, V.J.; Anda, R.F.; Nordenberg, D.; Williamson, D.F.; Spitz, A.M.; Edwards, V.; Marks, J.S. Relationship of childhood abuse and household dysfunction to many of the leading causes of death in adults: The Adverse Childhood Experiences (ACE) Study. *Am. J. Prev. Med.* **1998**, *14*, 245–258. [CrossRef]
19. Herbell, K.; Bloom, T. A qualitative metasynthesis of mothers' adverse childhood experiences and parenting practices. *J. Pediatr. Health Care* **2020**, *34*, 409–417. [CrossRef]

20. American Academy of Pediatrics. Adverse Childhood Experiences and the Lifelong Consequences of Trauma. 2014. Available online: https://cdn.ymaws.com/www.ncpeds.org/resource/collection/69DEAA33-A258-493B-A63F-E0BFAB6BD2CB/ttb_aces_consequences.pdf (accessed on 4 November 2024).
21. Balistreri, K.S.; Alvira-Hammond, M. Adverse childhood experiences, family functioning and adolescent health and emotional well-being. *Public Health* **2016**, *132*, 72–78. [CrossRef]
22. Bhatta, S.; Champion, J.D.; Young, C.; Loika, E. Outcomes of depression screening among adolescents accessing school-based pediatric primary care clinic services. *J. Pediatr. Nurs.* **2018**, *38*, 8–14. [CrossRef]
23. Masten, A.S.; Lucke, C.M.; Nelson, K.M.; Stallworthy, I.C. Resilience in development and psychopathology: Multisystem perspectives. *Annu. Rev. Clin. Psychol.* **2021**, *17*, 521–549. [CrossRef]
24. Schneider, M.; VanOrmer, J.; Zlomke, K. Adverse childhood experiences and family resilience among children with autism spectrum disorder and attention-deficit/hyperactivity disorder. *J. Dev. Behav. Pediatr.* **2019**, *40*, 573–580. [CrossRef]
25. Masten, A.S.; Obradović, J. Competence and Resilience in Development. *Ann. N. Y. Acad. Sci.* **2006**, *1094*, 13–27. [CrossRef] [PubMed]
26. Kwong, T.Y.; Hayes, D.K. Adverse family experiences and flourishing amongst children ages 6–17 years: 2011/12 National Survey of Children's Health. *Child Abus. Negl.* **2017**, *70*, 240–246. [CrossRef] [PubMed]
27. Lippman, L.H.; Moore, K.A.; McIntosh, H. Positive indicators of child well-being: A conceptual framework, measures, and methodological issues. *Appl. Res. Qual. Life* **2011**, *6*, 425–449. [CrossRef]
28. Connell, A.M.; Goodman, S.H. The association between psychopathology in fathers versus mothers and children's internalizing and externalizing behavior problems: A meta-analysis. *Psychol. Bull.* **2002**, *128*, 746–773. [CrossRef]
29. Goodman, S.H.; Rouse, M.H.; Connell, A.M.; Broth, M.R.; Hall, C.M.; Heyward, D. Maternal depression and child psychopathology: A meta-analytic review. *Clin. Child Fam. Psychol. Rev.* **2011**, *14*, 1–27. [CrossRef]
30. Bussey, K.; Bandura, A. Social cognitive theory of gender development and differentiation. *Psychol. Rev.* **1999**, *106*, 676–713. [CrossRef]
31. Child and Adolescent Health Measurement Initiative (CAHMI). National Survey of Children's Health (2 Years Combined Data Set): Child and Family Measures, National Performance and Outcome Measures, and Subgroups, SPSS Codebook. Available online: https://www.childhealthdata.org/learn-about-the-nsch/nsch-codebooks (accessed on 15 June 2022).
32. U.S. Census Bureau. NSCH Guide to Multi-Year Analysis. 2021. Available online: https://www2.census.gov/programs-surveys/nsch/technical-documentation/methodology/NSCH-Guide-to-Multi-Year-Estimates.pdf (accessed on 20 June 2022).
33. Treat, A.E.; Sheffield Morris, A.; Williamson, A.C.; Hays-Grudo, J.; Laurin, D. Adverse childhood experiences, parenting, and child executive function. *Early Child Dev. Care* **2019**, *189*, 926–937. [CrossRef]
34. Karatekin, C.; Hill, M. Expanding the original definition of adverse childhood experiences (ACEs). *J. Child Adolesc. Trauma* **2019**, *12*, 289–306. [CrossRef]
35. Herbell, K.; Breitenstein, S.M.; Melnyk, B.M.; Guo, J. Family resilience and flourishment: Well-being among children with mental, emotional, and behavioral disorders. *Res. Nurs. Health* **2020**, *43*, 465–477. [CrossRef]
36. McGowan, E.C.; Oyeku, S.O.; Lim, S.W. Family, neighborhood and parent resilience are inversely associated with reported depression in adolescents exposed to ACEs. *Acad. Pediatr.* **2023**, *23*, 773–781. [CrossRef]
37. Barnhart, S.; Bode, M.; Gearhart, M.C.; Maguire-Jack, K. Supportive neighborhoods, family resilience and flourishing in childhood and adolescence. *Children* **2022**, *9*, 495. [CrossRef] [PubMed]
38. Muthén, L.K.; Muthén, B.O. *Mplus User's Guide*, 8th ed.; Muthén & Muthén: Los Angeles, CA, USA, 2017.
39. Hu, L.T.; Bentler, P.M. Cutoff criteria for fit indexes in covariance structure analysis: Conventional criteria versus new alternatives. *Struct. Equ. Model. Multidiscip. J.* **1999**, *6*, 1–55. [CrossRef]
40. Schulz, S.; Nelemans, S.A.; Oldehinkel, A.J.; Meeus, W.; Branje, S. Examining intergenerational transmission of psychopathology: Associations between parental and adolescent internalizing and externalizing symptoms across adolescence. *Dev. Psychol.* **2021**, *57*, 269–283. [CrossRef] [PubMed]
41. Thompson, A.J.; Henrich, C.C. Cross-lagged effects between parent depression and child internalizing problems. *J. Fam. Psychol.* **2022**, *36*, 1428–1438. [CrossRef]
42. Griffith, J.M.; Young, J.F.; Hankin, B.L. Longitudinal Coupling of Depression in Parent-Adolescent Dyads: Within- and Between-Dyad Effects Over Time. *Clin. Psychol. Sci.* **2021**, *9*, 1059–1079. [CrossRef]
43. Yirmiya, K.; Motsan, S.; Kanat-Maymon, Y.; Feldman, R. From mothers to children and back: Bidirectional processes in the cross-generational transmission of anxiety from early childhood to early adolescence. *Depress. Anxiety* **2021**, *38*, 1298–1312. [CrossRef]
44. Bentley, N.; Hartley, S.; Bucci, S. Systematic Review of Self-Report Measures of General Mental Health and Wellbeing in Adolescent Mental Health. *Clin. Child Fam. Psychol. Rev.* **2019**, *22*, 225–252. [CrossRef]
45. Deighton, J.; Croudace, T.; Fonagy, P.; Brown, J.; Patalay, P.; Wolpert, M. Measuring mental health and wellbeing outcomes for children and adolescents to inform practice and policy: A review of child self-report measures. *Child Adolesc. Psychiatry Ment. Health* **2014**, *8*, 14. [CrossRef]

children

MDPI

Systematic Review

Effectiveness of Digital Mental Health Interventions for Children and Adolescents

José María Fernández-Batanero [1,*], José Fernández-Cerero [1], Marta Montenegro-Rueda [2] and Daniel Fernández-Cerero [3]

[1] Department of Teaching and Educational Organization, University of Seville, 41013 Sevilla, Spain; jfcerero@us.es
[2] Department of Didactics and School Organisation, University of Granada, 52005 Melilla, Spain; mmontenegro@ugr.es
[3] Department of Stomatology, University of Seville, 41009 Sevilla, Spain; dfcerero@us.es
* Correspondence: batanero@us.es

Abstract: Background/Objectives: Children's mental health is an issue of growing global concern, with a significant impact on children's emotional, social and cognitive development. In recent years, digital apps and platforms have emerged as innovative tools to address mental health challenges. This systematic review aims to evaluate the effectiveness of these technologies in supporting children's and adolescents' mental health. Methods: A systematic search of PubMed, PsycINFO, Scopus and Web of Science databases was conducted. Results: The results suggest that digital apps and platforms have significant potential to support children's mental health. However, their effectiveness depends on factors such as app design, parental involvement and cultural adaptation. Conclusions: The inclusion of gamified elements and integration with traditional mental health strategies can enhance outcomes.

Keywords: mental health; digital technology; digital intervention; children; adolescents; emotional well-being

1. Introduction

Child mental health is a global priority in the current context, marked by increasing challenges related to accelerated social change and technological pressures [1]. It is estimated that one in five children and adolescents worldwide experience a mental health disorder, posing a considerable challenge to families, communities and health systems [2]. These problems, exacerbated by factors such as unequal access to health resources, the stigma associated with psychological disorders, and natural disasters such as the COVID-19 pandemic, have led to a significant increase in the incidence of anxiety, depression and related mental health disorders in children and adolescents [3]. In this context, technologies emerge as promising tools to address children's mental health needs, but their implementation and effectiveness still raise crucial questions that require in-depth and critical analysis.

The accelerating advance in digital technologies, including mobile apps, online platforms and artificial intelligence-based solutions, has transformed the healthcare landscape, offering new opportunities for child mental health assessment, intervention and monitoring [4]. Recent studies indicate that these technologies can improve access to mental health services, especially in regions where resources are limited [5]. On the other hand, digital resources play a key role in mental health prevention and education by providing accessible information for both children and their families. Through these digital tools, it is possible to promote knowledge about emotional well-being and teach effective coping strategies in various situations [6]. However, significant challenges remain, such as the lack of rigorous scientific validation of many commercially available apps, ethical concerns related to data privacy, and unequal access due to digital divides [7]. In this sense, while technology brings multiple benefits in the field of mental health, its implementation should not be considered an absolute substitute for professional intervention. It is essential that these digital tools are integrated with traditional services, enabling more comprehensive and effective care for patients, especially in cases that require a specialised clinical approach [8].

Despite the increasing proliferation of technological interventions, evidence on their effectiveness and long-term sustainability remains fragmented and, in many cases, limited [9]. For example, while some studies highlight the positive impact of technology-based interventions on reducing symptoms of anxiety and depression [10], others point to a lack of standardisation in the design and evaluation of such tools, making it difficult to compare and generalise results [11]. This disparity of results underscores the urgent need to consolidate existing knowledge across the literature to identify trends, gaps and priority areas for future research. These gaps not only hinder theoretical advancement but also compromise the effectiveness and equity of technological interventions in clinical practice.

A review of the literature in this field is therefore necessary to address these challenges and contribute to the development of a more robust conceptual and empirical framework. Thus, this study seeks to critically synthesise the available evidence on the effectiveness of technologies in supporting children's mental health, highlighting both their strengths and limitations. Through a comprehensive analysis of recent studies, it aims to identify consistent patterns, highlight the most promising innovations, and propose priority areas for future research. This approach will not only clarify the state of the art, but also inform decision-making by researchers, health specialists and policy makers. The review is framed in a historical moment of growing interest in the intersection between technology and mental health, which makes it particularly relevant and timely. The review is framed in a historical moment of growing interest in the intersection between technology and mental health, which makes it particularly relevant and timely. We have conducted a systematic review study that aimed to evaluate the effectiveness of apps and digital platforms as interventions to improve the mental health of children and adolescents. Although this is a well-studied topic, it is a valuable update, addressing the specific gap in this particularly rapidly developing field of digital health apps, adding studies with more up-to-date technologies.

This research aligns with contemporary debates in psychology, psychiatry and technology, including the role of interdisciplinary approaches in the design of digital interventions [12]. For example, the integration of user-centred design principles and participatory research methodologies has been highlighted as a key strategy for improving the uptake and effectiveness of mental health technologies [13]. Furthermore, the 'digital psychology' framework provides a conceptual basis for understanding how human interactions with digital technologies can influence mental health and well-being [14].

On the other hand, the effectiveness that technologies can have, not only in clinical settings, but also in educational settings, has been demonstrated [15]. Therefore, the use of video games and gamification strategies has proven to be an effective alternative to facilitate access and improve continuity in psychological treatments for children and adolescents. In this sense, initiatives such as 'Harry's PathwaysToCare' have been created with the purpose of guiding young people in the process of seeking and using mental health services [16]. However, despite their advantages, the implementation of these technologies in the professional mental health setting remains limited. This is largely due to a lack of understanding of how they work and concerns related to the security and privacy of user data [17].

Following this line, the present study pursues the following objectives:

(1) To evaluate the effectiveness of various technologies on mental health in children and adolescents;
(2) To identify the advantages and limitations of these technologies for psychological well-being;
(3) To propose a framework for future research on the implementation of technologies for child and adolescent mental health.

To this end, the study answers the following research questions:

RQ1: What evidence exists on the effectiveness of digital technologies on the mental health of children and adolescents?

RQ2: What are the main challenges and barriers in the use of digital technologies for psychological well-being?

RQ3: What guidelines can guide future research on the implementation of mental health technologies for children and young people?

2. Methods

2.1. Review Methodology

This systematic review was conducted in accordance with the Preferred Reporting Items for Systematic Reviews and Meta-Analyses (PRISMA) guidelines [18] (Supplementary Materials S1). The implementation of these guidelines ensures a clear and comprehensive methodology, promoting transparency and rigour in the study selection process for systematic reviews. A search was conducted to identify studies exploring the efficacy of technologies on child and adolescent mental health.

2.2. Formulation of the Research Question

The search query was conducted using the PICO model [19] which includes four core elements: person or problem (P), indicator intervention (I), comparison (c) and outcome (O). The following aspects were considered: P—child or adolescent students; I—mental health; C—digital intervention or tool and O—impact of digital tools on mental health.

2.3. Search Strategy

The search was conducted in recognised academic databases, including PubMed, Scopus, Web of Science and PsycINFO, to identify studies published between 2020 and 2024. The delimitation of the study period to the years 2020–2024 was in response to several factors. Firstly, the COVID-19 pandemic represented a turning point in the development and implementation of digital mental health interventions, accelerating the adoption of technologies and generating a significant increase in the research and application of these strategies. The purpose of the study is to analyse effectiveness in a scenario characterised by the increasing digitisation of mental health care, largely driven by the conditions imposed since 2020 following the pandemic.

Keywords related to mental health, digital technology, digital interventions, children, adolescents and emotional well-being were used. Boolean operators (AND, OR) were applied to optimise the retrieval of relevant studies. In addition, reference lists of selected studies were reviewed to identify additional relevant publications.

2.4. Inclusion and Exclusion Criteria

Based on the inclusion and exclusion criteria, a number of guidelines were established to ensure that the selected studies were relevant and met the objectives of the review.

The inclusion criteria were as follows:

- Published between 2020 to 2024;
- Publications in scientific articles;
- Publications in English;
- Related to the field of study.

The exclusion criteria were as follows:

- Published outside the established time interval;
- Published in a format other than a scientific article (congress, thesis, etc.);
- Published in a language other than English;
- Research not related to the field of study.

2.5. Selection of Studies and Selection Process

Study selection was performed in several stages. First, the search results were combined using the desktop reference manager Mendeley and duplicate studies were removed. Second, two researchers independently screened the titles and abstracts of articles identified in the initial search to discard studies that did not meet the inclusion criteria. Subsequently, a full-text review of the pre-selected studies was conducted to confirm relevance and data extraction.

To ensure the reliability of the process, the inter-rater agreement index was calculated using Cohen's Kappa coefficient, yielding a value of 0.95, indicating a high level of inter-rater agreement. Any discrepancies were resolved by discussion between the researchers or, if necessary, with the intervention of a third evaluator. The results can be visualised in Figure 1.

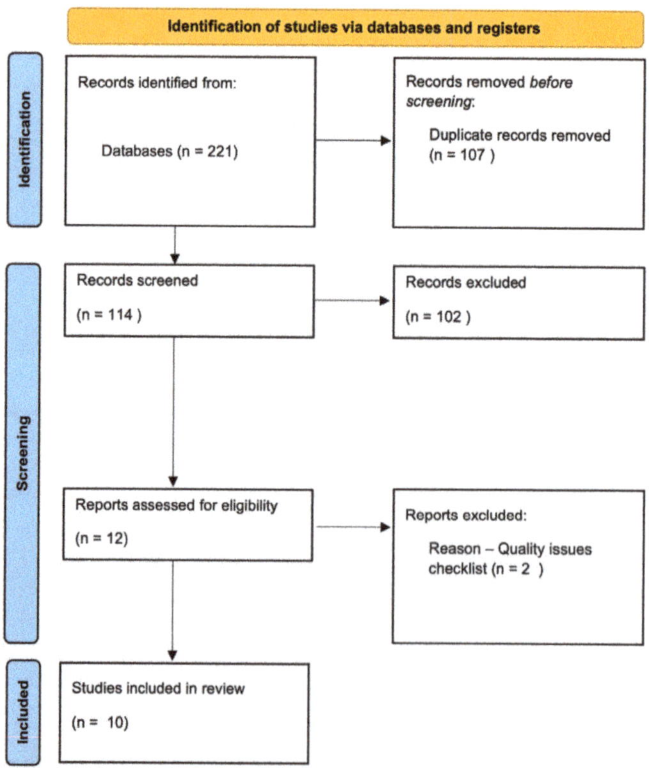

Figure 1. Flow chart.

2.6. Methodological Quality Assessment

Two reviewers independently determined the methodological quality of the selected studies using the critical appraisal tools for non-randomised studies of the Joanna Briggs Institute (JBI) at the University of Adelaide (Australia) [20]. This tool is designed to determine the robustness and validity of research, as well as to assess the methodological quality of a study and to determine the extent to which a study has excluded or minimised the possibility of bias in its design, conduct and/or analysis. The version for quantitative studies was adapted, with the cut-off point being 4 for acceptance for inclusion in this review (Supplementary Materials S2) [20].

To assess the risk of bias in the non-randomised studies included in this review, the Risk of Bias in Non-randomised Studies of Interventions (ROBINS-I) tool recommended by Cochrane was used. This tool allows us to identify and classify bias in seven key domains: confounders, participant selection, intervention classification, deviations from the intended intervention, missing data, outcome measurement and selection of reported outcomes. Each domain was assessed with a risk rating of low (green), moderate (yellow), high (orange) or critical (red) bias, providing a comprehensive assessment of the overall risk of each study. The application of this tool ensures greater transparency and methodological rigour in the synthesis of findings, allowing the robustness of the evidence analysed to be contextualised (Supplementary Materials S3) [21].

2.7. Data Extraction and Data Analysis

The following information was extracted from the included studies: authors, date of publication, methodological design, population size and characteristics, type of digital intervention implemented, country of implementation and main findings. To ensure consistency in data extraction, a standardised template incorporating the variables mentioned above was used.

Data analysis was conducted at two levels: descriptive and thematic. First, a quantitative analysis was conducted to examine the distribution of studies in terms of frequency of publication by year, types of digital interventions and mental health conditions addressed. Secondly, a qualitative analysis was conducted to identify patterns in the effectiveness of digital interventions. Study results were categorised according to reported effects on child and adolescent mental health. To do this, a response categorisation process was applied, where quantitative data were transformed into qualitative categories to facilitate analysis and interpretation. Segmentation and clustering techniques were used to identify patterns and groupings within the numerical responses. SPSS statistical software (v.29 for MacOS) was used to group results into clusters with significant similarities, improving understanding of key trends in digital mental health interventions.

3. Results

A search of four databases was conducted, resulting in 211 records. Of these, 10 articles were included in the review (Table 1). Finally, in order to extract relevant data to help answer our research questions, the selected studies were analysed and their data extracted using a standardised template that included information on methodological design, population, digital intervention and main findings.

The number of published studies on digital mental health fluctuated between 2020 and 2024, reflecting the impact of the global pandemic on interest and development in this topic. In 2020, only one study was identified, which is consistent with the time required to design and implement research after the onset of the health crisis. In 2021, the number of publications increased to four, suggesting a growth in attention to and exploration of digital mental health interventions. Subsequently, in 2023 and 2024, the number of studies decreased to two, which could indicate a stabilisation phase in scientific output. This pattern highlights how research responded to emerging needs driven by the pandemic and how, in recent years, the publication of studies appears to have reached a point of normalisation (Supplementary Materials S3).

Table 1. Information on included studies.

Author/Year	Methodological Design	Sample and Gender	Population and Age Group	Mental Health Condition(s)	Digital Intervention	Findings (Benefits and Limitations)	Country
Nahreen Zannat and Murni Mahmud, 2024 [22]	Quantitative	10 families. No gender is specified.	Children from 4 to 10 years old	Anxiety, stress and behavioural changes.	APP: Calm & Care	The app proved effective in addressing issues such as anxiety and stress stemming from the pandemic, promoting greater engagement and enthusiasm among children. It also facilitated active parental involvement through tools such as a dashboard to monitor progress and coordinate counselling sessions, all under strict privacy and security measures.	Bangladesh
Høgsdal, 2023 [23]	Quantitative	45 participants (25 girls and 17 boys)	Teenagers between 11 and 16 years old.	Stress and difficult emotions or situations	Applications: Opp and or NettOpp	The study indicates that young people are satisfied with both apps (Opp and NettOpp) to increase their knowledge about mental health and help them deal with stress and difficult situations. It also increases awareness about cyberbullying.	Norway Canada
Shi et al., 2021 [24]	Quantitative	131 participants (106 were female, 22 were male, and 3 identified themselves as non-binary).	Teenagers between 17 and 29 years old	Mental health and well-being support	Digital platform: Thought Spot	This platform helps transition-aged youth seek help from mental health and wellness resources. Participants highlighted its visual appeal, functionality, and usefulness; however, many stop using it within a short period of time (3 weeks).	Canada
Martínez et al., 2021 [25]	Quantitative	The study included 199 participants, of whom 106 were women and 93 were men.	Teenagers between 13 and 17 years old	Depression	Application: Take care of your spirit	Post-intervention results show a reduction in depressive and anxious symptoms in adolescents through digital interventions.	Chile
Osborn et al., 2020 [26]	Quantitative	103 students (gender not specified)	Teenagers between 13 and 18 years old	Stress, anxiety, depression..	Platform: Shamiri-Digital	The digital intervention produced a greater reduction in depressive symptoms in adolescents. Therefore, a brief digital and computer-based intervention may reduce depressive symptoms in adolescents in sub-Saharan Africa.	Kenya
Srivastava et al., 2020 [27]	Quantitative	21 adolescents (gender not specified)	Adolescents between 13 and 19 years	Depression	Web application: Smartteen	Smartteen is India's first computer-assisted intervention for the treatment of depression in adolescents. Preliminary results suggest that it is feasible, acceptable and effective in reducing depressive symptoms and helps save therapist time.	India
Gonsalves et al., 2021 [28]	Quantitative	248 adolescents (124 males and 124 females).	Teenagers between 13 and 18 years old	Stress	Application: POD Adventures	Results showed improvements in mental health symptoms, stress and well-being. Participants found POD Adventures easy to use, engaging and helpful in solving their problems.	India
Rahayu et al., 2024 [29]	Quantitative	Not specified	Children between 13 and 18 years old	Anxiety and depression	Not specified	The use of mobile apps for adolescent mental health has great potential to improve access to and effectiveness of services. These apps can provide useful support, education, and interventions to help adolescents manage their mental health problems. Therefore, their implementation should be part of a comprehensive strategy to promote youth well-being.	Indonesia

Table 1. *Cont.*

Author/Year	Methodological Design	Sample and Gender	Population and Age Group	Mental Health Condition(s)	Digital Intervention	Findings (Benefits and Limitations)	Country
Amer, N et al., 2023 [30]	Quantitative	5 participants (4 women and 1 man)	Young Arabs (no age range specified)	Depression, anxiety and stress	Sokoon	The tool proved to be practical, well-received and effective in reducing symptoms of anxiety and depression as it is based on cognitive behavioural therapy through gamification. In addition, it offers an accessible and culturally adapted alternative.	Egypt
Charvet et al., 2021 [31]	Quantitative	35 participants (28 women and 7 men).	Teenagers between 14 and 23 years old	Anxiety	Personal Zen	Was shown to be feasible and effective in reducing anxiety in paediatric patients with multiple sclerosis. Participants showed significant improvements in negative affect and anxiety following the intervention.	USA

Looking at the geographical origin of the studies collected, a large percentage of the articles come from South and Southeast Asia, with countries such as India, Indonesia and Bangladesh showing growth and interest in dealing with technologies and the mental health of users. On the other hand, studies were also found from countries from other continents such as Europe (Norway), South America (Chile), Africa (Kenya and Egypt) and North America (Canada and the United States). This global picture not only shows the universality of interest in digital mental health but also suggests that innovative solutions developed in these diverse contexts can be shared and adapted globally.

Figure 2 illustrates the distribution of study topics in digital mental health interventions, focusing on five main categories, each of which represents a significant area of research within the field of mental health. Depression, anxiety and stress each occupy 27.8% of the total number of studies, reflecting the high priority that these areas represent in current research. This balance shows that researchers are devoting similar resources to explore how digital interventions can help manage these disorders, which are prevalent and have a considerable impact on the world's population. On the other hand, we find emotional support (11.1%) and behavioural changes (5.6%). These studies address how digital interventions can influence behaviour modification, an essential aspect of improving overall well-being and managing mental health conditions.

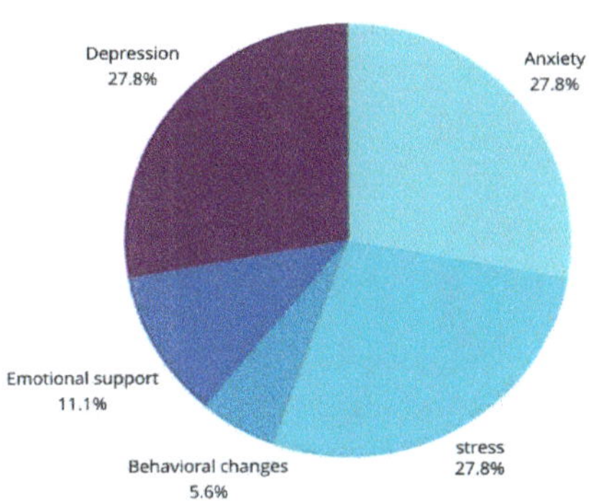

Figure 2. Distribution according to study topics.

Addressing the main findings of the collected studies, the results have been categorised into five main areas:

- Reduction in Anxiety and Stress: This section refers to digital interventions designed to help reduce anxiety and stress levels in young people. They often include relaxation techniques, cognitive behavioural therapy, and guided activities aimed at relieving emotional and psychological tension.

- Increase in Mental Health Awareness and Management: Focuses on increasing mental health awareness among young people and their caregivers. This may include education about the symptoms of different psychological disorders, strategies for managing them, and the importance of seeking professional help when necessary. Apps and platforms often provide informative resources and self-assessments.
- Active Participation in Mental Health: This outcome highlights the importance of active and engaged participation of users in their own mental health process. Interventions may include interactive modules, emotion diaries, and discussion forums that allow users to actively engage in their wellness journey.
- Reduction in Depressive Symptoms: This section addresses specific interventions to reduce symptoms associated with depression, such as persistent sadness, lack of interest in daily activities, and concentration problems. These interventions are often guided by psychological therapy principles and supported by regular follow-up.
- Improvements in General Well-being: Refers to interventions that aim to improve the general well-being of individuals, focusing not only on clinical aspects, but also on improving quality of life. This may include promoting healthy habits, developing social skills and strengthening emotional resilience

Based on the results obtained after analysing the main findings, it stands out that interventions focused on anxiety and stress reduction have shown a high effectiveness, reaching 87%. These interventions usually include programmes that implement stress management techniques and mindfulness, proving to be effective tools to help young people control their anxiety levels. On the other hand, interventions that promote increased knowledge and management of mental health show an effectiveness of 85%, focusing their action on educating young people about mental health problems and strategies for their management, thus increasing their awareness and skills to manage their own mental health.

Active participation in mental health, which includes interactive tools and progress monitoring, has proven to be especially effective with 89% effectiveness, encouraging greater engagement of youth in their treatment. The category with the highest reported effectiveness, at 90%, is the reduction in depressive symptoms. These interventions have shown positive results in helping adolescents regain interest in daily activities and improve their overall mood. Finally, interventions aimed at improvements in general well-being, ranging from promoting healthy lifestyles to developing social skills and emotional resilience, have shown 86% effectiveness. These programmes seek not only to reduce the symptoms of specific disorders but also to promote a comprehensive improvement in the quality of life of young people. In this sense, digital interventions in child and adolescent mental health are effective tools on a variety of fronts, offering significant support in the management and improvement of mental health. However, the findings reveal challenges for its implementation in both clinical and educational contexts (Figure 3). The figure shows the percentage distribution of the main barriers to the implementation of technologies in the health of young people. It can be seen that the training and acceptance of professionals represents the greatest limitation (30%), suggesting the need for training strategies to improve the adoption of these technologies in the clinical setting. This is followed by user commitment (25%) and scientific evidence and clinical validation (20%), indicating that adherence of young people and the lack of robust studies on the efficacy of these technologies remain major challenges. To a lesser extent, accessibility (15%) and data privacy and security (10%) also constitute barriers, although with less relative impact compared to the previous factors. These findings highlight the importance of addressing both professional training and scientific evidence to foster effective integration of technologies in youth health, as well as the importance of continuing to develop and implement technologies tailored to the mental health needs of this population.

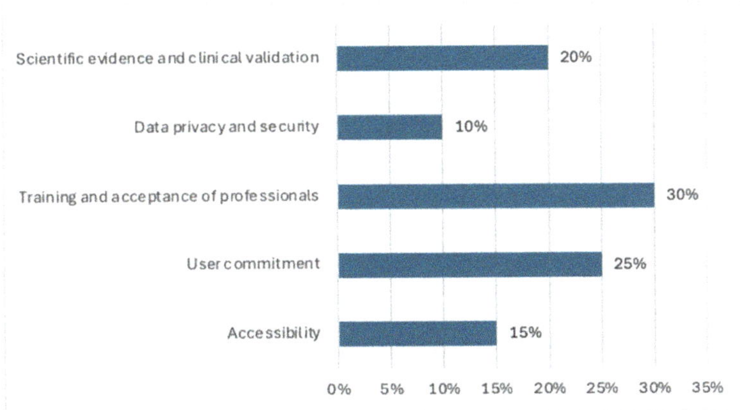

Figure 3. Challenges of implementing technologies in mental health interventions.

4. Discussion

The following are the discussions organised according to the research questions posed above:

RQ1: What evidence exists on the effectiveness of digital technologies in intervening and supporting child and adolescent mental health?

The study of previous research has confirmed the positive effect of the use of digital tools for the improvement of children and adolescent mental health. The literature review has shown that their application generates significant benefits in several areas. On the one hand, the efficacy of digital interventions for childhood anxiety, encompassing mobile applications, virtual reality and online therapies, has been the subject of study. The results indicate that these tools can facilitate access and standardisation of treatment, although further ethical and practical regulation is still required [32]. Following this line, other studies conducted research in which they evaluated the effectiveness of a digital platform designed for the treatment of anxiety and depression in adolescents. Through various methodologies and digital tools, they analysed the evolution of participants who used the platform as part of their mental health intervention. The results showed a significant improvement in their anxiety symptoms, suggesting that digital interventions can be an effective tool to expand access to psychological treatments in this population [33], as well as school-based interventions to reduce anxiety in children and adolescents that generate small but significant benefits, although their long-term impact remains limited [34]. However, it has also been reflected that it not only helps to reduce stress and anxiety, but also the symptoms of depression that individuals may have. Therefore, the use of digital tools has shown a significant reduction in depressive symptoms. These facts are supported by numerous studies [35].

On the other hand, following the results obtained in the present study, it is evident that the use of digital technologies in interventions to improve the mental health of adolescents provides greater awareness and management of mental health. In this sense, various studies support the results such as those carried out by Chen et al. [36], where their findings indicated that digital interventions, including mobile applications, virtual reality and educational games, have a moderate but significant effect both in improving emotional well-being and in managing and raising awareness of mental health of adolescents. In addition, these tools have proven useful in addressing problems such as anxiety, depression and bullying. Therefore, other research, through literature reviews, analysed the effectiveness of digital interventions in the emotional regulation of adolescents. Some found that digital games were particularly effective in reducing negative emotional experiences in young people at risk of anxiety, although most studies are in early stages of development [37]. The effectiveness of self-directed digital interventions, such as mobile applications, has also been evaluated in adolescents aged 11 to 18 years, with the aim of determining their impact on emotional regulation, the reduction in psychopathology and the improvement of academic and social functioning [38].

Finally, the use of digital tools has proven to be a promising tool for improving the emotional well-being of children and adolescents, especially in the development of social skills and in strengthening emotional resilience. One study analysed the effectiveness of a digital intervention designed to improve emotional regulation and social communication skills in children with difficulties in these areas. After 14 weeks of intervention, participants demonstrated significant improvements in their ability to manage emotions and establish social relationships, with effects sustained up to six months later [39].

RQ2: What are the main challenges and barriers in the use of digital technologies for psychological well-being?

The analysis of the studies selected for the review revealed the main barriers and challenges in the use and employment of digital technologies for psychological well-being. Below are the main aspects that hinder their adoption:

- Accessibility: While digital applications and platforms can improve access to mental health, significant digital gaps persist. In particular, children and adolescents in low-income communities may lack access to electronic devices or a stable internet connection, which limits their participation in digital interventions [5]. This digital disparity reduces equity in access to mental health services and represents a significant obstacle in the implementation of technological solutions on a large scale [29].
- User Engagement: Despite their proven effectiveness, many of these digital tools experience low user retention. For example, the study by Shi et al. [24] on the Thought Spot platform showed that although young people perceive its functionality and usefulness as positive, most abandon the application within a short period of three weeks. This phenomenon is due, in part, to the lack of motivation and the design of the interventions, which do not always align with the preferences and needs of adolescents [26].
- Training and Acceptance by Professionals: The integration of digital tools into traditional models of psychological and psychiatric care requires that mental health professionals be trained in their use and trust in their effectiveness. However, the lack of specific training and resistance to change can hinder their adoption in clinical settings [17]. It is essential that digital technologies are accompanied by training programmes for mental health professionals, thus ensuring their proper implementation [8].
- Data Privacy and Security: The use of digital apps and platforms for mental health involves the collection and storage of highly sensitive data, raising ethical and legal concerns regarding privacy and security. One example is the Calm & Care app, which incorporated security mechanisms to ensure safe monitoring by parents (Nahreen Zannat & Mahmud, 2024). However, not all apps offer adequate security measures, which can lead to user mistrust and hinder widespread adoption [22].
- Scientific Evidence and Clinical Validation: Although studies indicate that digital interventions can reduce anxiety, stress and depression in children and adolescents, the

lack of long-term clinical trials and qualitative studies limits the rigorous validation of these interventions [9]. For example, the Cuida tu Ánimo app demonstrated positive results in reducing depressive symptoms in adolescents, but its long-term effectiveness has not yet been confirmed with follow-up studies [25]. Standardisation in the design and evaluation of these tools is key to ensuring their applicability and reliability in clinical contexts [11].

Thus, we must bear in mind that despite the enormous potential of digital technologies to improve child and adolescent mental health, their adoption and long-term sustainability depend on addressing a number of challenges. Overcoming these barriers will require coordinated efforts between researchers, mental health professionals, and technology developers, in order to optimise the effectiveness and equity of these tools in clinical and educational practice.

RQ3: What guidelines can guide future research on the implementation of mental health technologies for children and young people?

Based on the results obtained, future research on the implementation of mental health technologies for children and young people should be guided by the following key aspects:

- Used as a complement to traditional therapy: Applications such as Cuida tu Ánimo have been shown to reduce depressive symptoms in adolescents [25]. These tools can be used as support between therapy sessions, offering practical exercises and educational resources that encourage treatment continuity and patient adherence.
- Remote monitoring and follow-up: Tools like Calm & Care allow parents and professionals to monitor the progress of young people, facilitating early intervention and personalization of treatment [22]. This is especially beneficial for managing fluctuating symptoms and optimising therapeutic strategies.
- Automation and efficiency for therapists: Gamification in mental health apps, as seen in tools such as Smartteen, incorporates game elements to improve user motivation and engagement. Studies such as Srivastava et al. [27] have shown that incorporating self-help and automated monitoring modules can effectively reduce depressive symptoms and optimise therapists' time. These gamification elements, such as rewards and goals, encourage regularity and persistence in users. However, not all aspects of gamification are equally effective. For example, while rewards may increase participation in the short term, they may not sustain motivation in the long term without the support of more in-depth therapeutic interventions. In addition, scoring and competition systems may generate anxiety in some users, counteracting the potential benefits. It is crucial to identify and apply those gamification elements that align the objectives of the application with the specific psychological needs of the users, avoiding those that may introduce new stressors or diminish the effectiveness of the treatment.
- Education and awareness: Platforms like Thought Spot and POD Adventures have shown an increase in mental health awareness and stress management, being useful in school programmes [24,28]. Integrating these tools into educational curricula can strengthen mental health literacy and reduce the stigma associated with psychological disorders.
- Personalization of interventions: Gamification and interactive approaches, such as those used in Sokoon, can increase engagement and improve therapeutic outcomes [30]. The ability to tailor digital experiences to each user's individual needs can improve adherence and motivation in treatment.
- Public health strategies: Governments and organisations can integrate these tools into mental health prevention and care campaigns in school, community, and clinical

settings [10]. By providing access to validated digital resources, early detection of disorders can be improved and timely intervention facilitated.

Digital interventions can improve the accessibility and effectiveness of traditional models of psychological and psychiatric care if their challenges are addressed, ensuring an adapted, scientifically validated implementation aligned with the needs of users and mental health professionals. Combining digital approaches with traditional interventions can strengthen mental health care systems, facilitating equitable access and continuous improvement in treatments.

This finding reinforces the applicability of our results for mental health professionals, educators, and policymakers, highlighting the importance of integrating digital solutions into existing mental health frameworks to maximise their impact and effectiveness.

5. Conclusions

The findings of this systematic review show that digital interventions for child and adolescent mental health have a significant impact on reducing symptoms of anxiety, stress, and depression, as well as improving general well-being and mental health literacy. The inclusion of interactive tools, gamification, and remote monitoring strategies has been shown to improve user adherence and engagement, facilitating access to psychological interventions in various contexts. However, the effectiveness of these interventions largely depends on factors such as the quality of the design, integration with traditional mental health approaches, and parental involvement. Despite positive results, challenges in their implementation, such as acceptance by professionals, accessibility in vulnerable populations and data privacy, continue to be barriers that limit their widespread impact. The integration of these tools into health and education systems requires a multidisciplinary approach that considers their scientific validation, scalability and alignment with traditional psychological care models.

5.1. Limitations

While this study provides a comprehensive synthesis of the effectiveness of digital interventions in children's mental health, it has some limitations that should be considered. First, the review focused only on studies published in English and in scientific articles, which could have excluded relevant research in other languages or formats.

Only quantitative studies have been included in this systematic review in order to objectively assess the effectiveness of digital interventions on child and adolescent mental health. This methodological decision is based on the need for measurable and comparable data to analyse the impact of these technologies in terms of symptom reduction, improved psychological well-being and other standardised indicators. Quantitative studies, in particular randomised controlled trials and longitudinal studies, offer greater methodological rigour and allow causal relationships to be established, which is essential to determine the real effectiveness of these interventions. Likewise, the exclusion of qualitative studies responds to the review's objective of synthesising evidence based on objective and replicable metrics, facilitating the possibility of statistical analysis and meta-analysis. However, it is recognised that qualitative studies can provide valuable information on user experience and challenges in implementing these technologies, so future research could complement these findings with a mixed approach that considers both types of evidence. While the use of the PICO model to formulate the research question is appropriate and has allowed the study to be clearly structured, it is important to recognise that the reliance on quantitative studies may limit the analysis of subjective factors, such as user experience when interacting with digital mental health interventions. In this sense, future research could benefit from a mixed approach, incorporating qualitative methodologies such as in-depth interviews or case studies to better understand the perception, usability and adherence of these tools in children and adolescents.

Although the registration of systematic reviews on platforms such as PROSPERO is a recommended practice to improve transparency and prevent duplication of studies, in this case such registration was not performed because PROSPERO prioritises systematic reviews of clinical interventions and randomised controlled trials, while this review focuses on digital interventions without a direct clinical intervention. Nevertheless, a rigorous methodological approach has been followed, using PRISMA guidelines and quality assessment tools such as JBI and ROBINS-I, ensuring the transparency and reliability of the review process.

5.2. Future Lines of Research

Based on the findings and limitations identified, future research should focus on several key aspects. First, it is necessary to conduct longitudinal studies that allow the sustainability of the effects of digital interventions to be evaluated in the long term. Likewise, it is recommended to expand qualitative research to better understand the barriers and facilitators in the adoption of these tools by users and mental health professionals. In addition, it is essential to explore strategies to improve user retention and engagement, including the personalization of interventions and the use of artificial intelligence to adapt content to individual needs. Finally, further analysis is required on the implementation of these technologies in low-resource contexts, ensuring their accessibility and equity in access to mental health care.

Given that the studies analysed in this review focus on quantitative methodologies, future research should explore qualitative approaches to assess in depth the user experience and health professionals' perception of these digital interventions. Furthermore, the application of the Cochrane model in future systematic reviews would improve the assessment of the quality of evidence and the consistency of the results, facilitating their integration into clinical and educational practice.

Supplementary Materials: The following supporting information can be downloaded at: https://www.mdpi.com/article/10.3390/children12030353/s1, Supplementary Materials S1 (Table S1: Checklist item), Supplementary Materials S2 (Table S2: Johanna Briggs Checklist (JBI)) and Supplementary Materials S3 (Table S3: Risk of bias ROBINS-I of the included studies; Figure S1: Distribution by year of publication).

Author Contributions: Conceptualization, J.M.F.-B., J.F.-C., M.M.-R. and D.F.-C.; methodology, J.M.F.-B., J.F.-C., M.M.-R. and D.F.-C.; software, J.M.F.-B., J.F.-C., M.M.-R. and D.F.-C.; validation, J.M.F.-B., J.F.-C., M.M.-R. and D.F.-C.; formal analysis, J.M.F.-B., J.F.-C., M.M.-R. and D.F.-C.; investigation, J.M.F.-B., J.F.-C., M.M.-R. and D.F.-C.; resources, J.M.F.-B., J.F.-C., M.M.-R. and D.F.-C.; data curation, J.M.F.-B., J.F.-C., M.M.-R. and D.F.-C.; writing—original draft preparation, J.M.F.-B., J.F.-C., M.M.-R. and D.F.-C.; writing—review and editing, J.M.F.-B., J.F.-C., M.M.-R. and D.F.-C.; visualisation, J.M.F.-B., J.F.-C., M.M.-R. and D.F.-C.; supervision, J.M.F.-B., J.F.-C., M.M.-R. and D.F.-C.; project administration, J.M.F.-B., J.F.-C., M.M.-R. and D.F.-C.; funding acquisition, J.M.F.-B. All authors have read and agreed to the published version of the manuscript.

Funding: The publication is part of the project PID2022-138346OB-I00, funded by MICIU/AEI/10.13039/501100011033/ERDF, EU.

Institutional Review Board Statement: Not applicable.

Informed Consent Statement: Not applicable.

Conflicts of Interest: The authors declare no conflicts of interest.

References

1. World Health Organization (WHO). *Mental Health Atlas 2020*; World Health Organization: Geneva, Switzerland, 2021. Available online: https://www.who.int/publications-detail-redirect/9789240036703 (accessed on 10 March 2025).
2. Kieling, C.; Baker-Henningham, H.; Belfer, M.; Conti, G.; Ertem, I.; Omigbodun, O.; Rahman, A. Child and Adolescent Mental Health Worldwide: Evidence for Action. *Lancet* **2019**, *378*, 1515–1525. [CrossRef] [PubMed]
3. Singh, S.; Roy, D.; Sinha, K.; Parveen, S.; Sharma, G.; Joshi, G. Impact of COVID-19 and Lockdown on Mental Health of Children and Adolescents: A Narrative Review with Recommendations. *Psychiatry Res.* **2020**, *293*, 113429. [CrossRef] [PubMed]
4. Fleming, T.; Merry, S.; Stasiak, K.; Hopkins, S.; Patolo, T. Digital Tools for Youth Mental Health: Review and Future Directions. *Front. Psychiatry* **2022**, *13*, 898523.
5. Gratzer, D.; Torous, J. Digital Mental Health Tools: Opportunities and Challenges. *Can. J. Psychiatry* **2021**, *66*, 5–7. [CrossRef]
6. Tai, Y. Analysis of the current status of children's mental health. In *SHS Web of Conferences*; EDP Sciences: Les Ulis, France, 2024. [CrossRef]
7. Torres-Rodríguez, A.; Griffiths, M.D.; Carbonell, X. The Ethical Challenges of Digital Mental Health Interventions. *Ethics Inf. Technol.* **2021**, *23*, 341–352.
8. Sanderson, C.; Kouzoupi, N.; Hall, C. Technology Matters: The human touch in a digital age—A blended approach in mental healthcare delivery with children and young people. *Child Adolesc. Ment. Health* **2020**, *25*, 120–122. [CrossRef] [PubMed]
9. Christensen, H.; Griffiths, K.M.; Farrer, L. Evidence on the Effectiveness and Sustainability of Digital Health Interventions. *J. Med. Internet Res.* **2019**, *21*, e13073. [CrossRef]
10. Hollis, C.; Falconer, C.J.; Martin, J.L.; Whittington, C.; Stockton, S.; Glazebrook, C.; Davies, E.B. Annual Research Review: Digital Health Interventions for Children and Young People with Mental Health Problems—A Systematic and Meta-Review. *J. Child Psychol. Psychiatry* **2020**, *61*, 858–877. [CrossRef]
11. Reynolds, J.; Griffiths, K.M.; Christensen, H. Limitations and Challenges in Digital Health Interventions: The Case of Mental Health Apps. *JMIR mHealth uHealth* **2021**, *9*, e26100.
12. Holmes, E.A.; O'Connor, R.C.; Perry, V.H.; Tracey, I.; Wessely, S.; Arseneault, L.; Ballard, C.; Christensen, H.; Silver, R.C.; Bullmore, E.; et al. Multidisciplinary research priorities for the COVID-19 pandemic: A call for action for mental health science. *Lancet Psychiatry* **2020**, *7*, 547–560. [CrossRef]
13. Klasnja, P.; Pratt, W.; Edwards, K. *Personal Health Informatics*; MIT Press: Cambridge, MA, USA, 2020.
14. Torous, J.; Roberts, L.W. The ethical use of mobile health technology in clinical psychiatry. *JAMA Psychiatry* **2017**, *74*, 437–438. [CrossRef] [PubMed]
15. Fernández-Cerero, J.; Fernández-Batanero, J.M.; Montenegro-Rueda, M. Possibilities of Extended Reality in education. In *Interactive Learning Environments*; Taylor & Francis: Abingdon, UK, 2024; pp. 1–15. [CrossRef]
16. Boydell, K.; Pignatiello, A. Special Series on the Use of Technology in the Delivery of Child and Youth Mental Health Services and Supports. *J. Can. Acad. Child Adolesc. Psychiatry* **2016**, *25*, 68. [PubMed]
17. Cliffe, B.; Croker, A.; Denne, M.; Stallard, P. Clinicians' use of and attitudes towards technology to provide and support interventions in child and adolescent mental health services. *Child Adolesc. Ment. Health* **2019**, *25*, 95–101. [CrossRef]
18. Page, M.J.; McKenzie, J.E.; Bossuyt, P.M.; Boutron, I.; Hoffmann, T.C.; Mulrow, C.D.; Shamseer, L.; Tetzlaff, J.M.; Akl, E.A.; Brennan, S.E.; et al. The PRISMA 2020 statement: An updated guideline for reporting systematic reviews. *Rev. Española Cardiología* **2021**, *74*, 790–799. [CrossRef]
19. Pollock, A.; Berge, E. How to do a systematic review. *Int. J. Stroke* **2018**, *13*, 138–156. [CrossRef] [PubMed]
20. Aromataris, E.; Munn, Z. *JBI Manual for Evidence Synthesis*; Joanna Briggs Institute: Adelaide, Australia, 2020.
21. Ciapponi, A. Herramientas ROBINS para evaluar el riesgo de sesgo de estudios no aleatorizados. *Evid. Actual. Práctica Ambulatoria* **2022**, *25*, e007024. [CrossRef]
22. Zannat, N.; Mahmud, M. Calm & care: A child-centred digital therapy platform for mental health. *J. Digit. Syst. Dev.* **2024**, *2*, 30–49. [CrossRef]
23. Høgsdal, H.; Kaiser, S.; Kyrrestad, H. Adolescents' Assessment of Two Mental Health-Promoting Mobile Apps: Results of Two User Surveys. *JMIR Form. Res.* **2023**, *6*, e40773. [CrossRef]
24. Shi, J.; Lo, B.; Wong, H.W.; Hollenberg, E.; Sanches, M.; Abi-Jaoudé, A.; Chaim, G.; Cleverley, K.; Henderson, J.; Johnson, A.; et al. Assessing the usability and user engagement of Thought Spot—A digital mental health help-seeking solution for transition-aged youth. *Internet Interv.* **2021**, *24*, 100386. [CrossRef]
25. Martínez, V.; Espinosa-Duque, D.; Jiménez-Molina, Á.; Rojas, G.; Vöhringer, P.A.; Fernández-Arcila, M.; Luttges, C.; Irarrázaval, M.; Bauer, S.; Moessner, M. Feasibility and Acceptability of "Cuida tu Ánimo" (Take Care of Your Mood): An Internet-Based Program for Prevention and Early Intervention of Adolescent Depression in Chile and Colombia. *Int. J. Environ. Res. Public Health* **2021**, *18*, 9628. [CrossRef]

26. Osborn, T.L.; Rodriguez, M.; Wasil, A.R.; Venturo-Conerly, K.E.; Gan, J.; Alemu, R.G.; Roe, E.; Arango, G.S.; Otieno, B.H.; Wasanga, C.M.; et al. Single-session digital intervention for adolescent depression, anxiety, and well-being: Outcomes of a randomized controlled trial with Kenyan adolescents. *J. Consult. Clin. Psychol.* **2020**, *88*, 657–668. [CrossRef]
27. Srivastava, P.; Mehta, M.; Sagar, R.; Ambekar, A. Smartteen—A computer assisted cognitive behavior therapy for Indian adolescents with depression—A pilot study. *Asian J. Psychiatr. Apr.* **2020**, *50*, 101970. [CrossRef]
28. Gonsalves, P.P.; Hodgson, E.S.; Bhat, B.; Sharma, R.; Jambhale, A.; Michelson, D.; Patel, V. Intervención de resolución de problemas guiada basada en aplicaciones para la salud mental de los adolescentes: Un estudio de cohorte piloto en escuelas de la India. *BMJ Salud Ment.* **2021**, *24*, 11–18.
29. Rahayu, T.; Supriyanti, S.; Kasim, J.; Munazar, M.; Vandika, A. Use of Mobile Applications for Monitoring Adolescent Mental Health. *J. World Future Med. Health Nurs.* **2024**, *2*, 264–275. [CrossRef]
30. Amer, N.; Shohieb, S.; Eladrosy, W.; Elbakry, H.Y.; Elrazek, S. Sokoon: Una aplicación de terapia cognitivo-conductual basada en la gamificación: Una aplicación para la depresión, el estrés y la ansiedad. *Int. J. Gaming Comput. Mediat. Simul.* **2023**, *15*, 1–26. [CrossRef]
31. Charvet, L.; George, A.; Cho, H.; Krupp, L.; Dennis-Tiwary, T. Mobile Attention Bias Modification Training Is a Digital Health Solution for Managing Distress in Multiple Sclerosis: A Pilot Study in Pediatric Onset. *Front. Neurol.* **2021**, *12*, 719090. [CrossRef] [PubMed]
32. Khanna, M.; Carper, M. Digital Mental Health Interventions for Child and Adolescent Anxiety. *Cogn. Behav. Pract.* **2022**, *29*, 60–68. [CrossRef]
33. Huffman, L.G.; Lawrence-Sidebottom, D.; Huberty, J.; Roots, M.; Roots, K.; Parikh, A.; Guerra, R.; Weiser, J. Using Digital Measurement-Based Care for the Treatment of Anxiety and Depression in Children and Adolescents: Observational Retrospective Analysis of Bend Health Data. *JMIR Pediatr. Parent.* **2023**, *6*, e46154. [CrossRef]
34. Hugh-Jones, S.; Beckett, S.; Tumelty, E.; Mallikarjun, P. Indicated prevention interventions for anxiety in children and adolescents: A review and meta-analysis of school-based programs. *Eur. Child Adolesc. Psychiatry* **2020**, *30*, 849–860. [CrossRef]
35. Yang, Y.; Wang, H.; Sha, W.; Guo, X.; Deng, W.; Wang, J.; Fu, C. Short Video-Based Mental Health Intervention for Depressive Symptoms in Junior High School Students: A Cluster Randomized Controlled Trial. *Psychol. Res. Behav. Manag.* **2023**, *16*, 4169–4181. [CrossRef]
36. Chen, T.; Ou, J.; Li, G.; Luo, H. Promoting mental health in children and adolescents through digital technology: A systematic review and meta-analysis. *Front. Psychol.* **2023**, *15*, 1356554. [CrossRef]
37. Reynard, S.; Dias, J.; Mitic, M.; Schrank, B.; Woodcock, K. Digital Interventions for Emotion Regulation in Children and Early Adolescents: Systematic Review and Meta-analysis. *JMIR Serious Games* **2021**, *10*, e31456. [CrossRef] [PubMed]
38. Thomson, A.; Lawrence, E.; Oliver, B.; Wright, B.; Hosang, G. Self-directed digital interventions for the improvement of emotion regulation—Effectiveness for mental health and functioning in adolescents: Protocol for a systematic review. *BMJ Open* **2024**, *14*, e081556. [CrossRef] [PubMed]
39. MacEvilly, D.; Maguire, K.; Brosnan, G.; Gaffney, L. Enhancing children's emotional regulation and social communication through group intervention–evidence of impact in an Irish outpatient Child and Adolescent Mental Health Service. *Child Lang. Teach. Ther.* **2024**, *40*, 56–76. [CrossRef]

MDPI AG
Grosspeteranlage 5
4052 Basel
Switzerland
Tel.: +41 61 683 77 34

Children Editorial Office
E-mail: children@mdpi.com
www.mdpi.com/journal/children

www.ingramcontent.com/pod-product-compliance
Lightning Source LLC
Chambersburg PA
CBHW061546210926
51850CB00009B/2017
* 9 7 8 3 7 2 5 8 6 2 4 0 5 *